A Short Textbook of
Preventive Me(
for the Tropics

UNIVERSITY MEDICAL TEXTS

General Editors

SELWYN TAYLOR DM, MCh, FRCS, Hon FRCS(Ed). Hon FCS(SA).

Dean Emeritus, Royal Postgraduate Medical School, Consulting Surgeon,
Hammersmith Hospital

HOWARD ROGERS MA, MB, BChir, PhD. MRCP

Reader in Clinical Pharmacology, Guy's Hospital Medical School

---

A selection of titles in the University Medical Texts Series is given below.
A complete list is available from the Publisher.

A Short Textbook of Medicine
J. C. HOUSTON CBE, MD, FRCP
C. L. JOINER MD, FRCP
J. R. TROUNCE MD, FRCP

A Short Textbook of Surgery
SELWYN TAYLOR DM, MCh, FRCS,
Hon FRCS(Ed), Hon FCS(SA)
L. T. COTTON MCh, FRCS

A Short Textbook of Chemical Pathology
D. N. BARON MD, DSc, MRCP, FRCPath

A Short Textbook of Medical Microbiology
D. C. TURK DM, MRCPath
I. A. PORTER MD, FRCPath
B. I. DUERDEN BSc (Med Sci), MD, MRCPath
T. M. S. REID BMed Biol, MB, ChB, MRCPath

A SHORT TEXTBOOK OF
PREVENTIVE MEDICINE
FOR THE TROPICS

Second Edition

ADETOKUNBO O. LUCAS
O.F.R., B.Sc.(Durh.), M.D.(Newcastle), D.P.H.(Belf.),
D.T.M. & H.(Eng.), F.R.C.P.(Lond.), S.M.Hyg.(Harv.),
F.M.C.P.H.(Nig), F.F.C.M.(U.K.).
Formerly Professor of Preventive and Social Medicine,
University of Ibadan

HERBERT M. GILLES
B.Sc., M.D.(Malta), M.Sc.(Oxon), F.R.C.P.(Lond.), F.F.C.M.(U.K.),
F.M.C.P.H.(Nig.), D.T.M. & H., M.D.
(Hon. causa, Karolinska Institutet, Stockholm),
Professor of Tropical Medicine and Dean,
Liverpool School of Tropical Medicine, Liverpool
President of the Royal Society of
Tropical Medicine and Hygiene

HODDER AND STOUGHTON
LONDON   SYDNEY   AUCKLAND   TORONTO

TO
KOFO AND MEJRA

British Library Cataloguing in Publication Data

Lucas, Adetokunbo O.
  A short textbook of preventive medicine for
  the tropics.—2nd ed.—(University medical texts)
  1. Medicine, Preventive—Tropics
  I. Title   II. Gilles, Herbert M.
  614.4′4′0913   RC961.5

  ISBN 0 340 33818 0

First published 1973
Eighth impression 1982
Second edition 1984
Third impression 1986

Typeset in 10/11 pt Times (Monophoto) by Macmillan India Ltd., Bangalore.

Printed and bound in Great Britain
for Hodder and Stoughton Educational,
a division of Hodder and Stoughton Limited,
Mill Road, Dunton Green, Sevenoaks, Kent
by Richard Clay (The Chaucer Press) Ltd, Bungay, Suffolk

EDITOR'S FOREWORD

The advances in our knowledge of the causes and treatment of tropical diseases in the Seventies have meant that the second edition of this valuable little book has had to be almost completely rewritten.

The eighties will probably be remembered as the time of a worldwide economic freeze and it is therefore all the more encouraging that so many governments and private organisations have increased their efforts to help the developing countries. The problems of poor nutrition and disease in the third world are on so vast a scale that preventive and social medicine, or community medicine, has a much greater impact than straightforward therapeutics. Yet treatment, of necessity, is prominent in this book and it is in the field of chemotherapy, of tropical disease in particular, that so many breakthroughs have occurred in the last few years. In this regard the new edition is completely updated.

Nutrition now has its proper place in the text and the rearrangement of the contents is not only logical but helps the reader to a good grasp of the subject. As the Foreword to the first edition pointed out this is quite one of the most important of the Medical Unibooks and I hope that it continues to lighten the burden of those in training who turn to it for guidance. I often use my own copy for reference and when I do so I never cease to wonder at the authors' skill in covering such a vast subject so succinctly.

Selwyn Taylor

Cover illustration: showing an electronmicrograph of a longitudinal section through three vertebrate cardiac muscle cells. Courtesy of Y. Uehara, G. R. Campbell and G. Burnstock, Department of Anatomy, University College, London.

PREFACE

The second edition of this book contains several changes. Naturally, we have taken advantage of the new edition to correct errors that have been identified in the first issue, to incorporate new information in sectors where there have been significant advances and to draw attention to areas which require more emphasis. Thus, for example, the section on smallpox takes note of the fact that the disease has been finally eradicated. The new thinking on the organisation of health services with particular emphasis on the role of primary medical care has necessitated the complete re-writing of this section.

This book is not intended to be, and could not be, an extensive treatise on the subject but we hope that it will provide useful guidance on how preventive medicine can contribute to the health of people in the tropics. Perhaps the most important concept to be grasped is the relationship between health and environmental conditions including human behaviour and other social factors. The basic strategy of preventive medicine is to identify the most significant factors with particular emphasis on the elements that can be most easily modified in order to prevent disease and promote health. Many examples illustrate the link between the environment and the occurrence of certain communicable diseases but the role of physical factors in the environment includes hazards from chemical pollutants and other toxic agents. The important role of human behaviour needs to be stressed including such issues as personal hygiene, diet, sexual habits, smoking and the use of drugs to mention only a few.

In order to emphasise repeatedly the important role of the environment and behaviour on health, it is useful to think of the simple slogan 'HEALTH, HABITAT and HABIT'.

A. O. Lucas
H. M. Gilles

CONTENTS

	Editor's Foreword	v
	Preface	vii
1	The Tropical Environment	1
2	Health Statistics	6
3	Epidemiology	26
4	Infections through the Gastro-intestinal Tract	44
5	Infections through Skin and Mucous Membranes	102
6	Arthropod-borne Infections	161
7	Airborne Infections	228
8	Nutritional Disorders*	258
9	The Organisation of Health Services	270
10	Family Health	288
11	Environmental Health	303
12	Health Education	320
13	Other Aspects of Public Health	324
	Index	343

* by Anne P. Burgess, formerly Senior Lecturer, and Dr H. J. L. Burgess, formerly Professorial Lecturer, Department of Nutrition, Institute of Public Health, University of the Philippines.

CHAPTER 1

THE TROPICAL ENVIRONMENT

Man's total environment includes all the living and non-living elements in his surroundings. It consists basically of three major components: physical, biological and social. Man's relationship to his environment is reciprocal in that the environment has a profound influence on man whilst, at the same time, man extensively alters his environment to suit his needs and desires.

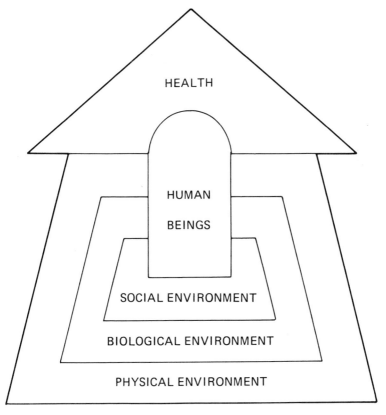

Fig. 1.1 Man's relationship with his environment

(a) Physical Environment

This refers to the non-living part of the environment—the air, soil, water, minerals; the temperature, humidity and other physical characteristics. The physical environment is extremely variable in the tropics covering arid deserts, savannahs, upland jungle, cold dry or humid plateaux, marshlands, high mountain steppes or tropical rain forest.

Climatic factors such as temperature and humidity have a direct effect on man, his comfort and his physical performance. The influence of the physical environment on the biological environment has an indirect effect on man. It determines the distribution of plants and animals which provide him with materials for food, clothing and shelter; it determines the natural distribution of the predators which prey on him and other animals which compete with him for food; and it determines the prevalence and distribution of parasites and their vectors.

Man alters the natural characteristics of his physical environment sometimes on a small scale but often on a very large scale. He may clear a small patch of bush, build a hut and dig a small canal to irrigate his vegetable garden; or he may build large cities, drain swamps, irrigate arid zones, dam rivers and create large artificial lakes. Many such changes have proved beneficial to man but some aspects of these changes have created new hazards.

(b) Biological Environment

All the living things in an area—the plants, animals and micro-organisms—constitute the biological environment. All these living things are interdependent on each other and they are ultimately dependent on their physical environment. Thus, the photosynthetic plants trap energy from the sun and circulate it among the living things in the area. Nitrogen-fixing organisms convert atmospheric nitrogen into the nitrates which are essential for plant life. A mammal may obtain its nourishment by feeding on plants (herbivore) or on other animals (carnivore) or both (omnivore). Under natural conditions, there is a balanced relationship between the growth and the size of the population of a particular species, on the one hand, and its sources of food and prevalence of competitors and predators, on the other hand.

Man deliberately manipulates the biological environment. He cultivates useful plants to provide food, clothing and shelter, and he raises farm animals for their meat, milk, leather, wool and other useful products. He hunts and kills wild animals and other predators, and he destroys insects which transmit disease or which compete with him for food.

In many parts of the tropics, insects, snails and other vectors of disease abound and thrive. This is partly because the natural environment favours their survival but also because, in some of these areas, relatively little has been done to control these agents.

(c) Social Environment

This represents the part of the environment which is entirely man-made. In essence it represents the situation of man as a member of society: his family group, his village or urban community, his culture including beliefs and attitudes, the organisation of society, politics and government, laws and the judicial system, the educational system, transport and communication, and social services including the health services.

There is much variation in the extent of technical development in the various countries in the tropics. Some of these countries are now highly developed whilst others are still in the early stages of technical development. Some of the developing countries show certain common features—limited central organisation of services, scattered populations living in small self-contained units, low level of economic development, limited educational facilities, and inadequate control of common agents of disease. Some of these communities are still held tightly in the vicious circle of ignorance, poverty and disease.

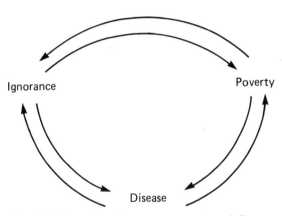

Fig. 1.2 The cycle of ignorance, poverty and disease

Many areas in the tropics are in transition. Rapid economic development and the growth of modern industries is causing mass migrations from rural to urban areas. Faster means of transportation, progress in education, the control and eradication of major endemic diseases, and other developments are effectively breaking the chains of disease, poverty and ignorance. At the same time new problems are emerging, including those resulting from the social and psychological stresses imposed by these bewildering changes and their destructive effects on traditional family life and communal relationships.

In these transitional societies there have been marked changes in the pattern of diseases. Communicable diseases which were formerly the predominant causes of disability, disease and death are now being replaced by non-communicable diseases and conditions. Malnutrition in the form of the deficiency of specific nutrients is being succeeded by problems resulting from over-indulgence, thus obesity is replacing marasmus as the predominant nutritional problem. Alcoholism and drug abuse are emerging as manifestations of social stresses and tensions.

THE ECOLOGICAL APPROACH TO PREVENTIVE MEDICINE

In preventive medicine, it is useful to consider the reciprocal relationship between man and his total environment. In the search of the causes of diseases, it is not sufficient merely to identify the specific agent of disease such as a virus or a parasite, but it is desirable to identify the influence of environmental factors on the interaction between man and the specific agent. For example, the typhoid bacillus (*Salmonella typhi*) is known to be the causative agent of disease but the occurrence of outbreaks of typhoid disease is determined by various environmental factors; water supply, methods of sewage disposal, prevalence of typhoid carriers, personal habits of the people (cleanliness), use of raw water, etc., attitude to and use of medical services, including vaccination. Similarly, a specific nutritional deficiency such as ariboflavinosis should not be viewed merely as a discrete metabolic defect but it should be seen in the context of the food habits of the community including food taboos, level of education and income of the population and local agriculture.

From this ecological approach, one can derive a rational basis for the control of diseases within the population. The control of typhoid is then seen not solely in terms of treating the individual patient with an antibiotic but also in terms of water supply, sewage disposal, food hygiene and vaccination. Malnutrition is managed not only by giving pills containing concentrated nutrients but also by giving suitable advice about diet and promoting the cultivation of nutritional foods both commercially by farmers and privately in home gardens; in more complex situations it may extend to promotion of welfare services such as unemployment benefits and food supplements for the needy.

The health worker should seek suitable opportunities for improving the health of the people through action on the environment. It is important that these lessons should be repeatedly emphasised.

The individual and the family can do much about the cleanliness of home and its immediate surroundings thereby reducing the occurrence of a number of infectious diseases. Domestic accidents, especially in such high risk areas as the kitchen and the bathroom, can be prevented by careful attention to the environment in the home. The individual needs to recognise HOW the environment in the home affects the health of his family, WHY he must act to improve the situation and WHAT he and his family can do to deal with the problem.

The *community* should be approached as a whole to deal with the widespread problems which affect many families, and also for help with those problems which require actions beyond the means of individual families. For example, certain environmental situations result from cultural habits which are common in the local community, e.g. collection and storage of water, disposal of human and other wastes, and the preparation of meals.

An adequate supply of safe water for each family and, especially in large villages and in urban areas, the disposal of waste often requires organisation at the community level. In most developing countries, modern development projects and urbanisation are introducing new risks. It is therefore necessary to ensure that these new initiatives should be carefully examined at the community level with regard to the siting of new projects and regulations to ensure that they are safely managed with minimal risk to the environment.

At the *national and international* level, large scale projects such as the creation of man-made lakes, irrigation projects and mining of minerals including oil, require careful assessment of their environmental impact. The adverse effects can best be minimised by careful planning so that as far as possible protective measures can be incorporated into the design of these projects.

FURTHER READING

WHO Tech. Rep. Ser. No. 586: *Health Hazards from New Environmental Pollutants.*

CHAPTER 2

HEALTH STATISTICS

The assessment of the health of the individual is made on clinical grounds by medical history, physical examination, laboratory tests and other special investigations. Theoretically, the health of a whole community can be assessed by conducting repeatedly a detailed clinical assessment of each individual. In practice, the health of the community is assessed less directly by the collection, analysis and interpretation of data about important events which serve as indicators of the health of the community—deaths (mortality data), sickness (morbidity data) and data about the utilisation of medical services.

Vital Statistics

These are records of certain vital events, births, deaths, marriages and divorces.

Health Statistics

These include vital statistics, and other data pertinent to health. Health statistics are derived from a variety of sources:

(a) *Notification* of diseases—infectious, industrial and other notifiable diseases.
(b) *Institutions*—records from hospitals, health centres, dispensaries, etc.
(c) *Special programmes*—school health service; control and eradication programmes of specific diseases, e.g. tuberculosis, yaws, smallpox, measles.
(d) *Epidemiological Surveys*—information is obtained from the whole community or from a sample by:
　(i) questionnaire—e.g. sickness survey
　(ii) physical examination—e.g. nutrition survey
　(iii) special investigation—e.g. mass miniature radiography (MMR), sputum, immunological tests.
(e) *Utilisation of medical services*—useful data can be obtained from:
　(i) Attendance at out-patient clinics—apart from the records of general out-patient clinics where sick patients are treated, pertinent statistical data can be obtained from special clinics such as antenatal clinics, child welfare, family planning.

(ii) The distribution and sales of drugs and vaccines can also yield valuable information.

(f) *Data initially collected for other purposes*—a variety of such data can give useful indication of some aspects of the health of the community:

(i) Routine medical inspection, e.g. pre-employment, insurance, army recruits.

(ii) Sickness absence records from schools, industry and other institutions may for example indicate an acute epidemic such as influenza.

COLLECTION OF DATA

A variety of mechanisms are used for the collection of the data which form the basis of health statistics. In order that health statistics from various communities can be compared, standardisation is essential nationally and desirable internationally:

1 Census of the Population

This is required to provide the essential population base for calculating various rates. The census usually includes not only a total count of the population but also a record of the age and sex distribution, and also some other personal data.

National censuses
In most countries, censuses are held periodically, usually every ten years.

Local censuses
The public health worker may need to conduct a census on a small scale in a local area where census data are unobtainable or not sufficiently accurate for a proposed epidemiological survey. For some studies, the census is conducted on the basis of the number of persons who are actually present on the census date in the defined area; this *de facto* population may include temporary residents and visitors but may exclude permanent residents who happen to be away. For other studies, especially where a longitudinal survey is planned, the census enumerates all persons who are normally resident in an area, i.e. this *de jure* population would exclude temporary residents and visitors but will include permanent residents who are temporarily away.

Population pyramid
The age and sex structure of the population is often displayed in the form of a histogram showing the percentage distribution of each sex at 5-year-age intervals. The shape is roughly pyramidal; the base representing the younger age-group, tapers to a narrow peak in the old age-group. In most developing countries the pyramid is typically broad, with

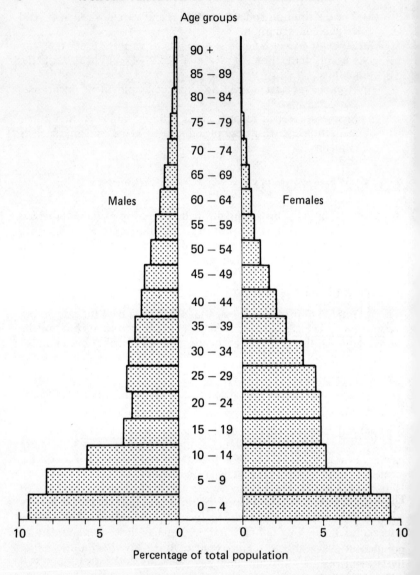

Fig. 2.1 Population pyramid of a developing country (Malumfashi, Nigeria 1977)

a rapid tapering off in the older age-groups. This represents the characteristic feature of a relatively young population. The shape of the pyramid is determined by the high birth rate and high child death rate in these communities (Fig. 2.1). In the more developed countries, the

Age groups

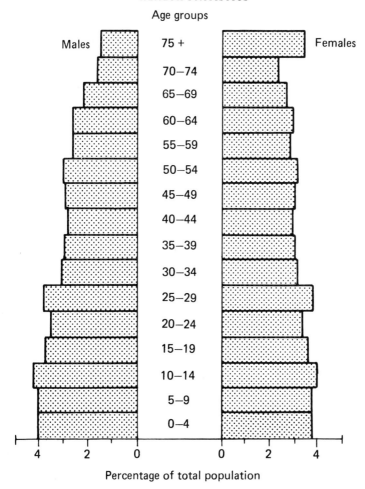

Males   75 +   Females

70—74

65—69

60—64

55—59

50—54

45—49

40—44

35—39

30—34

25—29

20—24

15—19

10—14

5—9

0—4

4   2   0   0   2   4

Percentage of total population

Fig. 2.2 Population pyramid of a more developed country (England and Wales, 1975)

population pyramid shows more gradual decline, indicating the relatively older population with a low death rate in childhood (Fig. 2.2).

2 Registration of Births and Deaths

The registration of births and deaths is compulsory in the developed countries but only in some of the developing countries. Births and deaths are two important events which can be clearly recognised by lay persons and as such the data can be collected by literate laymen. In addition to recording the fact of death, it is useful to establish the cause of death. The certification of the cause of death is done at various levels of sophistication, ranging from simple diagnoses that can be made by auxiliaries to more difficult diagnoses that can only be obtained from elaborate investigations of the patients by highly trained personnel and post-mortem examination by competent pathologists. In many developing countries there is difficulty in obtaining a complete registration of births and deaths. Even where the local laws make such registrations compulsory, the enforcement of these regulations is difficult and unpopular. Various devices have been tried to improve the quality of the data:

(a) *Registration centres*
These should be conveniently sited so that each person has reasonable access to the registration centre in his district. The registration centre should be adapted to the local social structure, using such persons as village heads, compound heads, religious scribes, or any other institutions that are appropriate in the particular area.

(b) *Rewards and penalties*
In some countries the population is induced to register births by attaching rewards to the possession of birth certificates. For example, the government free primary school may be available only to children whose births have been registered. By and large, unduly harsh penalties against defaulters are not to be recommended because such actions may antagonise the public and alienate them from other public health programmes and personnel.

(c) *Education*
Regardless of the method of registration that is adopted, the success of the scheme will depend on being able to get appropriate and sufficient information to the general public about the programme. They must know why the procedure is considered necessary and they must know of the benefits to them as individuals and communities.

3 Notification of Diseases

In every country there is a list of certain diseases, cases of which must be reported to the appropriate health authority.

The national reporting of diseases primarily includes communicable diseases, but in addition there are specific regulations about the reporting of certain industrial diseases. The notification of acute epidemic diseases is designed to provide the health authorities with information at an early stage so that they can take urgent action to control outbreaks of these infections. For example, the early notification of a case of typhoid would enable the health authorities to confine the epidemic to the smallest possible area in the shortest possible time. The notification of chronic and non-epidemic infections provides information which can be used in the long term planning of health services and also in the assessment and monitoring of control programmes. Various factors limit the usefulness of notification of diseases in the control of diseases:

(a) *Incomplete reporting* of diagnosed cases. This may be from the ignorance or negligence on the part of the health worker.

(b) *Missed diagnoses*—these would include atypical cases, mild and sub-clinical infections. In certain diseases a high proportion of infected persons who harbour the agent do not feel or appear ill, and yet they may transmit infection, i.e. they are 'carriers'.

(c) *Concealment of cases*—this may result from fear of consequences such as forcible confinement in an institution in an isolation hospital or ostracism in diseases which carry a social stigma in the community, e.g. leprosy, venereal diseases.

(d) *Over diagnosis*—because of mistaken diagnosis, some of the re-ported cases may prove not to be due to the particular disease.

4 International Notification of Diseases

A few diseases are subject to notification on the basis of international agreement. These internationally notifiable diseases which were some-times also known as quarantinable or 'convention' diseases are governed by International Sanitary Regulations. Formerly, six diseases were included—smallpox, plague, cholera, yellow fever, louse-borne typhus and louse-borne relapsing fever. The current situation is that plague, cholera and yellow fever are still notifiable to the World Health Organisation. Although global reporting of a few selected diseases has been helpful in the control of some infections that tend to spread rapidly across national boundaries, the limitations of this approach have been recognised. There has therefore been more emphasis on improving national programmes for the surveillance of diseases rather than relying mainly on the legal requirements of international notifications.

5 Improvement of Notifications

1 Simple forms
The notification form should be as simple as possible. In some communities with low levels of literacy, the notification has been achieved by the use of appropriate colour coded cards which already contain the address of the health office and the particular village. The village head can therefore notify a case of an infectious disease merely by dropping one card of the appropriate colour in the post box.

2 Education
As in other aspects of public health, the cooperation of the public depends on providing them with sufficient information, in this case telling them how notification of diseases can help the individual and the community.

3 *Feed-back*

The data that are compiled should be made available to all those who contributed information. They can thereby see how the information is being used.

6 Data from Medical Institutions

Hospitals, health centres, clinical laboratories and other medical institutions provide easily accessible sources of health statistics, but such institutional data must be used and interpreted most cautiously. The pattern of disease as seen in hospitals and in other medical institutions is distorted by many factors of selection which operate from the patient's home to the point at which he is seen and his condition diagnosed in an institution. With regard to the patient, his action depends on his awareness that he is sick and his knowledge that relief is available at a particular institution. He then makes his choice of treatment, from various alternatives which are available to him:

(a) self-treatment
(b) home medication with traditional drugs or patent medicine
(c) treatment by traditional healers
(d) treatment by quack or other unqualified persons
(e) modern medical treatment by a private medical practitioner or at the dispensary, health centre or hospital.

Factors in the institutions which influence the pattern of disease include the following:

(a) the types of services offered by the institution
(b) accessibility of the institution including such factors as the distance from the patient's home and the fees charged
(c) the special interests and reputation of the personnel.

Thus, for example, the establishment of a bacteriological laboratory in a hospital might lead to an increase in the frequency with which certain diseases such as typhoid is being diagnosed. The appointment of a specialist obstetrician in a hospital may lead to a concentration of difficult obstetric problems in the hospital as a result of referrals from other doctors and self-selection by patients who have heard of the specialist's reputation. A free clinic may attract large numbers of patients, including relatively large numbers of the poor, whereas an expensive private clinic will be used mainly by the rich and those who have financial provision through insurance.

Another defect of institutional data is that although the numerator (i.e. number of cases) is known, the denominator (i.e. the population at risk) is not easy to define. Comparisons from community to community on the basis of institutional data are difficult and fraught with the danger that erroneous conclusions may be based on the distorted pattern of hospital data.

In spite of these limitations and dangers, the information that is derived from medical institutions can supplement data from other sources. Useful data can be obtained from the following sources:

(a) *General out-patient clinics*—dispensaries, health centres, hospitals.
(b) *Special clinics*—infant and child welfare, school health, ante-natal, industrial, specific diseases—tuberculosis, leprosy.
(c) *Hospitals*—records of in-patients and deaths, autopsy records, laboratory reports.

ANALYSIS AND PRESENTATION OF DATA

Health statistics may be presented as absolute numbers but they are often expressed as rates, i.e. the number of events are related to the population involved, and in order to simplify comparisons, rates are usually expressed in relation to an arbitrary total e.g. 1000, 100 000 or 1 000 000.

$$\text{RATE} = \frac{\text{Number of persons affected or number of events}}{\text{Population at risk}} \times 1000$$

Rates which are calculated with the total population in an area as the denominator are known as *crude* rates.

The rates which are calculated with the particular segments of the population at risk as the denominator, are called *specific* rates.

Some Commonly Used Rates in Public Health

Crude rates

CRUDE BIRTH RATE =
$$\frac{\text{Number of live births reported during the year}}{\text{Mid-year population}} \times 1000$$

CRUDE DEATH RATE =
$$\frac{\text{Number of deaths reported during the year}}{\text{Mid-year population}} \times 1000$$

NATURAL INCREASE RATE =
$$\frac{\text{Number of live births minus number of deaths}}{\text{Mid-year population}} \times 1000$$

Crude rates from different populations cannot be easily compared, especially where there are striking differences in the age and sex structure of the population. Thus, the crude death rate may be relatively high in a population which has a high proportion of elderly persons compared with the rate in a younger population. Thus, if the death rate is to be used as an indicator of the health status of a population, adjustment of the crude rate is required. This adjustment may be in the form of:

(a) *Standardised rates*—there are rates which have been adjusted to correct for the age and sex structure or other peculiarities of the population. The adjustment is made to a standard population.

(b) *Specific rates*—these rates are calculated using data from specified segments of the population.

AGE-SPECIFIC AND SEX-SPECIFIC DEATH RATES =

$$\frac{\text{Number of deaths in persons in a specified age and sex group}}{\text{Number of persons in the specified age and sex group}} \times 1000$$

The death rate in a total population may be analysed separately for each sex in one-year age-groups, or more conveniently in 5- or 10-year age-groups.

Some Commonly Used Specific Rates

(a) *Specific rates* relating to infants and children:

INFANT MORTALITY RATE =

$$\frac{\text{Number of deaths in infants under 1 year}}{\text{Number of live births during the year}} \times 1000$$

NEONATAL MORTALITY RATE =

$$\frac{\text{Number of deaths in infants under 1 month of age}}{\text{Number of live births during the year}} \times 1000$$

POST-NEONATAL MORTALITY RATE =

$$\frac{\text{Number of deaths in infants between 1 month and 1 year}}{\text{Number of live births during the year}} \times 1000$$

(b) *Specific rates* relating to pregnancy and the puerperium:

STILL BIRTH RATE =

$$\frac{\text{Number of foetal deaths of 28 or more completed weeks of gestation}}{\text{Number of live births and still births}} \times 1000$$

PERINATAL MORTALITY RATE =

$$\frac{\text{Number of still births and deaths under 1 week}}{\text{Number of live births and still births}} \times 1000$$

MATERNAL MORTALITY RATE =

$$\frac{\text{Number of maternal deaths due to pregnancy, child birth and puerperal conditions}}{\text{Total number of live births and still births}} \times 1000$$

FERTILITY RATE =

$$\frac{\text{Number of births in a year}}{\text{Number of women between the ages of 15 and 49 years in the population}} \times 1000$$

The Use of Vital Statistics

These various rates are used to reflect the health status of a community; some relate to the community as a whole but others deal more specifically with special groups. Thus, the standardised death rate gives an indication of the overall health condition of the community, but the specific mortality rates in the most susceptible age-groups have in practice proved to be more sensitive indicators. The infant mortality rate is widely accepted as one of the most useful single measures of the health status of the community. The infant mortality rate may be very high (200–300/1000 live births) in communities where health and social services are poorly developed. Experience has shown that it can respond dramatically to relatively simple measures. Thus, with the establishment of maternal and child health services, the infant mortality rate may fall from being very high (200–300/1000 live births) to a moderate level (50–100/1000 live births). In the most advanced nations the rate is low (below 20/1000 live births). Even in these developed communities, the infant mortality rate shows striking differences in the different socio-economic groups; it may be as low as 10 deaths/1000 live births in the upper socio-economic group whilst it is 40 deaths/1000 live births in the lower socio-economic group of the same country.

The infant mortality rate is usually subdivided into two segments: the neonatal and the post-neonatal death rates. The neonatal death rate is related to factors operating on the foetus *in utero*, and also during and immediately after delivery. Thus, neonatal mortality rate is related to maternal and obstetric factors. On the other hand the post-neonatal mortality rate is related to a variety of environmental factors and especially to the level of child care. Improvement in maternal and child health services brings about a fall in both the neonatal and the post-neonatal death rates, but the fall occurs more dramatically in the latter rate. Thus, at high infant mortality rates (200 deaths/1000 live births), most of the deaths occur in the post-neonatal period but at very low levels (20 deaths/1000 live births), a high proportion of the deaths are neonatal and are mainly due to such problems as congenital abnormalities and immaturity.

In developed countries, the first year of life represents the period of highest risk in childhood and the death rate is very low in the older children. In many tropical developing countries, although the first year does represent the period of highest risk, a high mortality rate persists in the older children. Thus, the infant mortality rate taken by itself underestimates the loss of child life. The child death rate, which measures deaths in the 1–4 year age-group, is used to complete the picture.

Vital statistics can be used to study specific health problems and aspects of the health services. Thus, the maternal death, the still birth and the perinatal mortality rates are of value in studying obstetric problems and obstetric services.

The Presentation of Data

Statistical data can be summarised and presented in graphic form or non-graphically. In each case the aim is to produce a precise and accurate demonstration of the data, summarised to simplify and accented to draw attention to the most important features.

Numerical presentation may at its simplest be no more than an arrangement of the figures in order of magnitude, so that the range of the data from the smallest to the largest is clearly displayed. Simple statistical calculations can indicate salient features of the data. For example, a series of values can be summarised by calculating statistics such as:

(a) *Mean, median or mode*—each is a single value which is representative of the series of figures, i.e. an average.

(b) *Range or standard deviation*—these are measures of dispersion which show the degree of variability within the series of values.

Data can be presented in tabular form. Often the raw data are classified, compressed and grouped into a frequency distribution. For example, rather than showing the individual ages of persons, data may be classified into 5-year or 10-year age-groups, with a record of the number of persons in each group. For tabular presentation, data are sorted, arranged, condensed and set out in such a way as to bring out the essential points. For effective presentation, a few simple rules must be observed:

(a) The title of the table should clearly describe the material contained within the text. Three elements commonly feature in the title:
   (i) What? The material contained in the table.
   (ii) Where? Location of the study.
   (iii) When? Time of the study.

(b) Each *column* and each *row* should be clearly labelled; the units of measurement must be stated. If a rate is used, the base of measurement and the number of observations must be stated.

(c) The *totals* for columns and rows should be shown where appropriate.

(d) *Abbreviations* and *symbols* should be explained in footnotes except when they are well known and universally familiar (e.g. £, $, etc.).

Graphic Representation of Data

Statistical data can be summarised and displayed in the form of graphs, geometric figures or pictures. The aim of the graphic representation is to provide a simple, visual aid such that the reader will rapidly appreciate the important features of the data. The following examples will be described:

   (*a*) Bar diagram   (*b*) Histogram   (*c*) Pie diagram   (*d*) Graph.

(a) *Bar diagram*

In a bar diagram, the data are represented by a series of bars (i.e. slender rectangles). Each item in the group is represented by a bar, the *length* of the bar is proportional to the value of the item. It is particularly useful in representing discrete variables (Fig. 2.3).

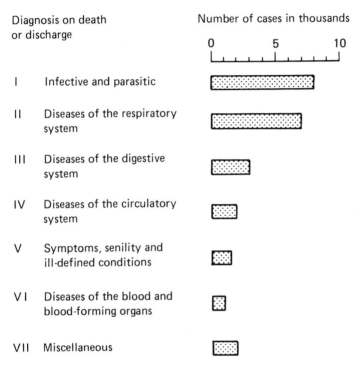

Fig. 2.3 Bar diagram

(b) *Histogram*
A histogram represents a frequency distribution in the form of adjoining rectangles which represent the frequency of each variable. The class intervals of the frequency distribution are shown on the horizontal axis, the frequencies are shown on the vertical axis (Fig. 2.4).

(c) *Pie diagram*
This consists of a circle which is divided into sectors which are proportional to the value of each variable (Fig. 2.5).

(d) *Graphs*
The simplest graph shows two variables: one on the horizontal axis and the other on the vertical axis (Fig. 2.6).

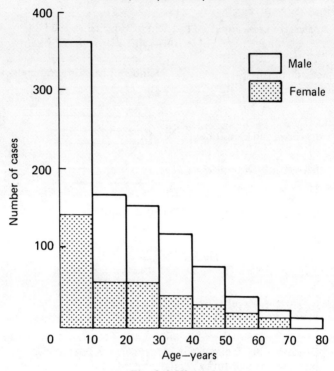

Fig. 2.4 Histogram

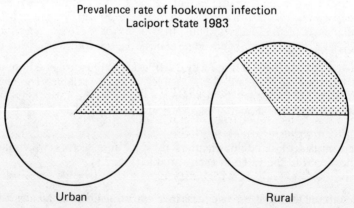

Fig. 2.5 Pie diagram (tinted area indicates proportion of population infected)

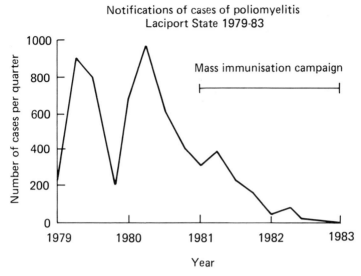

Notifications of cases of poliomyelitis
Laciport State 1979-83

Fig. 2.6 Graph

MORBIDITY STATISTICS

In addition to vital statistics, data about the occurrence of sickness within the community can provide more detailed assessment of the health of the community. Morbidity data are, however, more difficult to collect and interpret than the records of births and deaths (Fig. 2.7).

(i) Births and deaths are easily recognisable events which can be recorded by lay persons. Success in the collection of morbidity statistics depends on the extent to which individuals recognise departures from health and also on the availability of facilities for the diagnosis of the illnesses. Thus, the quality of morbidity statistics depend on the extent of coverage and the degree of sophistication of the medical services.

(ii) Whereas each vital event of birth and death can occur only on one occasion in the lifetime of any persons, sickness may occur repeatedly in the same person. In addition one person may, at one and the same time, suffer from several disease processes.

The various sources of morbidity data have been listed in the introductory section of this chapter.

Statistical Analysis of Morbidity data

In describing the pattern of sickness in a community, various morbidity rates are calculated. These fall into four major groups;

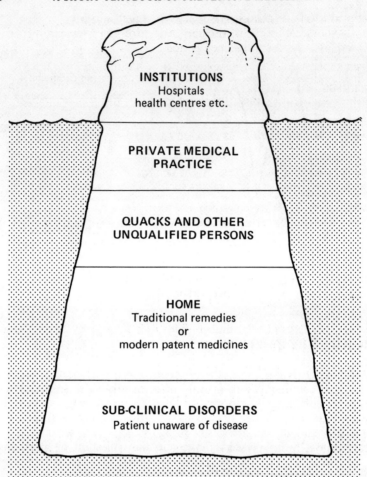

Fig. 2.7 The iceberg phenomenon. Data from institutions such as hospitals represent an unknown proportion and in some conditions, a very small proportion of the cases in the community. Institutional cases are often no more than the tip of the iceberg; the nature and extent of the larger mass beneath the surface can be discovered by well-designed epidemiological studies

1 Incidence rates

These describe the frequency of occurrence of new cases of a disease or spells of illness. The incidence rate may be defined in terms of *numbers of persons* who start a spell of sickness in the defined period, or alternatively, in terms of the spells of illness during the period:

INCIDENCE RATE (PERSONS) =

$$\frac{\text{Number of persons who start a spell of illness during the defined period}}{\text{Average number of persons exposed to risk during the period}} \times 1000$$

INCIDENCE RATE (SPELLS) =

$$\frac{\text{Number of spells of illness which start during the defined period}}{\text{Average number of persons exposed to risk during the period}} \times 1000$$

2 *Prevalence rates*
The prevalence rate of illness can be defined as the number of persons who are currently sick at a specific point in time.

POINT PREVALENCE RATE (PERSONS) =

$$\frac{\text{The number of persons who are sick at a given time}}{\text{Average number of persons exposed to risk}} \times 1000$$

3 *Duration of illness*
The average duration of illness can be measured per completed spell of illness, per sick person, or per person.

4 *Fatality rate*
The fourth element is the number of deaths in relation to the number of new cases of a particular disease.

THE CASE FATALITY RATE =

$$\frac{\text{Number of deaths ascribed to a specified disease}}{\text{Number of reported cases of the specified disease}} \times 1000$$

This is in part a measure of the severity of the illness.

Statistical Classification of Diseases and Causes of Death

The use of standard classification of diseases and injuries has greatly aided the statistical analysis of morbidity and mortality data. Through the United Nations and the World Health Organisation, an internationally recommended classification has been evolved, and it is periodically revised. Although this classification may be extended or modified to suit local and national conditions, the essential structure for international comparisons must be preserved.

The cause of death can be defined as 'the morbid condition or disease process, abnormality, injury or poisoning leading directly or indirectly to death. Symptoms or modes of dying such as heart failure, asthenia, etc., are not considered to be the causes of death for statistical purposes'.

These causes of death are classified broadly under seventeen main sections:

I Infective and Parasitic Diseases
II Neoplasms

  III Allergic, Endocrine System, Metabolic and Nutritional Diseases
  IV Diseases of the Blood and Blood-forming Organs
   V Mental, Psychoneurotic and Personality Disorders
  VI Diseases of the Nervous System and Sense Organs
 VII Diseases of the Circulatory System
VIII Diseases of the Respiratory System
  IX Diseases of the Digestive System
   X Diseases of the Genito-urinary System
  XI Deliveries and Complications of Pregnancy, Childbirth and the Puerperium
 XII Diseases of the Skin and Cellular Tissue
XIII Diseases of the Bones and Organs of Movement
XIV Congenital Malformations
 XV Certain Diseases of Early Infancy
XVI Symptoms, Senility and Ill-defined Conditions
XVII Accidents, Poisonings and Violence

Two alternative classifications of items included in Group XVII have been provided:

E XVII Alternative Classification of Accidents, Poisonings and Violence (External Cause)

N XVII Alternative Classification of Accidents, Poisonings and Violence (Nature of Injury)

The E and N classifications are independent and either or both can be used.

The more detailed classification includes over 600 categories of diseases, 153 external causes of injury and 189 categories showing the nature of the injury. Shorter lists are available: an Intermediate list of 150 cause groups A (list) and two Abbreviated lists of 50 causes each (list B and C).

In the rural areas of the tropics where facilities are limited and autopsies infrequent, e.g. in many provincial hospitals, the use of individual headings gives an impression of precision to diagnoses which is often not justified. The use of cause groups (A list) in these circumstances permits a more valid estimate of the size of the problem, e.g. diarrhoeal diseases; it focuses on the necessity for corrective action and makes it easier to detect change over a period of time.

Certification of the Cause of Death

This is usually provided by the physician who was in attendance on a sick patient during his last illness. The certificate is made out on a form which is usually based on the International form of medical certificate of cause of death. This form is in two parts (Fig. 2.8).

In many developing countries, only a small proportion of deaths occur under the supervision of trained doctors. In the other cases, a certificate of death may be provided by other categories of staff

	CAUSE OF DEATH	Approximate interval between onset and death
I Disease or condition directly leading to death	(*a*) .... due to (or as a consequence of)	....
Antecedent causes Morbid conditions, if any, giving rise to the above cause, stating the underlying condition last	(*b*) .... due to (or as a consequence of) (*c*)	....
II Other significant conditions contributing to the death, but not related to the disease or condition causing it	....	....

I This does not mean the mode of dying, e.g. heart failure, asthenia, etc. It means the disease, injury, or complication which caused death.

Fig. 2.8 International form of medical certificate of cause of death

including health auxiliaries. Attempts have been made to evolve for the use of such staff simple classifications of causes of death, based mainly on symptoms and broad descriptions. Such methods of recording crude causes of death can be of great value if the data are interpreted with care. Such statistics should, however, be tabulated separately from certifications from qualified physicians.

THE USE OF HEALTH STATISTICS

There is a tendency to over-emphasise the collection of statistics and to pay insufficient attention to its use. Much information collected at great cost remains unused in the achives of health departments. A few examples illustrate how statistics can be used in a dynamic way to identify and deal with problems affecting the health of the community.

The delivery of health care at the primary level generates a lot of raw data. At the health post, the dispensary, the maternal and child welfare clinic and the general practitioner's clinic, data can be collected and used in a simple but effective manner. For example, the pattern of diseases seen at the clinic can be summarised using simple classification in broad diagnostic groups. In this way the proportion of attendances due to common problems—diarrhoeal diseases, acute respiratory infections, minor injuries—can be monitored. A sudden change can call attention to an epidemic, and trends over time can also be observed. At a health centre, for example, each service unit should be encouraged to collect and display statistics on high priority problems. The curative section should show graphs of cases of acute diarrhoea in a simple graph so that comparisons can be made day by day, week by week, and month by month. They should also be alert to draw attention to any sudden increase in the number of cases. The child welfare clinic should display the number of children they have immunised so that by comparing with the number of children born the coverage can be assessed over time. The graphs could also show the number of children commencing the vaccination programme and the number completing the course. No specific list can be prescribed for all centres but each centre should select a few priority problems for careful scrutiny. These data can form the basis of discussions among the staff and with the community on the strategy for dealing with specific problems.

In addition to the collection of data for local use, the primary health care unit should also pay attention to the need to contribute accurate data for use at the district and national level. A community physician in charge of a district should use the data provided by peripheral units to obtain an indication of the pattern of diseases and operation of the health services. Trends which may not be apparent in one local unit may become obvious on compilation of data from several dozen districts. For example, an outbreak of diarrhoeal disease may be confined to a small area involving one or two villages but an increase in the number of cases over a wider area may call attention to a more serious problem.

At the district level, the officer in charge should also select data that would give information about the health problems within the district. Apart from the data on diseases, the information about the operation of the health services within the district should also be examined.

What proportion of children are being immunised community by community? What proportion of pregnant women receive ante-natal care and how many deliver their babies under supervision? Scrutiny of such information would enable the district officer to assess the performance of the health teams, and to gauge the community response.

At the *national* level, the statistical unit serving the Ministry of Health can be a most valuable resource for decision making. Data that are carefully collected, evaluated and interpreted should form the basis of defining the priorities for health care, for allocating resources and for monitoring progress. Such national data can be analysed to show distribution by geography, and other relevant variables. National health data can also be compared with data from other countries especially with countries that have a similar ecological setting.

FURTHER READING

WHO Tech. Rep. Ser. No. 559: *New Approaches in Health Statistics.*

CHAPTER 3

EPIDEMIOLOGY

Originally, the term 'epidemiology' meant 'the study of epidemics', but the techniques which were originally used in the study and control of epidemics have also been usefully applied in the study of non-communicable diseases. In its modern usage, the term epidemiology refers to the study of the distribution of disease in human populations against the background of their total environment. It includes a study of the patterns of diseases as well as a search for the determinants of diseases.

The modern definition of epidemiology includes three important elements:

(a) All Diseases Included

The term is no longer restricted to the study of infections but it includes cancer, malnutrition, road accidents, mental illness and other non-communicable diseases. Epidemiological techniques are also being applied to the study of the operation of health services.

(b) Populations

Whereas clinical medicine is concerned with the features of disease in the individual, epidemiology deals with the distribution of disease in populations, communities or groups.

(c) Ecological Approach

The frequency and distribution of disease are examined against the background of various circumstances in man's total environment—physical, biological and social. This is an ecological approach; the occurrence of disease is examined in terms of the interrelationship between man and his total environment.

THE DISTRIBUTION OF DISEASE

Three major questions are usually asked in epidemiology:
WHO? What is the distribution of the disease in terms of *persons*?
WHERE? What is the distribution of the disease in terms of *place*?
WHEN? What is the distribution of the disease in terms of *time*?

Answers to these questions provide clues to the factors which determine the occurrence of the disease.

THE EPIDEMIOLOGICAL TOOL—THE RATE

The basic tool of epidemiology is the rate—it relates the number of cases to the population at risk. In order to compare populations of different sizes easily, the rate is usually expressed as the number of events in an arbitrary total, e.g. 1000 or 100000.
Two main types of rates are calculated:

1 *Incidence rate*
This indicates the occurrence of new cases within a stated period:

$$\text{INCIDENCE RATE} = \frac{\text{Number of new cases in a stated period}}{\text{Population at risk}} \times 1000$$

2 *Prevalence rate* (Point Prevalence Rate)
This is the number of cases which are present within the population at a particular point in time.

$$\text{PREVALENCE RATE} = \frac{\text{Number of current cases at a specified time}}{\text{Population at risk}} \times 1000$$

Incidence, Prevalence and Duration

There is obviously some relationship between the rate at which new cases occur and the number of cases present at any particular point in time. The third factor to be considered is the *duration* of the illness. The prevalence rate would rise:
(a) if the incidence of illness increases but the average duration remains unchanged.
(b) if the incidence rate remains unchanged but the average duration of the illness increases.
Thus, the prevalence rate is dependent on the combination of these two factors, incidence rate and duration of illness. Under certain conditions where no marked changes are occurring in these factors, there is a simple mathematical relationship:

Prevalence rate = Incidence rate × Average duration

This relationship changes if the incidence rate is rapidly altering as during an acute epidemic or if the average duration of the illness is changing perhaps in response to treatment.

EPIDEMIOLOGICAL METHODS

There are three main types of epidemiological studies:

1 Descriptive Epidemiology

The distribution of disease is described in terms of the three major variables: People, Place and Time. This is the first phase of epidemiological studies in which one answers the questions:

'Who is affected? In what place? And at what time?'

The answers to these questions together with knowledge of the clinical and pathological features of the disease and information about the population and its environment, assist in developing hypotheses about the determinants of the disease. These hypotheses can be tested by analytical studies.

Various characteristics of persons, place and time are used in descriptive epidemiology:

People

    Age, sex, marital status;

    Race, ethnic group, religion;

    Occupation, education, socio-economic status;

    Personal habits—use of alcohol and tobacco.

Place

    Climatic zones;

    Country, region, state, district;

    Urban or rural;

    Local community, city wards;

    Precise location in an institution.

Time

    Year, season, day;

    Secular trends, periodic changes;

    Seasonal variations and other cyclical fluctuations.

Some of these and other variables may be used to describe the distribution of the disease.

2 Analytical Epidemiology

Two types of study are employed:

(a) *Case history studies* ('*retrospective studies*'): '*case control studies*'.

For case history studies, a group of affected persons are compared with suitably matched control groups of non-affected persons.

For example, in a study designed to test the hypothesis that cigarette smoking is an important factor in the causation of cancer of the lung, a number of patients with this disease ('cases') were questioned about their smoking habits. Similar questions were asked from a group of patients who had cancer at other sites (controls). This enquiry showed significant differences in the smoking habits of cases compared with controls. This was a case history study in that the subjects were selected on the basis of being *affected* or *non-affected persons.*

(b) *Cohort studies*

For cohort studies, a group of persons who are exposed to the suspected aetiological agent are compared with matched control subjects who have not been similarly exposed. For example, in a further study on cancer of the lung, a large group of persons were questioned about their smoking habits. The incidence rate of cancer of the lung among the smokers (exposed) was compared with the rate among non-smokers (non-exposed). Thus in this cohort study the subjects were selected on the basis of *exposure* or *non-exposure.*

Compared with cohort studies, case history studies have the advantage of being relatively quick, easy and cheap. A significant number of cases can be assembled for the case history study and a variety of hypotheses can be rapidly screened. The more promising ones can be further examined by the more laborious, time-consuming and expensive cohort studies. The latter have the advantage of giving a more direct estimation of the risk from exposure to each factor.

3 Experimental Epidemiology

This involves studies in which one group which is deliberately subjected to an experience is compared with a control group which has not had a similar experience. Field trials of vaccines and of chemoprophylactic agents are examples of experimental epidemiology. In such trials, one group receives the vaccine or drug, whilst the control group is given a placebo; alternatively, a new vaccine or drug may be compared with a well-established agent of known potency. The opportunities for experimental epidemiology in man are not numerous; often it is not feasible to carry out such controlled trials especially on things that are related to personal behaviour.

Epidemiological Data

As in clinical medicine, epidemiological data may be obtained in the form of answers to questions, physical examination of persons and results of laboratory and special investigations. In assessing the value of a particular method the following qualities should be considered:

(a) *Sensitivity*—ability of the test to detect the condition when it is present. A highly sensitive test will be positive whenever the condition is present; a less sensitive test will be positive in a proportion of cases, but will give a *false negative* case in others.

(b) *Specificity*—ability of the test to differentiate cases in which the condition is present from those in which it is absent. A highly specific test will be positive only when the relevant condition is present but a less specific test will give *false positive* results.

(c) *Repeatability*—the extent to which the same result is obtained when the test is repeated on the same subject or material. The variation which occurs on repeating the test may be due to the following:
  (i) Variation in the thing being measured
  (ii) Limitation in the accuracy of the instrument
  (iii) Observer error or variation.

There may be variations in the findings of one observer when he measures or classifies the same object on repeated occasions, i.e. *intra-observer variation or error*. There may be differences between the findings of two observers when they measure or classify the same object, i.e. *inter-observer variation or error*.

Observer variation and error can be minimised by:
  (i) Carefully standardising the procedures for obtaining the measurements and classifications.
  (ii) Defining the criteria in clear objective terms.
  (iii) Training all the participants in the methods to be adopted to ensure uniform standard techniques.
  (iv) Providing standard reference material such as photographs or standard X-ray films for direct comparison.
  (v) Taking measurements and making the classifications without knowledge of the status of the patient, whether he is a 'case' or a control subject. In the double-blind technique, subjects are randomly allocated to treatment and control groups; neither the subjects nor the observers know to which groups each subject is assigned. Thus, there is 'blind' assignment of subjects as well as 'blind' assessments of the results.

EPIDEMIOLOGY OF COMMUNICABLE DISEASES

Communicable diseases are characterised by the existence of a living infectious agent which are transmissible. Apart from the infectious agent, two other factors, the host and the environment, affect the epidemiology of the infection:

Agent: The Seed
Host: The Soil
Route of transmission: The Climate.

Infectious Agents

These may be viruses, rickettsiae, bacteria, protozoa, fungi or helminths. The biological properties of the agent may play a major role in its epidemiology.

In order to surive a parasite must be able to do the following:
(a) Multiply
(b) Emerge from the host

(c) Reach a new host

(d) Infect the new host.

The ability of the infective agent to survive in man's environment is an important factor in the epidemiology of the infection. Each infective agent has its precise habitat on which it depends for its survival. The term *reservoir of infection* is used to describe this natural habitat of the infective agent. The term 'reservoir' implies the following:

(i) *Habitat*—the infective agent lives and multiplies there.

(ii) *Survival*—the infective agent primarily depends on the reservoir for its survival. The reservoir may be man, animal or non-living material.

1 Reservoir in Man

This includes a number of important pathogens which are specifically adapted to man—the infective agents of measles, smallpox, typhoid, meningococcal meningitis, gonorrhoea and syphilis. The human reservoir includes both active cases and carriers.

Carriers

A carrier is a person who harbours the infective agents without showing signs of disease but is capable of transmitting the agent to other persons. Convalescent carriers are persons who continue to harbour the infective agent after recovering from the illness. They may excrete the agent for only a short period; or they may become chronic carriers, excreting the organism continuously or intermittently over a period of years. A healthy carrier is a person who remains well throughout the infection. In some cases, the infected person excretes the pathogens during the incubation period, before the onset of symptoms or before the characteristic features of the disease (e.g. the measles rash or glandular swelling in mumps) are manifested; these are known as *incubatory carriers* or precocious carriers.

Carriers play an important role in the epidemiology of certain infections: poliomyelitis, meningococcal meningitis, typhoid and amoebiasis:

(a) The number of carriers may far outnumber the sick patients.

(b) The carrier and his contacts do not know that he is infected, hence neither of them will take precautions to avoid transmission of the infection.

(c) The carrier is not debilitated by his infection and he can continue with his normal daily routine, moving freely from place to place, making contacts over a wide area. On the contrary, the sick patient's contacts may be restricted to close family contacts, friends and visitors.

(d) Chronic carriers may serve as a source of infection over a very long period and as a means of repeatedly re-introducing the disease into an area which is otherwise free of infection.

2 Reservoir in Animals

Some infective agents which affect man have their reservoir in animals. The term *zoonosis* is applied to those infectious diseases of vertebrate animals which are transmissible to man under natural conditions:

(a) Where man uses the animal for food, e.g. taeniasis.
(b) Where there is a vector transmitting the infection from animals to man, e.g. plague (flea), viral encephalitis (mosquito).
(c) Where the animal bites man, e.g. rabies.
(d) Where the animal contaminates man's environment including his food, e.g. salmonellosis.

Health workers should collaborate closely with veterinary authorities in identifying and dealing with these problems.

3 Reservoir in Non-living Things

Many of these agents are basically saprophytes living in soil, and fully adapted to living free in nature. Biologically, they are usually equipped to withstand marked environmental changes in temperature and humidity. Apart from the vegetative forms, some develop resistant forms such as spores which can withstand adverse environmental conditions, e.g. Clostridial organisms, the infective agents of tetanus (*Clostridium tetani*), gas gangrene (*C. welchii*) and botulism (*C. botulinum*).

THE SOURCE OF INFECTION

This term refers to the immediate source of infection, i.e. person or object from which the infectious agent passes to a host. This source of infection may or may not be a portion of the reservoir. For example, man is the reservoir of typhoid infection; a cook who is a carrier may infect food that is served at a party; that item of food is the source of infection in that particular outbreak.

MODE OF TRANSMISSION

This refers to the mechanism by which an infectious agent is transferred from one person to the other or from the reservoir to a new host. Transmission may occur by:

(a) *Contact*, either directly, person to person, or indirectly through contaminated objects. Contact infections are more likely to occur where there is crowding, since this increases the likelihood of contact with infected persons. Hence they tend to be more marked in urban than in rural areas, and they are associated with overcrowding in household.

(b) *Inhalation*—through airborne infection. Poor ventilation, over-crowding in sleeping quarters and in public places are important factors in the epidemiology of airborne infections.

(c) *Infection*—through the contamination of hands, food or water.

(d) *Penetration of skin*—directly by the organism itself (e.g. hookworm larvae, schistosomiasis) by the bite of a vector (e.g. malaria, plague) or through wounds (e.g. tetanus).

(e) *Transplacental infection*—congenital infection, e.g. syphilis, toxoplasmosis.

HOST FACTORS

The occurrence of infection and its outcome are in part determined by host factors. The term immunity is used to describe the ability of the host to resist infection. Apart from determining the occurrence of infection, the host's immune responses also modify the nature of the pathological reaction to infection. Allergic reactions in response to infection may significantly contribute to the clinical and pathological reactions.

Resistance to infection is determined by non-specific and by specific factors:

(i) Non-specific Resistance

This depends on the protective covering of skin which resists penetration by most infective agents, and the mucous membranes, some of which include ciliated epithelium which mechanically scavenges particulate matter. Certain secretions—mucus, tears and gastric secretions—contain lysozymes which have anti-bacterial activity; in addition, the acid content of gastric secretion also has some anti-microbial action. Reflex responses such as coughing and sneezing also assist in keeping susceptible parts of the respiratory tract free of foreign matter.

(ii) Specific Immunity

Specific immunity may be due to genetic or acquired factors.

(a) *Genetic*

Certain infective agents which infect other animals do not infect man, and vice versa. This species-specificity is, however, not always absolute and there are some infective agents which regularly pass from animals to man.

There are also variations in the susceptibility of various races and ethnic groups, e.g. Negroes tend to have a high level of resistance to vivax malaria infection.

Specific genetic factors have been associated with resistance to infection, e.g. persons who have haemoglobin S are more resistant to infection with *Plasmodium falciparum* than those with normal haemoglobin AA.

(b) *Acquired immunity*

Acquired immunity may be active or passive. In active immunity the host manufactures antibodies in response to an antigenic stimulus. In passive immunity, the host receives pre-formed antibodies. Active immunity may be naturally acquired following clinical or subclinical infection; or it may be induced artificially by administering living or killed organisms or their products. The new born baby acquires passive immunity by the transplacental transmission of antibodies; in this way the newborn babies of immune mothers are protected against such infections as measles, malaria and tetanus in the first few months of life. Passive immunity is artificially induced by the administration of antibodies from the sera of immune human beings (homologous) or animals (heterologous). Protection from passive immunity tends to be of short duration, especially when heterologous serum is used.

Factors affecting Host Immunity

The resistance of the host to infection is affected by such factors as age, sex, pregnancy, nutrition, trauma and fatigue.

(i) *Age*

For some infections, persons at both extremes of age tend to be most severely affected, i.e. children and the elderly. Some infections predominate in childhood; this usually occurs in situations in which most children become infected and thereby acquire lifelong immunity. Other infections predominate in adults; this may be determined by exposure, e.g. industrial (e.g. anthrax), sexual (e.g. gonorrhoea). Age may also influence the clinical pathological form of an infection, e.g. miliary tuberculosis is more likely in children whilst cavitating lung lesions are more likely in adults.

(ii) *Sex*

Some infective diseases show marked differences in their sex incidence; this is apart from infections which specifically affect the genital and other sex organs. Such infections as poliomyelitis and diphtheria often show a preponderance in females.

(iii) *Pregnancy*

Pregnancy increases susceptibility to certain infections; these occur more frequently, show more severe manifestations and have a worse prognosis than in non-pregnant women of a similar age-group, e.g. viral infections such as poliomyelitis; bacterial infections such as pneumococcal infection; and protozoal infection such as malaria and amoebiasis. It does not appear that there is uniform depression of resistance to all infections. Certain infections, e.g. typhoid and meningococcal infection, do not occur more frequently nor show greater clinical severity in pregnant women.

(iv) *Nutrition*

Good nutrition is generally accepted as an important measure in enhancing resistance to infection. Severe specific deficiency of vitamin A renders the cornea and the skin more liable to infection. In addition to such specific effects it has been noted that poorly nourished children are more liable to succumb to gastro-enteritis and measles. The relationship has not been definitely established in the case of some other infections; it seems likely that some of the infections are not adversely affected by nutrition.

(v) *Trauma and fatigue*

Stress in the form of trauma and fatigue may render the host more susceptible to infections. One classical example is the effect of trauma and fatigue on poliomyelitis. The paralytic form of the disease may be precipitated by violent exercise during the prodromal period or by trauma in the form of injections of adjuvanted vaccine; paralysis tends to be most severe in the limb into which the vaccine was injected or which was subjected to most fatigue.

Herd Immunity

The level of immunity in the community as a whole is termed 'herd immunity'. When herd immunity is low, introduction of the infection is likely to lead to severe epidemics. For example, the introduction of measles into an island population which had no previous experience of the infection resulted in massive epidemics. On the other hand, when herd immunity is high, the introduction of infection may not lead to a propagated spread. A disease may be brought under complete control when a high proportion of the population has been immunised; even though a small proportion remains non-immune the transmission of infection may virtually cease.

Incubation Period (See Fig. 3.1)

This is the interval of time from the infection of the host to the first appearance of symptoms and signs of the disease. In practice, it is not easy to determine precisely the time of infection and hence incubation period is measured from the time of first exposure to the onset of the first symptoms. Each infection has its characteristic range, varying from a few hours to several years.

Knowledge of the incubation period of an infection can be used in the control of infections as well as in the clinical assessment of patients.

(a) *Tracing the source of infection*

Investigation of likely sources can concentrate on the relevant period in relation to the onset of symptoms. For example, in tracing the likely source of a case of smallpox, one would want to know of the patient's movements and his contacts with sick persons 7–21 days before the onset of symptoms. In a case of syphilis, the suspects would include all his sexual partners in the three-month period preceding the appearance of the chancre.

(b) *Period of surveillance or quarantine of contacts*
The surveillance or quarantine of contacts is maintained for the period of time equal to the usual maximal incubation period of the infection.

(c) *Immunisation*
Certain infections can be prevented by immunisation of the host during the incubation period, e.g. (i) *Passive immunisation* with immune globulin can prevent or modify an attack of measles in a child who has been in contact with the infection; (ii) *Active immunisation* with smallpox vaccine early in the incubation period can protect a contact from smallpox infection.

(d) *Identifying point source epidemics*
An outbreak resulting from a simple common exposure (a point source epidemic) will give rise to cases which will all be present within the incubation period of the infection. Propagation of the epidemic apart from this single exposure would be indicated by the occurrence of cases later than the known extreme length of the incubation period.

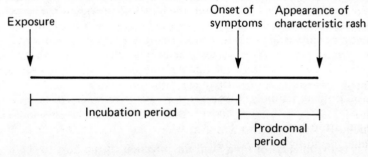

Fig. 3.1 Point source epidemic

(e) *Prognosis*
In some infections, the prognosis is related to the incubation period. For example, the shorter the incubation period, the worse the prognosis of tetanus.

Prodromal Period (see Fig. 3.1)

The prodromal period is the interval between the onset of symptoms of an infectious disease and the appearance of the characteristic manifestation such as a skin rash. For example, in measles, the infection presents with fever and coryza, but the characteristic rash appears about four days later.

CONTROL OF COMMUNICABLE DISEASES

A programme for the control of a communicable disease should be based on a detailed knowledge of the epidemiology of the infection and on effective public health organisation to plan, execute and evaluate the programme. The epidemiological information should include knowledge of the distribution of the infection in the local area, of the major foci of infection and of the overall effect of the infection on the population.

The programme must include some mechanism for:
(a) recognising the infection and the confirmation of the diagnosis
(b) notifying the disease to the appropriate authority
(c) finding the source of infection
(d) assessing the extent of the outbreak by finding other cases and the other exposed persons.

(a) *Recognition of the infection*
This is in the first instance the responsibility of the physicians and auxiliary personnel who are treating the patients. For the early recognition of communicable diseases, it is necessary that physicians and medical auxiliaries should be able to recognise the clinical manifestations of the major infective diseases in the area. This is particularly important in the case of acute epidemic diseases such as smallpox, where prompt action is required to prevent the disastrous spread of infection. Thus, the medical auxiliary at the most peripheral unit should be able to initiate appropriate action which would lead to the early recognition of the outbreak of an epidemic. Laboratory services should be used to support clinical diagnosis. Ideally there should be a Public Health Laboratory system which can process specimens from patients and from the environment.

(b) *Notification of diseases*
A notifiable disease is one the occurrence of which must be reported to the appropriate health authority. The group includes the major epidemic diseases and other communicable diseases about which the health authorities require information. Some diseases are also notifiable internationally.

(c) *Identification of the source of infection*
Epidemiological investigations are directed to finding the source of infection. This involves analysis of the information about the time sequence of the occurrence of cases and the history of the movements of the patients. Knowledge of the incubation period of the infection is of great value in interpreting the data.

(d) *Assessment of the extent of the outbreak*
This involves finding other infected persons in addition to those who
have been notified, and identifying others who also have been exposed to
the risk of infection: the contacts of known patients and others who have
been exposed to a common source such as a polluted stream.

METHODS OF CONTROLLING COMMUNICABLE DISEASES

Basically, there are three main methods of controlling a communicable
disease:
1 eliminate reservoir of infection
2 interrupt the pathway of transmission
3 protect the susceptible hosts.

1 Elimination of the Reservoir

Where the reservoir is in man, the objective would be to find and treat all
infected persons, both patients and carriers, thereby eliminating sources
f infection. For some infections, segregation of infected persons through
isolation or quarantine may be required.

(a) *Isolation of patients*
Isolation is indicated in the control of acute epidemic diseases such as
cholera, or for chronic infections such as lepromatous leprosy. Isolation
of patients is indicated for infections which have the following
epidemiological features:
  (i) High morbidity and mortality
 (ii) High infectivity
(iii) No significant extra-human reservoir
(iv) Infectious cases easily recognisable
 (v) No significant reservoir or carriers.

(b) *Quarantine*
This refers to the limitation of movement of persons who have been
exposed to infection. The restriction continues for a period of time equal
to the usual longest duration of the incubation period of the disease.

(c) *The Zoonoses*
Where the reservoir of infection is in animals, the appropriate action will
be determined by the usefulness of the animals, how intimately they are
associated with man and the feasibility of protecting susceptible
animals. Where, as in the case of the plague rat, the animal is regarded as
a pest, the objective would be to destroy the animals and exclude them
from human habitations. Where, as in the case of rabies in an urban
area, pet dogs are susceptible, the approach would be to protect them
with rabies vaccine whilst destroying stray dogs. Animals that are used

as food should be examined and the infected ones eliminated. This examination may take place in life, e.g. tuberculin testing of cattle, or it may take place after slaughter during meat inspection.

Where the reservoir is in soil, elimination of the reservoir is not feasible but it may be possible to limit man's exposure to the affected area, e.g. in some areas, infection with *Histoplasma capsulatum* occurs in persons who go into bat-infested caves. Such exposure can be avoided.

2 Interruption of Transmission

This mostly involves improvement of environmental sanitation and personal hygiene. The control of vectors also depends largely on alterations in the environment and in addition the use of pesticidal agents.

3 Protection of the Susceptible Host

This may be achieved by active or passive immunisation. Protection may also be obtained by the use of anti-microbial drugs, e.g. chemoprophylaxis is used for the prevention of malaria, meningococcal meningitis and bacillary dysentery.

Mass campaigns are sometimes indicated for dealing with acute epidemics or as a method of controlling or eradicating endemic diseases. Any vaccine or drug for a mass campaign must be effective, safe, cheap and simple to apply. Following the emergency operation of a mass campaign, the programme should be integrated into the basic health services of the community.

SURVEILLANCE OF DISEASES

Surveillance of diseases means the exercise of continuous scrutiny of and watchfulness over the distribution and spread of infections and the related factors, with sufficient accuracy and completeness to provide the basis for effective control. This modern concept includes three main features:
(a) The systematic collection of all relevant data
(b) The orderly consolidation and evaluation of these data
(c) The prompt dissemination of the results to those who need to know, particularly those who are in a position to take action.

The surveillance of communicable diseases has two main objectives. The first objective is the recognition of acute problems which demand immediate action. For example, the recognition of an outbreak of a major epidemic infection such as smallpox or the fresh introduction of it into a previously uninfected area, must be recognised promptly so that infection may be confined to the smallest possible area in the shortest possible time. Secondly, surveillance is used to provide a broad assessment of specific problems in order to discern long term trends and epidemiological patterns. Thus surveillance provides the scientific basis for ascertaining the major public health problems in an area, thereby serving as a guide for planning, implementation and assessment of programmes for the control of communicable diseases. Surveillance is essential for the proper assessment of priorities in public health programmes.

Surveillance involves the collection, evaluation and correlation of epidemiological information which is kept in separate elements by different administrative and professional groups. The sources of data include the following:

(a) Registration of deaths
(b) Notification of diseases and the reporting of epidemics
(c) Laboratory investigations
(d) Investigation of individual cases and epidemics
(e) Epidemiological surveys
(f) Distribution of the animal reservoir and the vector
(g) Production, distribution and care of vaccines, sera and drugs
(h) Demographic and environmental data.

Effective surveillance depends on the synthesis of all the data derived from the sources which are relevant to the particular problem. The detailed organisation of surveillance varies from country to country, but the basic feature is the mechanism by which pertinent epidemiological data are brought together, to be evaluated, correlated and interpreted by competent epidemiologists, thereby providing the logical basis for effective action. Most major control and eradication programmes now place considerable emphasis on surveillance in making the initial assessment and in evaluating the progress of the programme.

The techniques of surveillance are now being applied to such problems as the environmental hazards associated with atmospheric pollution, ionising radiation and road traffic accidents; to non-communicable diseases such as cancer, atheroma and other degenerative diseases; and to social problems such as drug addiction, juvenile delinquency and prostitution.

EPIDEMIOLOGY OF NON-INFECTIOUS DISEASES

Epidemiological methods have been widely applied in the study of non-infectious diseases. Such studies have yielded many fruitful results, especially in providing the basis for taking effective preventive action long before the specific aetiological agent is identified and long before the mechanism of the pathogenesis of the disease are understood. For example, Lind in the eighteenth century demonstrated that the occurrence of scurvy is associated with lack of fresh fruits in the diet of sailors. He was able to take effective action in preventing scurvy by the use of lime juice more than 150 years before the recognition of vitamin C as the specific factor involved. Epidemiological studies have made important contributions to knowledge of the aetiology of various diseases including the following examples:

(a) *Nutritional disorders*—scurvy, beri-beri, pellagra, dental caries, goitre.
(b) *Cancer at various sites*—skin, lungs, penis, cervix uteri, breast, bladder, leukaemia.
(c) *Congenital abnormalities*—Down's syndrome, thalidomide poisoning.
(d) *Intoxications*—chronic beryllium poisoning, alcoholic cirrhosis.
(e) *Mental illness*—puerperal insanity, neuroses, suicide.
(f) *Accidents*—home, road and industrial accidents.
(g) *Degenerative diseases*—tropical neuropathy, coronary artery disease, hypertension, arthritis.

Epidemiological Investigation of Non-infectious Diseases

For the study of infectious diseases, it is convenient to use the simple model of 'Agent', 'Mode of transmission' and 'Host'. This model needs to be modified in dealing with non-infectious diseases. Firstly, instead of a specific aetiological agent, the non-infectious disease may result from multiple factors. Secondly, since there is no infective agent being transmitted, it is more appropriate to replace this with 'environmental factors'. Thirdly, host factors cannot be analysed in terms of active or passive immunity but rather in terms of various host factors—genetic, social, behavioural, psychological, etc.—which modify the risk of developing these various diseases.

Risk factors

The concept of risk factors is increasingly used in the study of non-communicable disease. For example, many factors are associated with the occurrence of ischaemic heart disease including diet, exercise, and the use of cigarettes. From the public health point of view it is desirable to be able to assign different weights to each of these factors. How much does cigarette smoking contribute to the risk of the occurrence of ischaemic heart disease? Conversely how much change in the rate can be expected if a group alters its smoking habits. Similarly, the same question can be asked with regard to diet and exercise. Furthermore, there is the possibility that the effects of individual factors are not merely additive but may interact.

It is possible to obtain numerical estimates of the risk factors by the use of statistical methods including multiple regression and partial correlations.

Apart from the study of the aetiology of non-communicable diseases, the concept of risk factors has been applied to other health phenomena.

For example, in obstetric practice, the outcome of pregnancy is influenced by factors in the mother, in the environment and in the health care given to the mother and the newborn baby. Thus prenatal mortality rate is associated with such factors as the age of the mother, the number of previous pregnancies, her past obstetric history, her stature (especially her height and the size and shape of her pelvis), her state of health (especially the presence of diseases such as hypertension, diabetes, anaemia).

In some cases the risk factors relate directly to aetiological factors, such as cigarette smoking and cancer of the lung, but in other cases the risk factor identified may be a convenient, easily identified and measured indicator of an underlying factor. For example, the level of education of the mother can be identified as a risk factor in relation to the health status of the infant. The effect of the mother's education is indirect. It would have been more direct to measure her practices with regard to child care and specific indicators of mother care can be devised and validated. In many communities however the level of maternal education can serve as an index of important environmental, social and economic factors which affect the health of the child.

In spite of these apparent differences, the basic epidemiological approach is identical; the epidemiological investigation of non-communicable disease involves a study of the distribution of the disease (descriptive), a search for the determinants of the distribution (analytical), and deliberate experiments designed to test hypotheses (experimental). The basic strategy is to discover populations or groups in which the disease is relatively rare; these groups can then be compared and contrasted in the hope of discovering the probable causes of the disease. The effects of making alterations in these supposed factors can be examined by controlled trials.

THE USE OF EPIDEMIOLOGY

Epidemiology is a powerful tool of proven value in public health practice. The epidemiological approach should be more extensively used in defining and solving health problems in developing countries. Specialist epidemiologists have an important role in devising the epidemiological services, in training personnel and dealing with difficult problems especially at the district or national level. However, other health personnel who are not specialised in this discipline can and should use epidemiological methods in their work.

At the primary health care unit, epidemiological methods should be used to determine the most common causes of death, disease and disability, to find out which persons are at highest risk and to identify the determinant factors. Epidemiological methods should also be used to improve the health services. If for example data show that acute diarrhoeal diseases are among the commonest causes of death in a rural district, the most appropriate interventions can best be designed on the basis of epidemiological analyses of the problem. What is the distribution of the cases by age and sex? What is the geographical distribution? What is the seasonal distribution? Among the cases, what is the case fatality rate in different age groups? The data obtained at the health centre may not be sufficient to provide answers to these questions. A simple survey, house to house, will provide some of the missing data and also additional information about sources of water supply, cooking practices, food storage and other relevant matters. Such surveys could draw attention to polluted sources of water supply, to unhygienic practices in the home and to the need of promoting the use of simple oral rehydration for young children who have acute diarrhoea. Such studies do not call for elaborate protocols or for sophisticated statistical analyses and yet the findings can be very valuable in guiding and evaluating public health measures.

FURTHER READING

WHO Tech. Rep. Ser. No. 573: *The Veterinary Contribution to Public Health Practice.*
WHO Tech. Rep. Ser. No. 637: *Parasitic Zoonoses.*

CHAPTER 4

INFECTIONS THROUGH THE GASTRO-INTESTINAL TRACT

A number of important pathogens gain entry through the gastro-intestinal tract. Some of these cause diarrhoeal diseases (e.g. *Salmonella*, *Shigella*) whilst others pass through the intestinal tract to cause disease in other organs (e.g. poliomyelitis, infective hepatitis).

THE INFECTIVE AGENTS

The pathogens include viruses, bacteria, protozoa and helminths (Table 4.1).

Table 4.1 Examples of pathogens which are acquired through the gastro-intestinal tract

Viruses	Bacteria	Protozoa	Helminths
Poliomyelitis	*Salmonella typhi*	*Entamoeba histolytica*	*Ascaris lumbricoides*
Coxsackie	*Salmonella paratyphi*	*Giardia lamblia*	*Enterobius vermicularis*
	Cholera		
Infectious hepatitis	*Brucella* species		*Dracunculus medinensis*
	Pathogenic *Escherichia coli*		*Taenia solium*
			Taenia saginata

Physical and Biological Characteristics

In considering the epidemiology of these infections, it is useful to note some of the physical and biological properties of each infective agent. The organisms vary in their ability to withstand physical conditions such as high or low temperatures and drying; and they also differ in their susceptibility to chemical agents including chlorine. The vegetative form of *Entamoeba histolytica* is rapidly destroyed in the stomach but the cyst form survives digestion by gastric juices. Differences in the sizes of the organisms are also of epidemiological importance. Thus, simple filtration through a clay filter will eliminate most of the large organisms—bacteria, protozoa, and the eggs or larvae of helminths—from polluted water, but the filtrate will contain the smaller organisms such as viruses.

Mode of Transmission

Viruses, bacteria and cysts of protozoa are directly infectious for man as they are passed in the faeces, but in the case of helminths, the egg may become infectious only after maturation in the soil (e.g. *Ascaris*) or after passing through an intermediate host (e.g. *Taenia saginata*). The most important pattern of transmission is the passage of infective material from human faeces into the mouth of a new host and this is known as 'Faeco-oral' or 'Intestino-oral' transmission. It should be noted, however, that not all the pathogens which infect through the mouth are excreted in the faeces; for example, guinea-worm infection is acquired by mouth but the larvae escape through the skin. On the other hand, the ova of hookworm are passed in faeces but the route of infection is by direct penetration of the skin by the infective larvae.

The Faeco-oral Route of Transmission

The direct ingestion of gross amounts of faeces is uncommon, except in young children and mentally disturbed persons. Faeco-oral transmission occurs mostly through unapparent faecal contamination of food, water and hands—the three main items which regularly make contact with the mouth (Fig. 4.1). It should be noted that minute quantities of faeces can carry the infective dose of various pathogens. Thus, dangerously polluted water may appear sparkling clear, con-

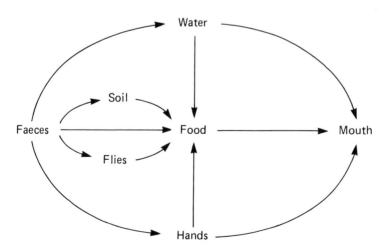

Fig. 4.1 Pathways of faeco-oral transmission

taminated food may be free of objectionable odour or taste, and apparently clean hands may carry and transmit disease.

As shown in the diagram, food occupies a central and important position. Not only can it be contaminated directly by faeces but also indirectly through polluted water, dirty hands, contaminated soil and filth flies. Water may be polluted directly by faeces; faecal material may be washed in from the polluted soil on the river bank. There are many opportunities for the contamination of hands: the person may contaminate his hands on cleaning after defaecation or in touching or handling contaminated objects including soil. Contamination of the soil with faeces plays an essential role in the transmission of certain helminths which must undergo a period of maturation before becoming infectious (e.g. *Ascaris*). Filth flies, in particular, the common housefly, spread faecal material and play a role in the transmission of gastro-intestinal infections. The housefly mechanically transfers faecal pollution:

(a) By carrying faeces on its hairy limbs
(b) By regurgitating the contents of its stomach on to solid food as a means of liquefying it ('Vomit drop')
(c) By defaecating on the food; its faeces may contain surviving organisms derived from human faeces.

Although flies are physically capable of transmitting these infections, it is not easy to determine how important they are in particular epidemiological situations and it is likely that their importance has been exaggerated in relation to the other mechanisms of transmission.

Epidemic Patterns in relation to the Mode of Transmission

Some of the infections which are acquired through the gastro-intestinal tract, characteristically occur in epidemic form, e.g. typhoid. The vehicle of infection may be water. The water-borne epidemic is typically explosive; it may affect people over a wide area who have no other traceable connection but the use of the same source of water supply. Food-borne outbreaks may be more localised, affecting persons from the same household or boarding institution, those who feed communally at a hotel, restaurant, aeroplane or staff canteen, or those who have taken part in a festive dinner or picnic.

Host Factors

Certain non-specific factors in the host play some part in preventing infection through the gastro-intestinal tract. Thus, the high acid content and the anti-bacterial lysozyme in the stomach, and the digestive juices in the upper part of the intestinal tract destroy potentially infective organisms but do not constitute an impenetrable barrier to infection. More significant is the specific immunity which can be derived from previous infections or from artificial immunisation. This immunity is in part related to specific antibodies in the sera of convalescent patients or artificially immunised persons. It has also been demonstrated that the intestinal mucosa may acquire resistance to certain pathogens such as cholera or poliomyelitis; this local resistance is mediated through fractions of immunoglobulins which are secreted by the mucosa.

Control of the Infections acquired through the Gastro-intestinal Tract

The most effective method of controlling these diseases can best be determined from a knowledge of the epidemiology of the infection with particular reference to the local community. The basic principles involved in the choice of method can be conveniently discussed with reference to Fig. 4.1. Control can operate at various levels:

1 *The infective agent*
  (a) Sanitary disposal of faeces
  (b) Elimination of human and animal reservoirs.
2 *The route of transmission*
  (a) Provision of safe water supply
  (b) Protection of food from contamination
  (c) Control of flies
  (d) Improvement of personal hygiene.
3 *The host*
  (a) Specific immunisation
  (b) Chemoprophylaxis
  (c) Specific treatment.

The measures listed in sections 1 and 2 relate to the improvement of environmental sanitation, and are mostly not specifically related to any particular infection. In general action can be taken (i) at the individual level, (ii) at the family level, (iii) at the community level, (iv) by investigating specific outbreaks, e.g. at school or parties, (v) by instituting surveillance charts in dispensary or primary health unit, and (vi) through health education.

1 VIRAL INFECTIONS

The most common viral infections transmitted through the gastro-intestinal tract are: (i) Poliomyelitis and other enteroviruses and (ii) Viral Hepatitis A (HAV).

Poliomyelitis and Other Enteroviruses

The enteroviruses, in addition to poliovirus, mainly include the *Coxsackie*, *Echo* (enteric cytopathogenic human orphan), *Reo* and *Rota* viruses. These viruses were first isolated from the faeces of patients during poliomyelitis investigations. Healthy persons may excrete enteroviruses for short periods, and in areas where standards of environmental sanitation are low they are prevalent among infants and young children. *Coxsackie viruses* are classified into two groups, A and B, and although frequently isolated from healthy persons they may cause a variety of human illnesses, e.g. herpangina, summer grippe, vesicular stomatitis, virus meningitis, etc. The presence of *Coxsackie* Group B virus can interfere with poliomyelitis virus multiplication, while a mixed *Coxsackie* Group A and poliomyelitis virus infection might result in a more severe paralysis.

Echo viruses are also excreted by healthy persons, particularly children, but may cause illnesses such as diarrhoea and virus meningitis. *Reo viruses* were first isolated from the faeces of healthy children but have been also found in children with diarrhoea and steatorrhoeic enteritis. By far the most important enterovirus in the tropics is poliomyelitis. In 1973, *rotavirus* was detected in the duodenal epithelium of infants with acute nonbacterial gastro-enteritis. Clinically, children aged six months to three years are susceptible with a peak incidence at 9–12 months, but older children and adults may excrete the virus. Data from community based studies in Guatemala and Bangladesh suggest that *rotavirus* accounts for approximately 10 to 20 % of all community diarrhoea cases. *Rotavirus* has been shown to be a common intestinal infection in animals and has been demonstrated as a cause of diarrhoea in mice, calves, piglets, chickens, kittens, goats and other animals. *It should be noted that the enteroviruses may interfere with oral poliomyelitis vaccination campaigns in the tropics.*

Poliomyelitis is an acute febrile illness classically resulting in a flaccid paralysis 'infantile paralysis'. The *incubation period* varies from 4 to 35 days with an average of about 10 days.

Medical Geography
The disease has a world-wide distribution; it is endemic in many areas of the tropics and subtropics but appears periodically in the form of epidemics. Poliomyelitis remains a serious problem in a large part of the developing world where the disease presents a constant threat to the childhood populations with consequences for social and economic development.

Virology
There are three distinct types of polio virus, type I (Brunhilde), type II (Lansing) and type III (Leon), which invade the central nervous system. The viruses grow well in tissue culture, they resist desiccation but are killed in half an hour by heat (60°C).

Epidemiology
Man is the reservoir of infection, the polio virus is excreted in the stools of infected cases, convalescent and healthy carriers. The virus is transmitted by food, water, or by droplet infection of flies. The incidence rates in males and females are similar. Trauma, excessive fatigue and

pregnancy during the period of acute febrile illness and intramuscular injections some time before the acute episode all seem to be provoking factors leading to paralysis. Tonsillectomy increases the risk of bulbar poliomyelitis. The mechanism of these various stresses is not clear.

In many areas of the tropics infection is hyperendemic and all of the known types of poliomyelitis virus (I, II and III) are prevalent. Within such communities the disease smoulders but epidemic outbreaks undoubtedly occur. The virus strains responsible for paralytic illness in any area may vary, and at different periods in the same area one type or other may predominate.

Poliomyelitis is a highly infectious disease and the alimentary tract is of prime importance as a portal of entry and exit of the virus, as it is with other enteroviruses. The factor of greatest importance in determining the incidence of paralytic poliomyelitis is the state of immunity of the affected population. In many tropical countries where sanitation is primitive and living conditions are crowded and poor, facilities for the spread of polio virus are good. Consequently infants have the opportunity of coming into contact with all three types of poliomyelitis virus early in life, and few of them reach pre-school age without having been infected with at least one strain, although, clinically, the infection is in most cases unapparent. Immunity is acquired early. In countries where the sanitary arrangements are good, the risk of contact with the virus at an early age is diminished and older persons are affected. Thus the most significant difference between the occurrence of poliomyelitis in the well-developed countries of the temperate zone and the less-developed areas of the tropics is in the distribution of cases in the various age-groups. Serum antibody surveys carried out among children in many parts of the tropics have shown that by the time they are 3 years old 90 per cent have developed antibodies against at least one type of poliomyelitis. Passive immunity is transmitted from mother to offspring and lasts for about 3–6 months.

Laboratory diagnosis
The virus is isolated from specimens of faeces, throat swabs or from throat and nasopharyngeal washings.

Control

High standards of hygiene and mass immunisation are the two most important measures of control.

(a) The individual
The disease is notifiable and isolation of individual cases is highly desirable. This measure by itself is not enough to control an epidemic because of the large numbers of asymptomatic carriers. All pharyngeal and faecal discharges of patients should be treated with disinfectants and disposed of as safely as possible. Contacts should be protected with oral polio vaccine and kept under observation for a period of three

weeks from the date of their last known contact. Tonsillectomy and dental extractions should be deferred when a poliomyelitis epidemic is present in the community and injections of any kind reduced to a minimum. Individuals should avoid over-exertion such as games, swimming, etc.

(b) *The community*

Crowds should be avoided during epidemics. Food should be protected from flies and sanitary disposal of faeces encouraged. Health education aimed at raising the standards of personal hygiene should be rigorously carried out. Rehabilitation for paralysed persons is essential. A 'lameness register' for all children entering school from the time an immunisation programme is initiated (see below) may serve as an indicator of the impact of the programme.

(c) *Immunisation*

Immunisation provides the most reliable method for the prevention of poliomyelitis and for controlling rapid spread during an epidemic. Two types of poliomyelitis vaccine are currently available: (i) the killed (Salk) vaccine which is given by injection and (ii) the attenuated (Sabin) vaccine which is given by mouth and through a mild infection induces protection against the disease. Unfortunately, evidence has accumulated that in many tropical countries the oral vaccine fails to provoke a satisfactory antibody response in a high percentage of recipients, probably because of interference by other enteroviruses (see pp. 47–8). Despite this, however, the Sabin vaccine does in practice appear to afford protection against the disease, especially when used in *mass immunisation* campaigns in the tropics. It is the most practical and economical method of rapidly immunising a large susceptible population and bringing an epidemic of poliomyelitis to an end. The simplest scheme for immunisation is to give 3 doses of the trivalent oral poliomyelitis vaccine at intervals of 4 weeks, and a fourth dose at school entry. For immunising small groups attending hospitals and clinics in the tropics the killed Salk vaccine might be preferable. Preparations are now available which incorporate killed poliomyelitis vaccine with triple antigen. A course of 3 injections given at 4-week intervals will thus provoke satisfactory immunity against tetanus, diphtheria, whooping cough and poliomyelitis. Children in the tropics should all be immunised against these diseases and expatriates irrespective of age should be protected against poliomyelitis before going out to the tropics.

Poliomyelitis—Summary

1 *Occurrence*—World-wide
2 *Organisms*—Polio virus I, II, III
3 *Reservoir of infection*—Man
4 *Modes of transmission*—Food, water, droplet

5 *Control*— (i) Isolation
(ii) Sanitary disposal of faeces
(iii) Health education
(iv) Immunisation

Infectious Hepatitis—Viral Hepatitis A (HAV)

The disease is characterised by loss of apetite, jaundice and enlargement of the liver. The *incubation period* varies from 15 to 40 days with an average around 20 days.

Medical geography
The disease is widespread but is probably more common in the tropics and subtropics; in these areas, most infections are acquired in childhood and many are subclinical.

Virology
Virus A is identified with infectious hepatitis (short-incubation hepatitis). HAV—Hepatitis A virus is in the range of 25–28 nm and is identified by immune electron microscopy. Other serological tests for hepatitis A virus are—(i) complement fixation, (ii) immune adherence haemagglutination, and (iii) radioimmunoassay.

Epidemiology
Man is the reservoir of infection, excreting the organism in the faeces and possibly urine. A viraemia also occurs. Faecal-oral spread is the most important mode of transmission by direct or indirect contact. Sporadic cases are probably caused by person-to-person contact, but explosive epidemics from water and food have also occurred. Food handlers can disseminate the infection. The ingestion of shellfish grown in polluted waters is attended by a risk of acquiring hepatitis A. Although in most parts of the tropics infective hepatitis is essentially a childhood disease, many adult patients are also seen and the disease is particularly severe in pregnancy. In many countries the incidence of infectious hepatitis is rising. Hepatitis has many epidemiological similarities to poliomyelitis and is a sensitive indicator of poor community hygiene. Violent exercise during the early stages of the disease seem to result in severe clinical attacks of hepatitis. In general, children tolerate hepatitis well and recover more rapidly than adults. A high frequency of glucose-6-phosphate dehydrogenase deficiency has been found among patients with hepatitis, and patients with the enzyme defect have a longer and more severe course. A high incidence of acute coma and an increased death rate was associated in Accra, Ghana, with immigration, shanty town residency, lower socio-economic status and pregnancy; a similar situation has been observed in India with regard to pregnancy. In the Ghana study, men required a longer time to recover from equivalent degrees of liver damage than women. Hepatitis is a recognized hazard for 'overlanders' who return from tropical countries by bus or hitch-hiking.

Control

If patients are in hospital they should if possible be barrier nursed as for any faeces-carried infection. Food handlers should not resume work until three weeks after recovery. All measures of personal and community hygiene useful in reducing the spread of infection should be encouraged.

Immunisation

Human immune serum globulin (ISG) is useful for persons going to the tropics where the disease is endemic. Even when it does not prevent infectious hepatitis, it does modify the severity in those persons who contract the disease. It is also extremely useful in protecting family contacts during epidemics (0.05 ml per kg, intramuscularly). The dose for those going to the tropics is 0.02 ml per kg of a 16 g per 100 ml solution and passive protection lasts for about 6 months. Recovery from a clinical attack creates a lasting active immunity.

Infectious Hepatitis—Summary

1 *Occurrence*—World-wide
2 *Organism*—Hepatitis A Virus (HAV)
3 *Reservoir of infection*—Man
4 *Modes of transmission*—Person to person, food, water
5 *Control*— (i) Personal and community hygiene
        (ii) Immunisation

Other types of viral hepatitis

Hepatitis B virus (HBV) causes long incubation hepatitis. HBV possesses at least 3 separate antigens: hepatitis B surface antigen (HBs Ag), hepatitis B core antigen (HBc Ag), and e antigen (HBe Ag). The HBe Ag is a valuable marker of the potential infectivity of HBs Ag-positive serum. Subdeterminants of both hepatitis B surface antigen and hepatitis B e antigen occur.

Another variant of acute hepatitis is referred to as Non-A : Non-B hepatitis with clinical symptoms similar to those of hepatitis B.

Serum hepatitis or hepatitis B (HBV) is *not* transmitted by the faeco-oral route and is only included here for convenience. The carrier state—defined as the presence of HBs Ag for more than six months—rises from 0.1 % in parts of Europe to 15 % in several tropical countries. Hepatitis B may be transmitted as a result of transfusion or by accidental inoculation of minute quantities of blood, e.g. repeated use of hypodermic needles without adequate sterilisation in particular with drug addicts, mass immunisation, tattooing and ritual scarification. Transmission may also occur by (1) insect bites (2) perinatally (3) mouth to mouth (4) during intercourse (5) and from the serous exudates of skin ulcers. The main prevention of hepatitis B lies in scrupulous aseptic technique for all injections—preferably the use of disposable syringes and needles. A hepatitis B vaccine is now available. On the basis of a possible causal relationship between hepatitis B virus and primary liver cancer, a strategy for the prevention of primary hepatocellular carcinoma using the vaccine is being worked out.

II BACTERIAL INFECTIONS

The most important bacterial infections that gain entry through the gastro-intestinal tract are: (i) The enteric fevers, (ii) Infant gastro-enteritis, (iii) The bacillary dysenteries, (iv) Cholera, (v) Brucellosis, (vi) Food poisoning.

Enteric Fevers

These infections are caused by members of the *Salmonella* group, *Salmonella typhi* and *S. paratyphi* A, B or C. They are one of the most common causes of a pyrexia of unknown origin. The *incubation period* is usually from 10 to 14 days.

Medical geography
The enteric fevers have a world-wide distribution although they are endemic only in communities where the standards of sanitation and personal hygiene are low.

Typhoid Fever

Bacteriology
S. typhi is a Gram-negative, aerobic, non-sporing, rod-like organism. The organism can survive in water for 7 days, in sewage for 14 days and in ice-cream for 1 month. In warm dry conditions most of the bacilli die in a few hours. Boiling of water or milk destroys the organism. There are many phage types of *S. typhi* and these have proved of great value in tracing the source of an epidemic. Outbreaks of chloramphenicol-resistant *S. typhi* Vi-Phage Type E1 have occurred in Mexico, South-East Asia and India.

Epidemiology
Typhoid fever presents one of the classical examples of a water-borne infection. All ages and both sexes are susceptible. Man is the only reservoir of infection. This may be an overt case of the disease, an ambulatory 'missed' case or a symptomless carrier. About 2–4 percent of typhoid patients become chronic carriers of the infection. The majority are faecal carriers. Urinary carriers also occur and seem more common in association with some abnormality of the urinary tract and in patients with *Schistosoma haematobium* infection. Although in most

patients the focus of persistent typhoid infection in carriers is in the gall bladder, in some, the deep biliary passages of the liver have also been incriminated. This seems particularly so in Hong Kong, where an association between *Clonorchis sinesis* and *S. typhi* carriers has been demonstrated. An association between *S. mausoni* infection and *S. typhi* has been reported from Egypt. Food handlers, especially if they are intermittent carriers, are particularly dangerous and have been responsible for many outbreaks of the disease. close contact with a patient whether family or otherwise, e.g. nurse, may result in infection being transmitted by soiled hands or through fomites such as towels.

Contamination of water—the cause of major outbreaks—can occur through cross-connection of a main with a polluted water supply, faecal contamination of wells, or faulty purification. Typhoid can also be spread by shell-fish, particularly oysters which mature in tidal estuaries and are thus exposed to contaminated waters. Milk-borne outbreaks occur either by direct contamination from a carrier or indirectly from utensils. Ice-cream, other milk products, ice, fruit, vegetables and salads may be infected directly from a carrier or indirectly. Flies or infected dust may be sources of infection. Food (e.g. tinned meat, vegetables infected from human faeces used as manure) can also cause epidemics.

Laboratory diagnosis
A leucopenia with a relative lymphocytosis is often seen. Blood or 'clot' culture during the first two weeks of the disease usually yields *S. typhi*. After about the tenth day the Widal test (O and H agglutinations) becomes positive and rises progressively—a rising titre rather than absolute values is necessary for diagnosis. The diazo test is a red coloration given by the froth of the urine of typhoid patients when mixed with the diazo reagents, despite its definite limitations it is a simple and useful diagnostic test in areas where laboratory facilities are minimal. It becomes positive during the second and third weeks. The Vi reaction is of help in the detection of the carrier state.

Control

The ultimate control of typhoid fever from a community depends on the sanitary disposal of excreta which will stop the dissemination of faecal matter from one person to another, the introduction of a permanent method of purification of water, and raising the standards of personal hygiene. In any outbreak of typhoid fever every attempt should be made to trace it to its ultimate source by the use of phage-typing, and serological tests, particularly for the presence of Vi antibody, to detect the chronic carrier.

(a) *The individual*
All typhoid patients should be barrier nursed in a general hospital or removed to an infectious diseases hospital. Cases should be immediately notified or if possible the room from where they came should be cleansed and disinfected. All fomites should be likewise disinfected. The treat-

ment of choice is still chloramphenicol 2 g daily for 14 days while trimethoprim-sulphamethoxazole is a valuable substitute. The patients should remain in hospital until, following treatment, stools and urine are bacteriologically negative on three occasions at intervals of not less than 48 hours. The above measures are not all feasible in many parts of the tropics and a compromise has often to be arrived at.

(b) *The community*
The chronic carrier is a difficult problem especially in the tropics, each one should be assessed in relation to his occupation and kept under as much surveillance as possible. In patients in whom the gall bladder is the definite site of infection, surgery (cholecystectomy) should be carried out. The prolonged administration of ampicillin (4 g daily for 1–3 months) has also been used successfully to treat *Salmonella* carriers; while a trimethoprim-sulphamethoxazole combination (Septrin) has given encouraging results.

If the water supply is suspect, e.g. by the simultaneous occurrence of a large number of cases in a limited area, boiling or hyperchlorination is required. If food is suspected, it should be traced back to its source and enquiries made as to any recent illness among persons handling the food; samples of the food should be taken for medical examination. Milk should be pasturised or boiled. The use of fresh human manure as fertiliser should be actively discouraged and vegetables boiled or cooked before consumption. Food should be protected from flies, the numbers of which should be reduced to a minimum.

(c) *Immunisation*
One attack of typhoid fever confers permanent immunity. Field trials in Yugoslavia, Poland, the USSR and Guyana have proved the value of typhoid vaccines, which have been shown to have a protective effect of nearly 90 per cent. Vaccines with a high content of Vi antigen are the most successful, and acetone-inactivated vaccines are superior to those killed by heat and phenol. One subcutaneous injection of 500 million killed *S. typhi* gives adequate protection. For primary immunisation of adults 0.5 ml subcutaneously on two occasions is given at a 4 weeks interval. One booster injection can be given every 5 years. Recent studies indicate that the live oral vaccine Ty 21a is safe, stable and effective against typhoid fever for at least 2 years.

The Paratyphoid fevers are food borne rather than waterborne. Infections and fatality is much lower than for typhoid fever. In other respects the diseases are very similar and the same preventive measures are generally applicable as for typhoid fever.

Enteric Fevers—Summary

1 *Occurrence*—World-wide
2 *Organisms*—S. typhi: S. paratyphi A, B, C

3 *Reservoir of infection*—Sick patient, convalescent, carrier (faecal,
             urinary)
4 *Modes of transmission*—Water, food, flies
5 *Control*— (i) Isolation, notification, search for source of infection
            (ii) Supervision of carriers
            (iii) Sanitary disposal of excreta
            (iv) Purification of water, control of flies, food hygiene
            (v) Immunisation
            (vi) Health education

Gastro-enteritis

Gastro-enteritis is one of the commonest causes of childhood mortality
in the tropics. Severe vomiting and diarrhoea leading to dehydration are
the cardinal features. The *incubation period* is usually from 1 to 5 days.

Medical geography

Infant gastro-enteritis has a world-wide distribution but is especially
common in the tropics.

BACTERIOLOGY Although gastro-enteritis in children can be due to a
  variety of causes, the bulk of infections in infants have been attributed
  to three groups of *Escherichia coli* or to viruses. The three groups of *E.
  coli* which have been recognised as important diarrhoeal pathogens
  are: (1) *enterotoxigenic E. coli* (ETEC) which produce enterotoxins,
  (2) *enteropathogenic E. coli* (EPEC) which have been responsible for
  frequent outbreaks of infantile diarrhoea in many parts of the world
  and of which the following specific serotypes—0111, 055, 026, 0229,
  0125, 0126, 0127 and 0128 seem to be the most frequent, and (3)
  enteroinvasive E. coli (EIEC) which have a pathogenesis similar to
  that of shigellosis.

    Echo, Coxsackie, Reo and Rota viruses cause diarrhoea in children
  (see p. 48).

    In 1977 *Campylobacters* sp. (*C. jejuni* and *C. coli*) were also
  recognised as a cause of acute gastro-enteritis in children and adults.

Epidemiology

Gastro-enteritis is much less common among infants who are breast fed.
Poverty, diet, fly infestation and ignorance of elementary hygiene are
responsible for the maintenance and spread of the disease. The
unfortunate newly acquired habit of early cessation of breast feeding
now gaining ground in the tropics and its substitution by bottle feeding
has contributed to an increased incidence of the disease among infants
and *is a retrograde step in more ways than one*. ETEC have been
responsible for outbreaks in Mexico, Morocco, Kenya, Brazil, Peru,
Bangladesh and India. There seem to be geographical differences in the
type of enterotoxin produced by strains. The incidence of infection is
highest in children under two years of age. ETEC have been isolated
from water and food sources; it is presumed that humans are the major

reservoir of infection. In a study on Bangladesh, 13% of household contacts of hospitalised cases were found to be infected with ETEC.

In developing countries EPEC are isolated from diarrhoea cases in the second six months of life. The aetiological significance of these isolations from sporadic cases of infantile gastro-enteritis is unclear and controversial.

There is some evidence that *Campylobacter* enteritis may be an important cause of diarrhoea in the developing countries although the magnitude of the problem has yet to be determined. *C. jejuni* enteritis is probably a zoonotic infection; consumption of contaminated poultry is a vehicle of infection; dogs may constitute another source of transmission.

Laboratory diagnosis
This is based on isolating the organism—an *E. coli* group, *Campylobacter* or an enterovirus from the faeces.

Control

(a) *The individual*
The child should be treated with the appropriate antibiotic whenever possible. Scrupulous attention to personal and general cleanliness is necessary for the prevention of gastro-enteritis. Breast feeding should be encouraged to be continued for as long as possible. If artificial feeding must be used, rigorous attention to the sterilisation of all utensils used for the preparation of the feed and of the bottles should be maintained. It is wiser in these instances to teach mothers how to feed their infants using a cup and spoon, since these are easier to keep clean than bottles. Personal cleanliness, e.g. hands and nails, must be enforced in all households containing infants and young children.

(b) *The community*
Control of flies is imperative; all food, feeding utensils especially bottles and teats must be stored in fly-proof surroundings. The sanitary disposal of faeces, and constant health education is necessary.

Gastro-enteritis—Summary

1 *Occurrence*—World-wide
2 *Organisms*— (i) *E. coli* groups
           (ii) Enteroviruses
           (iii) *Campylobacters*
3 *Reservoir of infection*—Man: Animals.
4 *Modes of transmission*— (i) Milk: Water: Food
                        (ii) Flies
5 *Control*— (i) Personal hygiene
          (ii) Sanitary disposal of faeces
          (iii) Encouraging breast feeding

  (iv) Sterilisation of milk bottles and other utensils
  (v) Control of flies
  (vi) Health education

Bacillary Dysentery

Bacillary dysentery is characterised by diarrhoea, fever and a sudden onset of abdominal pain. The *incubation period* is 1 to 7 days.

Medical geography

The infection has a world-wide distribution but it is commoner in tropical than in temperate climates.

Bacteriology

Species and varieties of the genus *Shigella* are numerous and they can be conveniently classified into four main subgroups:

1 *Sh. dysenteriae* of which there are 10 serotypes
2 *Sh. flexneri* of which there are 8 serotypes
3 *Sh. boydii* of which there are 15 serotypes
4 *Sh. sonnei* of which there are 15 colicen types

  The proportion of infections due to individual serotypes varies from country to country, and in the same country at different times. The organisms of greatest clinical importance are *Sh. dysenteriae, Sh. flexneri, Sh. boydii* and *Sh. sonnei*. Multiresistance, i.e. to sulfonamides, tetracycline, ampicillin and chloramphenicol, is prevalent in many developing countries. The dysentery bacilli are non-motile, Gram-negative organisms.

Epidemiology

Infection is derived from cases of the disease, from healthy convalescents (who can excrete organisms for up to 2 months or more); and from symptomless carriers who keep up infection in the community.

  The organisms, which are excreted in the faeces, may gain access to food through the soiled fingers of patients or carriers. Owing to the low infectious dose of *Shigella*, they may also pass from person to person by contact with inanimate articles, e.g. lavatory seats, door handles, crockery, bedding and clothes. Fly-borne infection is important in some parts of the tropics where these insects are numerous, e.g. the Middle East. Epidemics may occasionally result from the contamination of milk, ice-cream or water. Occupation (e.g. food handlers who are carriers) is an important factor in the social epidemiology of bacillary dysentery as well as of other faeces-transmitted diseases.

  Young children are more liable than older persons to acquire *Shigella* infections, and when infected to suffer from clinical disease. Diarrhoeal diseases surveys carried out in Mauritius, Sudan, United Arab Republic, Ceylon, Iran, Bangladesh and Venezuela showed that morbidity and mortality was highest among children under the age of 3. Diarrhoea was commonest during the weaning period and greater in bottle-fed than breast-fed infants. *Shigellae* were isolated both from children suffering from diarrhoea and from those having no diarrhoea.

Laboratory diagnosis
Direct microscopical examination of the faeces will reveal pus cells and sometimes red blood cells. The isolation of the specific organism from the faeces cultured as early as possible in the disease provides the best means of diagnosis. Fluorescent antibody techniques have been used for more rapid identification of the organisms.

Control

(a) *The individual*
The patient should be treated at home or in hospital and barrier nursed if possible. Strict personal hygiene should be encouraged among the family contacts or nursing personnel looking after the case and the stools should be treated with a disinfectant before disposal, clothing and bed linen should be similarly treated. If the disease is notifiable, the Medical Officer of Health should be informed.

(b) *The community*
The most valuable community measures are provision for the sanitary disposal of faeces, a pure water supply, food hygiene and control of flies. Health education to increase the standards of personal hygiene and stop the transmission of the disease within a family and from food handlers is essential. Hands *must* be washed before food is handled and facilities for this must be made available.

Bacillary Dysentery—Summary

1 *Occurrence*—World-wide
2 *Organisms*—Shigella dysentereae, S. flexneri, S. boydii and S. sonnei
3 *Sources of infection*—Sick patient, convalescent, carrier (especially food handler)
4 *Modes of transmission*— (i) Faecal contamination of food, water or fomites
(ii) Flies
5 *Control*— (i) Sanitary disposal of faeces
(ii) Pure water supply
(iii) Food hygiene
(iv) Control of flies
(v) Health education
(vi) Adequate treatment of patient

Cholera

This is a disease of rapid onset caused by *Vibrio cholerae* and characterised by vomiting; profuse dehydrating diarrhoea with 'rice water stools' and marked toxaemia. Muscular cramps, suppression of urine and shock occur later. The *incubation period* is 1 to 7 days. Cholera is a notifiable and internationally quarantinable disease. The global number of cholera cases reported to WHO in 1979 was 54 179 from 42 countries.

Medical geography

Classical cholera, caused by *Vibrio cholerae*, classical biotype (*V. cholerae* 01) is now virtually limited to the Indo-Pakistan subcontinent and notably in the deltas of the Ganges and Brahmaputra rivers. Cholera El Tor, caused by *Vibrio cholerae* El Tor biotype, was originally confined to a limited geographical area in the Celebes in Indonesia but has been spreading in a pandemic form since 1961 to Indonesia, Sarawak, the Philippines, Sabah, Taiwan, Korea, Hong Kong, the Chinese mainland, West New Guinea, Malaysia, Singapore, Burma, Thailand, India, Pakistan, Afghanistan, Iran, Bahrein, Nepal, Turkey and Iraq. It has been reported from Egypt, Libya, Tunisia, the southern USSR, Czechoslovakia and Spain, and has now firmly established itself in Africa, South of the Sahara.

Bacteriology

V. cholerae was discovered by Koch in 1883 and is a delicate Gram-negative organism. There are two biotypes, classical and El Tor. Each biotype contains three serotypes—Inaba, Ogawa and Hikojima. The El Tor biotype is named after the El Tor quarantine station in Egypt, where it was first isolated in 1920.

Epidemiology

The reservoir of infection is a sick person, a convalescent patient or a carrier through the faeces or vomit. For every typical case of the disease there may be 10–100 other symptomless persons excreting the vibrio.

Cholera may begin suddenly as a water-borne disease. In Calcutta, where cholera is endemic, the supply of filtered water falls short in summer and the people are found to use both unfiltered and tank water. Cholera also spreads by contaminated food (e.g. dates or shellfish), infected inanimate objects and by flies. Intrafamilial spread also occurs. Gastric acidity is a major factor in host resistance, the disease being more common in persons with hypochlorhydria. In order to flourish, cholera requires a combination of dense population and poor sanitation. For many years there was a tendency to overlook the role of symptomless carriers in the transmission of cholera, until it was shown that the carrier state in cholera El Tor may last for more than 12 years ('Cholera Dolores' in the Philippines) and that the vibrio can establish itself in the gall bladder.

Cholera El Tor has been proved capable of speedy and extensive spread over much wider areas than classical cholera, and in several such areas cases due to cholera El Tor have displaced those of classical cholera. In Calcutta, for instance, by the end of 1964 there was only one case of classical cholera for every ten or more cases of cholera El Tor. This epidemiological phenomenon is explained by the demonstration that the El Tor biotype eliminates the classical biotype in a few hours both *in vitro* and *in vivo*. Cholera has a seasonal pattern but the season varies from locality to locality and can change dramatically over a short time.

V. cholerae 01 has developed resistance to tetracycline in Tanzania and Bangladesh. The potential for spread of resistant strains to neighbouring countries is a matter of grave concern.

Immunity
Clinical cholera gives rise to a solid immunity for at least three years. This prolonged protection may either be due to the stimulation of local antibody response with persisting SIgA antibodies or to an mucosal immunological memory that can rapidly be boosted by reinfection.

Preliminary studies from the International Centre for Diarrhoeal Disease Research at Dacca indicate that B-Subunit (whole cell cholera vaccine) given either orally or intramuscularly induces a similar or higher immune mucosal response than clinical cholera.

Studies in children less than 2 years old in Bangladesh indicate that the injection of specific breast milk antibodies against cholera may protect against the development of severe symptoms.

Laboratory diagnosis
A definite diagnosis of cholera can be made only after isolation of *V. cholerae* from the faeces of patients. The faeces should be transported to the laboratory as rapidly as possible in alkaline peptone water (pH 9.0). Three methods are available for the rapid recognition of cholera vibrios: (i) the selective enrichment/fluorescent-antibody technique, (ii) the oblique-light technique and (iii) the gelatin-agar method. Microscopic examination of a stool specimen may show large numbers of vibrios.

Control

During epidemics the recognition of cases clinically is relatively easy, sporadic cases however can easily be missed and hence in endemic areas any case of severe gastro-enteritis must be considered as cholera until the contrary is proved.

(a) *The individual*
Early diagnosis, isolation and notification of cases is very important. A search for the source of infection should be made and steps taken to deal with that source when found. Concurrent disinfection of stools, fomites, house, linen, clothing, etc., should be carried out. The administration of antibiotics reduces the diarrhoeal period. Before the patient is discharged from hospital, two negative stool cultures are required and terminal disinfection of bedding, etc., must be carried out. *Oral*

rehydration has revolutionised the treatment of cholera and other acute diarrhoeal diseases.

The most suitable fluid for oral and nasogastric use is a glucose-salt solution which contains in one litre of water:

Sodium chloride (table salt)	3.5 grams
Sodium bicarbonate (baking soda)	2.5 grams
Potassium chloride	1.5 grams
Glucose (dextrose)	20.0 grams

Contacts must be traced, immunised (1 ml, 8000 million vibrios) and watched for 5 days or, if carriers, until two negative stools are obtained. Attendants of patients must be also immunised (1 ml), instructed to observe scrupulous cleanliness and disinfection of their hands and should be forbidden to consume food or drink in the patient's room or to go into the kitchen. Detailed surveillance of every person who might have the disease is desirable but rarely feasible in most of the cholera-prone countries.

(b) *The community*

Immediate steps must be taken to raise the existing standards of environmental sanitation and in particular to check all water supplies. Chlorination should be stepped up to 1.3 parts per million. Excreta and refuse disposal must be rigorously controlled and all other fly-breeding sources eliminated; if possible, houses should be sprayed with DDT. Bacteriological examination of pooled night-soil has been used to detect infections in Hong Kong, and from this source the infection can be traced backwards to its origin. The same method applied to latrines in Calcutta was not as successful. Food sanitation should be enforced and all public swimming-pools closed. People should be instructed to boil water, to eat only cooked foods and raise their standards of personal hygiene. Camps and hospitals for isolation cases should be improvised. Congregations of persons, e.g. in markets, places of prayer, etc., should be discouraged during epidemics. Control of travellers and pilgrims especially from endemic areas of cholera should be rigidly and continuously enforced. The establishment of treatment centres for diarrhoeal diseases is advocated. Countries must show a greater willingness to provide the WHO and their neighbours with a regular flow of information on their current states of cholera.

(c) *Immunisation*

All people at risk or travellers entering an endemic area must be vaccinated. Two injections given subcutaneously of 0.5 ml and 1.0 ml respectively at weekly intervals provide some protection. During epidemics, however, one injection of 1.0 ml is considered sufficient for mass immunisation and for contacts.

The efficiency of cholera vaccines in preventing disease has ranged from 0-80 per cent, averaging about 50 per cent. This level of induced immunity is of relatively little public health value. The highest level of protection is generally in the first three months and may continue for an additional three months. The available evidence suggests that both classical and El Tor vaccines will protect against either biotype.

The WHO epidemiological model of cholera indicates that the improvement of sanitation is the optimal means of controlling cholera and that vaccination is beneficial when applied together with sanitation. Cholera vaccine does not however prevent the development of the carrier state in household contacts.

Under International Sanitary Regulations, the validity of a cholera vaccination certificate extends for a period of 6 months, beginning 6 days after the first injection of the vaccine, or, in the event of a re-vaccination on the date of that re-vaccination.

Cholera—Summary

1 *Occurrence*—India/Pakistan subcontinent, S.E. Asia, the Near East, Africa, Southern and Central Europe
2 *Organisms*—*Vibrio cholerae*, classical and El Tor biotypes
3 *Reservoir of infection*—Man
4 *Modes of transmission*—Water, food, flies
5 *Control*— (i) Diagnosis, isolation, notification and antibiotics
        (ii) Search for source of infection
      (iii) Concurrent and terminal disinfection
      (iv) Environmental sanitation
       (v) Immunisation
      (vi) Health education, personal hygiene

Brucellosis

Brucellosis is one of the most important infections of animals which can affect man and which are referred to as Zoonoses. The human disease is characterised by fever, heavy night sweats, splenomegaly and weakness. The *incubation period* varies from 6 days to as long as 3 months.

Medical geography

The infection is widely distributed but is particularly prevalent in the countries around the Mediterranean Sea. Brucellosis is more prevalent in the tropics than is generally supposed and has been widely reported from Africa, South America and India.

Bacteriology

Human disease is attributed to *Brucella abortus*, *Br. suis* and *Br. melitensis* from cattle, swine and goat exposure respectively. *Brucella* are small, non-motile, non-sporing, Gram-negative coccobacilli. Apart from their different CO_2 requirements, the members of this group resemble each other closely in their cultural characters.

Epidemiology

Many animals can serve as sources of infection for man, among which the most important are cattle, swine, goats and sheep.

The modes of transmission are ingestion, contact, inhalation and inoculation from animals which are discharging *Brucella*. Infection by ingestion may occur by the gastro-intestinal route and by penetration of the mucous membrane of the oral cavity and throat. The transmission of *Brucella* by ingestion of contaminated milk, milk products, meat and meat products is well recorded. Viable *Brucella* may be present in the viscera and muscles of infected carcasses for periods of over 1 month. Camel meat and water are also vehicles of infection. Contact with infected material, e.g. placentae, urine, carcasses, etc., is a common mode of infection and brucellosis is an occupational disease of veterinarians, farmers, etc. Air-borne infection through the mucous membranes of the eye and respiratory tract can occur, while accidental inoculation has been recorded among veterinarians and laboratory workers. Brucellosis results in economic loss to animal husbandry. There is loss of protein food from animal abortion, premature births, infertility and reduced production of milk.

Laboratory diagnosis

The laboratory diagnosis of brucellosis includes bacteriological and serological methods as well as allergic tests. *Brucella* organisms can be cultured from the blood, bone marrow, synovial fluid, lymph nodes and other sources. A progressive rise of antibody titre occurs in acute brucellosis and the serum agglutination test nearly always gives significantly positive results in the presence of active infection. The interpretation of the agglutination test is not always easy since, owing to the occurrence of latent and past infections, a certain number of persons in countries where the disease is endemic have very high titres. The complement fixation test can also be used in the diagnosis of chronic brucellosis, while the intradermal test when positive only indicates a state of specific allergy and must be interpreted with great caution. It is a useful adjunct to other methods of diagnosis especially in epidemiological surveys.

Control

The main control of human brucellosis rests in the pasteurisation of milk and environmental sanitation of farms.

(a) *The individual*

Persons having contact with herds should observe high standards of personal hygiene. Exposed areas of skin should be washed and soiled clothing renewed. Employees in the slaughter houses should wear protective clothing when handling carcasses and these should be removed and disinfected after use. The antibiotic of choice for the specific treatment of brucellosis is tetracycline.

(b) *The community*

Pasteurisation of milk is the most important method of prevention of human brucellosis; when this is not possible all milk should be boiled before use. Health education and propaganda should be carried out. Infected animals should be segregated and possibly slaughtered. High standards of animal husbandry must be encouraged and, when possible, animals should be vaccinated.

(c) *Immunisation*
Vaccination in man is dangerous, a living vaccine 19-BA (a derivative of *Br. abortus* strain 19) has been used, however, in the USSR in persons at high risk of *Brucella* infection.

Vaccination of animals can result in control and even eradication of brucellosis among them. Living attenuated vaccines of *Br. melitensis*, and 19 *Br. abortus* have been widely and successfully used. Killed vaccines are also available.

Brucellosis—Summary

1 *Occurrence*—World-wide
2 *Organisms*—*Brucella abortus, B. melitensis, B. suis*
3 *Reservoir of infection*—Animals, e.g. cattle, goats, sheep and swine
4 *Modes of transmission*—Ingestion, contact
5 *Control*— (i) Pasteurisation of milk
             (ii) Elimination of brucellosis from herds

Bacterial Food Poisoning

Food poisoning in the tropics is commonly due to three species of bacteria: *Salmonella* spp. which are the most important, *Staphylococcus aureus* and *Clostridium welchii*.

1 Salmonella Food Poisoning

Salmonella food poisoning typically presents with diarrhoea, vomiting and fever. The *incubation period* is usually 12 to 24 hours.

Medical geography
This is world-wide, but infection is commoner in tropical communities with low hygiene standards.

Bacteriology
Salmonellae have been subdivided into many types, the majority being named after the place where they were first isolated. The commonest type causing food poisoning is *S. typhimurium* which is widely distributed in the animal, bird and reptilian kingdoms.

Epidemiology
The source of infection is usually *Salmonella*-infected animals, e.g. cattle, poultry, pigs, dogs, cats, rats and mice.

Meat is the common mode of transmission either as a result of illness in cattle or by contamination from intestinal contents in unhygienically maintained abattoirs. Other vehicles of infection are eggs and egg products, as a result of faecal contamination of the shell, and milk and milk products. Foodstuffs can be infected at any stage from the abattoir to the home by rats and mice, by human carriers of *Salmonellae* or subclinically infected persons during the processing or preparation of food. Typically explosive small epidemics occur among groups of people who have eaten of the same food.

Laboratory diagnosis
Serological agglutination methods are needed to identify the type of *Salmonella*, but the genus is readily recognised by standard bacteriological techniques.

Control

This is essentially a matter of food hygiene to be applied from the abattoir to the home.

(a) *The individual*
No individual should handle food stuffs except after thorough washing of hands. Any person suffering from diarrhoea should be debarred from handling or preparing food. High standards of personal hygiene must be maintained by any person connected with food whether cooked or uncooked.

(b) *The community*
Veterinary inspection of abattoirs must be thoroughly and scrupulously carried out and inspection of animals done both before and after slaughter. Carcasses of animals suffering from salmonellosis must be condemned from human consumption. The abattoirs should be hygienically maintained in order to avoid infection or contamination from intestinal contents. Meat and meat products should be thoroughly cooked and if possible refrigerated if they are to be served cold. If no refrigeration facilities are available, foods should be carefully stored away from rats, mice, flies and kept as cool as is feasible in the circumstances. Health education is needed to raise the general standards of personal and food hygiene.

Salmonella Food Poisoning—Summary

1 *Occurrence*—World-wide
2 *Organism*—*Salmonella* spp.
3 *Reservoir of infection*—Animals
4 *Mode of transmission*—Meat and meat products
5 *Control*— (i) Personal and food hygiene
        (ii) Inspection of abattoirs
        (iii) Health education of caterers and food handlers
        (iv) Refrigeration

2 Staphylococcus Food Poisoning

Staphylococcus food poisoning is characterised by an abrupt onset with nausea and vomiting sometimes accompanied by diarrhoea and shock. The *incubation period* is from 1 to 6 hours, i.e. very short, which is a differential point from *Salmonella* food poisoning.

Medical geography
The disease is world-wide.

Bacteriology
Certain strains of coagulase-positive staphylococci which produce a heat resistant enterotoxin are responsible for this type of food poisoning. They must be differentiated from the non-enterotoxin producing *Staphylococcus aureus* and *albus*.

Epidemiology
The source of infection is man, i.e. food handlers carrying the organism in the nose, throat, hand and skin lesions such as boils, carbuncles and whitlows. Food is contaminated either by droplet infection or by direct contact with infected cutaneous lesions. The mode of transmission is through manufactured semi-preserved foods eaten cold such as hams, tinned meats, sauces, custards, cream fillings of cakes and unpasteurised milk due to staphylococcal infection of cattle. A sudden outbreak of vomiting and diarrhoea in a group of persons who have partaken of the same meal within a few hours suggests staphylococcus food poisoning. Any occasion for mass feeding as occurs in funerals, weddings, schools and other institutions, is liable to result in staphylococcus food poisoning. In these instances food is often pre-cooked, stored and then served cold or after rewarming.

Laboratory diagnosis
If an unconsumed portion of the suspected food is still available this should be sent to the laboratory for examination of enterotoxin-producing staphylococci.

Control

This consists in the proper education of food handlers and high standards of food hygiene.

(a) *The individual*
All food handlers should be educated in personal hygiene and excluded from contact with foodstuffs if they suffer from purulent nasal discharges or pyogenic skin lesions until they are cured.

(b) *The community*
High standards of catering should be maintained and hygienic techniques for handling, preparation and storage of foods used. Whenever possible, cooked foods should be refrigerated and the adequate heat treatment of all milk and milk products is essential.

Staphylococcus Food Poisoning—Summary

1 *Occurrence*—World-wide
2 *Organisms*—Enterotoxin-producing staphylococci
3 *Reservoir of infection*—Man
4 *Mode of transmission*—Semi-preserved foods
5 *Control*— (i) Personal hygiene of food handlers
             (ii) Food hygiene and refrigeration

3 Clostridium welchii Food Poisoning

Clostridium welchii food poisoning presents with diarrhoea and pain, vomiting is not very common. The *incubation period* is 12 to 24 hours.

Medical geography
The condition is world-wide. A diffuse sloughing enteritis of the jejunum, ileum and colon known as '*enteritis necroticans*' or '*pigbel*' is very common in New Guinea.

Bacteriology
There are many serotypes of *Cl. welchii*. The rod-like organisms require anaerobic conditions in which to grow. They are Gram-positive and produce endospores. In New Guinea *Cl. perfringens* (*Cl. welchii*, type C) is thought to be associated aetiologically with 'pigbel'.

Epidemiology
The source of infection can be human, animal, or fly faeces, and the spores of *Cl. welchii* survive for long periods in soil, dust, clothes and in the environment generally. The carrier rate in human populations varies from 2 per cent to 30 per cent. The mode of transmission is by ingestion of meat which has been pre-cooked and eaten cold, or reheated the next day prior to consumption.

In New Guinea the disease in both epidemic and sporadic forms, is related to pig feasting, which is an integral and complex part of the indigenous cultures of all highland tribes. Males are affected more often than females. The fatality rates vary from nil to 85 per cent.

Laboratory diagnosis
Cl. welchii can be isolated from the stools of individuals suffering from the disease and from food remnants.

Control

A proper standard of food hygiene is the most effective method of controlling *Cl. welchii* food poisoning.

All meat dishes should be either cooked and eaten immediately or refrigerated until required. Reheating of foodstuffs should be avoided and in New Guinea special precautions should be taken when pig-feasting occurs. A successful vaccine has been developed with a clostridial toxoid prepared from type C cultures.

Clostridium Food Poisoning—Summary

1 *Occurrence*—World-wide, New Guinea (special type)
2 *Organism*—*Cl. welchii*
3 *Reservoir of infection*—Man, animals
4 *Mode of transmission*—Ingestion of meat
5 *Control*—Cooking and storage of meat, vaccination.

III PROTOZOAL INFECTIONS

The most important protozoal infections transmitted by the faeces/oral route are (i) amoebiasis, (ii) the flagellate infestations and (iii) toxoplasmosis.

Amoebiasis

Amoebiasis is caused by the protozoan *Entamoeba histolytica*. The parasite lives in the large intestine causing ulceration of the mucosa with consequent diarrhoea.

Medical geography
Amoebiasis has a world-wide distribution, but clinical disease occurs most frequently in tropical and subtropical countries. In temperate climates the infection is often non-pathogenic and symptomless.

Applied biology
The amoeba multiplies by binary fission. It lives in the lumen of the large intestine where under suitable conditions it invades the mucous membrane and submucosa. If red blood cells are available, the amoeba will ingest them. When diarrhoea occurs, amoebae are expelled to the exterior as such, and then are found in the freshly passed fluid stools. Amoebae are very sensitive to environmental changes, and so are short lived outside the body. When there is no diarrhoea and other conditions are favourable for encystation, the amoebae cease feeding, become spherical, secrete a cyst wall and the nucleus divides twice to form the characteristic mature four-nucleate cyst.

There are two other characteristic structures, a glycogen vacuole which acts as a carbohydrate reserve, and chromatoid bodies which are a ribosome store. Cysts kept cool and moist remain viable for several weeks.

The cyst is the infective form, and when ingested hatches in the lower part of the small intestine or upper part of the large intestine and a four-nucleate amoeba emerges from the cyst. After a series of nuclear and cytoplasmic divisions, each multinucleate amoeba gives rise to eight uninucleate amoebae, which establish themselves and multiply in the large intestine.

The sizes of the cysts produced by individual strains are uniform; they vary from $7 \mu m$ to $15 \mu m$ in diameter; they can be divided into two groups, those strains producing cysts over $10 \mu m$ and those below 10μ in diameter. The strains producing small cysts are now held to belong to a separate species, *E. hartmanni*. Infections with *E. hartmanni* are symptomless.

Epidemiology

Infection with *E. histolytica* occurs throughout both temperate and tropical climates, although the incidence of overt disease is high only in the tropics and subtropics. The disease is spread by cyst passers, who may be divided into two main groups:

(a) convalescents who have recovered from an acute attack
(b) individuals who can recall no clinical evidence of infection.

The latter possibly are the more common source of infection, even in countries with high standards of hygiene. Bad sanitation is more important than climate in the predominance of overt infection in the tropics. Carrier rates of *E. histolytica* among symptomless subjects have varied from 5 per cent in temperate areas with good hygiene to 80 per cent in some tropical communities. The parasite can be transmitted by direct contact through the contaminated hands of cyst carriers, e.g. in institutions; it is also transmitted indirectly by means of contaminated food, such as raw vegetables fertilised with fresh human faeces; and through the intermediaries of food handlers and flies. Infected water has occasionally been held responsible for the transmission of large outbreaks of the disease.

Although several animals harbour *E. histolytica*—monkeys, dogs, pigs, rats, cats—they are thought to be of no epidemiological importance in human infections. Amoebic dysentery is not infrequently a house or family infection. Among other factors influencing the epidemiology of the disease we have to consider the following: (i) age and sex, (ii) race, (iii) immunity and (iv) diet.

Any differences that have been reported in the incidence of the disease between males and females are probably related to exposure rather than a true sex susceptibility to the infection. The disease seems to appear in fulminating form in pregnant and puerperal women. This may be a corticosteroid effect. Amoebiasis in childhood is not uncommon. It usually occurs in the age-group nil to 6 years, as those between the ages of 7 and 16 years seem to enjoy a greater immunity to ill effects from *E. histolytica* infection than others.

All races are susceptible to the disease. Although the infection is often milder in Europeans, this is probably related to sanitary standards, diet, and freedom from debilitating disorders, rather than to a genuine racial factor. Reports from Madras indicate that amoebiasis was twenty times more frequent in Hindus than in Muslims, while in Durban the incidence and severity of amoebic dysentery is greater in Africans than in Indians or Europeans.

There is no evidence that amoebiasis confers any protective immunity and the infection can persist for many years after its establishment. The general condition of patients plays an important role; thus, severe cases of amoebiasis are often seen among soldiers on active service.

Laboratory diagnosis

The clinical diagnosis of amoebiasis has to be confirmed by identification of *E. histolytica*. During an attack of amoebic dysentery the motions are loose, offensive, and contain mucus and blood, faecal elements are always present. On microscopical examination motile amoebae, some with engorged red cells, will be found in the freshly passed stool or in specimens removed at sigmoidoscopy or proctoscopy.

In asymptomatic infections, and during remission, the stool is semiformed and contains *E. histolytica* cysts. They can be seen to contain one or more bar-shaped chromatoid bodies and staining with iodine reveals one to four nuclei and a glycogen mass. Repeated stool examinations (six specimens collected at weekly intervals) should be made before absence of infection can confidently be assumed. Concentration techniques for cysts are available, and cultural methods may assist diagnosis in scanty infections.

Until recently, immunological methods for the diagnosis of intestinal and extra-intestinal amoebiasis have been equivocal. Complement-fixation, precipitin, and intradermal tests have all been used with varying success. New techniques, e.g. latex agglutination and amoebic gel-diffusion tests, with improved antigens promise better results. The fluorescent antibody test has proved very reliable.

Control

The main control measure is the provision and use of sanitary disposal of faeces coupled with personal cleanliness.

(a) The individual

Raising the standards of personal hygiene through health education is the only method that can be applied to the individual, e.g. advice on washing of hands, especially after defaecation. Food handlers, e.g. cooks, are a specially important group to train. Adequate treatment of individual infections with metronidazole or other amoebicides reduces the reservoir of infection.

The community

The provision of a safe water supply and facilities for sanitary disposal of faeces are the main control measures applicable to the community. The use of human faeces as fertilisers should be discouraged. In areas where a pure water supply is not available, water should be boiled and raw vegetables and fruit thoroughly washed and dipped in boiling water. Food should be protected from flies.

Amoebiasis—Summary

1 *Occurrence*—World-wide
2 *Organism*—*E. histolytica*
3 *Reservoir of infection*—Man
4 *Modes of transmission*—Contaminated hands, food
5 *Control*— (i) Sanitary disposal of faeces
         (ii) Personal hygiene

Other Amoebae

Infection of the human gut may occur with other amoebae, namely *E. coli*; *Dientamoeba fragilis*; *Endolimax nana*; and *Iodamoeba butschlii*. There is controversy, however, concerning the actual pathogenicity of these organisms. *Naegleria fowleri* has been reported as causing a fatal necrotising meningo-encephalitis.

Flagellate and Other Intestinal Protozoa

A number of flagellate protozoa commonly parasitise the human intestine and genito-urinary tract, e.g. *Trichomonas hominis*; *Chilomastix mesnili*; *T. vaginalis*; and *Giardia lamblia*. The ones with real claims to pathogenicity are *G. lamblia* and *T. vaginalis* which are found both in the tropics and in temperate countries. *T. vaginalis* urethritis is common in males (see p. 135).

1 Giardiasis

Heavy infection with *G. lamblia* is often accompanied by diarrhoea or steatorrhoea.

Applied biology
The trophozoite lives in the upper part of the small intestine particularly the duodenum and jejunum. In appearance it resembles a half-pear split longitudinally measuring 12–18 μm in length. It reproduces itself by a complicated process of binary fission. The cysts—which are the infective forms—occur in the faeces, often in enormous numbers. They are oval in shape, contain at first two nuclei which divide, giving rise to four in the mature cyst.

Epidemiology
Man is the source of infection. *G. lamblia* is harboured by many animals, but these play little part in the epidemiology of human infections. The infection is transmitted by the ingestion of cysts, as a result of insanitary habits or contaminated food. It is common in children and in adults, sometimes causing symptoms of malabsorption in both, due to mechanical irritation rather than invasion of the mucous membrane. Giardia infections may persist for years and the parasite may invade the biliary tract. 'Overlanders' are particularly prone to acquire the infection.

Recent outbreaks have had the following features in common: they occur in communities in which (1) surface water (streams, rivers, lakes) not well water is used; (2) chlorination is the principal method for disinfecting water; and (3) water treatment does not include filtration. These outbreaks exemplify the increasing frequency with which Giardia is being implicated as the cause of water-borne outbreaks of diarrhoea. It is also evident that chlorine levels used in routine disinfection of municipal drinking water (0.4 mg/l free chlorine) are not effective against Giardia cysts, although hyperchlorination (5–9 mg/l free chlorine residual) may be successful.

Laboratory diagnosis
Diagnosis of infection is made by finding cysts of the parasite in formed stools and vegetative forms in fluid stools.

Control

The main control measures are the provision and use of a safe method of excreta disposal and the raising of personal standards of hygiene. Boiling is the most reliable method for killing Giardia cysts in water.

2 Trichomonas hominis and T. vaginalis

T. hominis inhabits the caecum and large intestine. The body is pear-shaped, 10–15 μm in length. The single ovoid nucleus is situated in the rounded-anterior end and there are three flagellae. There is no cystic phase. The presence of these flagellates in diarrhoeic stools has no pathogenic significance. *T. vaginalis* is found in the vagina and male urethra. It is larger than *T. hominis*, reaching 27 μm in length, and usually has five anterior flagella. No cysts are known. The flagellate is commonly found during the reproductive period in women, and men play an important part in the transmission of the infection. The incidence of infection in the vagina may be high and the presence of the parasite is associated with lowered vaginal acidity.

In the female vaginitis is usual and an anterior urethritis may occur. Posterior urethritis is rare and the bladder is never affected.

Diagnosis is made by finding the flagellate in vaginal and prostatic secretions or in the urine.

Control

This involves the treatment of both marriage partners simultaneously with metronidazole, 200 mg tds for 5 days.

3 Isosporiasis

The coccidia *Isospora belli* and *I. hominis* are widely distributed in the tropical world. No pathological accounts are available and the pathogenicity of these organisms is mild and controversial.

4 Balantidiasis

Balantidiasis in man has been recorded from most parts of the world, and is caused by infection with the ciliate protozoon, *Balantidium coli* which is a common parasite of the pig.

Applied Biology

The large ovoid cysts are passed in the faeces and contain the parasite which may be seen moving actively. The enclosed balantidium then loses its cilia, and sometimes two individuals are found in the same cyst. *B. coli* reproduces asexually by transverse fission. Transmission of infection takes place by ingestion of cysts, but the subsequent life cycle is not known.

Epidemiology

B. coli has been found in the intestinal contents of man and a large number of animals—wild boars, sheep, horses, rats, frogs, monkeys, etc., but domestic pigs are much the most important reservoir hosts. Infection in man is comparatively rare despite man's close contact with pigs in many countries, and in more than 50 per cent of human cases there may be no history of contact with pigs.

It is possible that man is most often infected by fingers, food, drinking water, or soil contaminated by pigs' faeces containing balantidia, usually in the encysted form. Handling of the intestines of infected animals or flies are other possible modes of transmission. Furthermore, the possibility of infection from green vegetables grown in soil fertilised by pig excrement must be borne in mind, especially as cysts may remain viable for weeks in moist faeces.

The reported incidence in man is very variable (0.5–5.1 per cent) and depends on whether freshly collected specimens of faeces are examined or not. Epidemics have been reported from mental institutions, and in Papua New Guinea a high incidence of infection has been recorded.

Laboratory diagnosis

The stools are bloody and mucoid. Examination of faeces will reveal the typical large ovoid cysts 45–60 μm in length containing the parasite. The trophozoites may also be seen in freshly collected stools. The protozoon is oval in shape and of variable size—20–30 μm in length by 40–60 μm in breadth. The body is clothed with a thick covering of cilia arranged in longitudinal rows. Both the direct and indirect fluorescent antibody techniques have recently been applied in the diagnosis of *B. coli*.

Control

High standards of personal hygiene must be maintained, especially among persons in close contact with pigs—gloves should be worn when handling the intestines of potentially infected animals. Green vegetables should be washed and dipped in boiling water. Environmental sanitation of piggeries should be encouraged. Sanitary disposal of faeces and purification of water are the main control measures for the community.

Toxoplasmosis

Toxoplasmosis is caused by the intracellular sporozoon *Toxoplasma gondii*. The infection may be congenital or acquired. Clinically there are four types of acquired toxoplasmosis: (i) asymptomatic, (ii) acute, (iii) glandular and (iv) chronic.

Medical geography
Toxoplasmosis has a world-wide distribution. In the tropics it is probably commoner than is generally realised.

Applied biology
The life cycle of *T. gondii* is similar to that of coccidian parasites and its taxonomic status is now considered to be a coccidian parasite related to the genus *Isospora*. When extracellular, the organism is crescent shaped, about 6 μm long. The cytoplasm stains blue with Giemsa and the eccentric nucleus red. In the intracellular stages *T. gondii* appears singly or in clusters within the reticulo-endothelial cells. Aggregations of the organisms may form pseudocysts. The cystic form of the parasite reaches 100 μm in diameter. Reproduction of the organism is by binary fission. Toxoplasma trophozoites and cysts characterise acute and chronic infections respectively, but cysts may form early in the acute stage and trophozoites may remain active for years in some chronic infections.

Epidemiology
Man is the main reservoir of human infection. The method of transmission of *T. gondii* from person to person is unknown except in congenital infections. Surveys of various populations have shown that a high incidence of asymptomatic infection occurs in the warm or hot humid areas, and a low incidence in the cold areas and hot dry areas. In general, there does not appear to be any differences in infection rate between urban and rural populations, between sexes or between races in the same environment. *T. gondii* is widely distributed in the animal kingdom, being particularly common in cats, dogs and rabbits. However, in spite of the circumstantial evidence indicating a possible transmission between animals and man, it is probable that both may become infected from a common source or sources. Ingestion of raw beef and pork meat are a recognised mode of infection and it has been demonstrated that infection was particularly high in a tuberculosis hospital in France, where the children were fed raw or underdone meat. Antibodies, however, are found just as frequently in vegetarians as in meat eaters in India. High infection rates have also been found in sewage workers, rabbit trappers, laboratory workers and nurses. The role of droplet infection and mechanical subcutaneous inoculation by biting, or

blood-sucking arthropods, in the transmission of toxoplasmosis, has yet to be proved. *Toxoplasma* can be transmitted inside the egg of the cat roundworm *Toxocara cati*, but this is not likely to be the main mode of infection in man.

Laboratory diagnosis

In the blood there may be a leucocytosis or leucopenia. An eosinophilia has been described. There may be a mild degree of anaemia and a leukaemoid reaction and atypical lymphocytes may be seen.

Toxoplasma may be isolated from blood, cerebrospinal fluid, saliva, sputum, lymph nodes, skin, liver and muscle by intraperitoneal injection of the biopsy or other material into mice, guinea-pigs or hamsters. Mice are most suitable as they do not suffer from toxoplasmosis as a laboratory infection.

A number of serological tests have been described for the detection of antibodies to *T. gondii*, the cytoplasm-modifying test of Sabin-Feldman (dye-test) is the one most widely used. It is a sensitive test which shows the presence of antibody in many of the normal adult population, and the most convincing method of diagnosing active toxoplasmosis is by the demonstration of at least a fourfold rise in titre, coupled with the isolation of toxoplasma in the tissues or body fluids by inoculation of mice.

Other serological tests in common use are:
 (i) complement-fixation tests
 (ii) direct agglutination test
(iii) haemagglutination test
(iv) fluorescent antibody test.

Recently a toxoplasma neutralisation test and a micro-agglutination test have been described.

Control

The most effective treatment for both man and animals is a combination of pyrimethamine and sulphonamides. Intimate contact with sick animals should be avoided, and ingestion of raw meat discouraged.

Toxoplasmosis—Summary

1 *Occurrence—World-wide*
2 *Organism—T. gondii*
3 *Reservoirs of infection*—Man, other mammals
4 *Modes of transmission*—Raw beef and pork
5 *Control*—(i) Personal hygiene
              (ii) Thorough cooking of meat of animal origin

IV HELMINTHIC INFECTIONS

Many important helminths are transmitted through the gastro-intestinal tract and the infections they give rise to can be classified as follows:

Nematodes	Cestodes	Trematodes	
Ascariasis	Taeniasis	Paragonimiasis—Lung fluke	
Toxocariasis	Diphyllobothriasis	Clonorchiasis	⎫
Trichuriasis	Hymenolepsiasis	Opisthorchiasis	⎬ Liver flukes
Enterobiasis	Hydatid disease	Fascioliasis	⎭
Dracontiasis		Fasciolopsiasis	⎫
Trichinosis		Heterophyiasis	⎬ Intestinal flukes
Angiostrongyliasis		Metagonimiasis	⎭
Gnathostomiasis			

Ascariasis

This disease, due to *Ascaris lumbricoides*, is often symptomless and infection is discovered incidentally; occasionally it causes intestinal obstruction in children.

Medical geography
A. lumbricoides, the large intestinal roundworm, has a world-wide distribution the incidence of which is largely determined by local habits in the disposal of faeces. Its highest prevalence is in the hot humid climates of Asia, Africa and tropical America.

Applied biology
The adult worms live in the small intestine. Their colour is yellowish-white and they may reach a length of 40 cm. The female is prolific, laying up to 200 000 eggs a day. The typical egg has a yellowish-brown mamillated appearance.

The eggs are passed in the faeces, and providing the environment is suitable a larva develops within the egg and becomes infective in about 10 days. After eggs containing larvae are swallowed by man, the young worms hatch, are set free in the small intestine and begin the migration. This takes them through the wall of the small intestine, and by way of the hepatic portal system to the liver. They are then carried by the bloodstream to the right heart and to the lungs, where they remain for several days, after which they migrate passively up the bronchi and trachea to the pharynx. They are now swallowed and re-enter the small intestine where they become sexually mature in about 2 months.

The migratory phase of larval development in the liver and lungs requires 8–15 days and is associated with fever, allergic dermatitis, eosinophilia and pneumonitis or pneumonia.

Epidemiology

Man is the reservoir of infection which is spread by faecal pollution of the soil. The eggs are swallowed as a result of ingestion of soil or contact between the mouth and various inanimate objects carrying the adherent eggs. Contamination of food or drink by dust or handling is also a source of infection. Eggs of *Ascaris* pass unaltered through the intestine of coprophagous animals and can thus be transported to locations other than human defaecation sites. The well-protected eggs withstand drying and can survive for very lengthy periods.

Although all age-groups show infection in endemic areas, the incidence and intensity are highest in the younger age-groups. Infants may be parasitised soon after birth by ova on the mother's fingers. In human subjects the observed differences in incidence and intensity at different ages are probably due to differences in behaviour and occupational activities between children and adults, as well as to the development of acquired resistance.

Ascaris eggs are resistant to cold and to disinfectants in the strengths in normal use. They are killed by direct sunlight and by temperatures above 45°C. Under optimum conditions eggs may remain viable for as long as 1 year. *A. suis*, which infects pigs, is morphologically identical and can mature in man, but cross-infection has not been proved. In epidemiological studies, serological tests (e.g. larval microprecipitation test) are useful to detect early infections as well as the lung manifestations of the larval stages of *Ascaris* infection.

The prevalence of ascaris infection in children can be usefully used as an index of faeco-oral transmission in a community.

Laboratory diagnosis

The microscopical diagnosis of ascariasis can be confirmed by examination of faeces samples. Because of their characteristic morphology and colour the ova can be found relatively easily in 'direct smears'. Concentration and quantitative techniques are available.

Control

The main method of control is the sanitary disposal of human excreta.

(a) *The individual*

Health education should be directed towards raising standards of personal hygiene especially among mothers, who should be encouraged to train young children not to defaecate indiscriminately.

(b) *The community*

A method of sanitary disposal of faeces, i.e. some type of latrine acceptable to the people and best suited to the terrain, should be introduced and the people encouraged to use it. Human faeces should not be used as fertiliser unless previously composted so that the resulting high temperature can kill the eggs. Sanitary facilities should be provided for persons who spend long hours at work out of doors and such persons, e.g. farmers, should be encouraged to use the facilities provided. Mass treatment of pre-school and school children may be undertaken using a single dose of one of the piperazine compounds (2 g-5 g) or levamisole (40 mg-80 mg).

Chemotherapy can be utilised as the short-term approach to control, fortified by improvements in personal hygiene and sanitation as the long-term solution for ascaris and the other faeco-orally transmitted helminth infections.

Evidence has accumulated that ascaris infection retards growth in children and clinical signs of protein-energy malnutrition increase in ascaris infected children and significantly decrease after deworming.

Ascariasis—Summary

1 *Occurrence*—Hot humid climates of the world
2 *Organism*—*A. lumbricoides*
3 *Reservoir of infection*—Man
4 *Modes of transmission*—Contaminated hands, food, drink
5 *Control*— (i) Sanitary disposal of faeces
        (ii) Personal hygiene
        (iii) Chemotherapy

Toxocariasis (visceral larva migrans)

Evidence has now accumulated that human disease due to larval migration of *Toxocara canis* and *T. cati* constitutes an important public health problem, and although the majority of reports to date have emanated from the more developed countries we believe that it is merely a question of time before these infections are widely reported from the tropics as a major cause of some of the otherwise unexplained clinical syndromes seen in these areas.

Medical geography

The majority of human cases have been reported from the eastern half of the United States, but the disease has been recognised in the Philippines, Mexico, Hawaii, Turkey, Puerto Rico and other countries. Toxocaral infection of dogs has been reported from Malta, Nigeria, Uganda, Kenya, Tanzania, Mexico and India.

Applied biology

T. canis and *T. cati* are parasites of dogs and cats and their presence in the human host is an abnormal migration of their larval phase.

Under favourable conditions, the eggs passed in the dog's faeces become infective in 2–3 weeks. From the swallowed eggs emerge the contained second-stage larvae which penetrate the intestinal walls and reach the liver. The majority of larvae remain in the liver but others may pass on to the lungs or other organs of the body, including the central nervous system and the eye. Occasionally the larvae complete their cycle of development in the human host, resulting in infection with adult *T. canis* or *T. cati*.

Epidemiology

The reservoir of infection is the dog, or less frequently the cat. Infection is acquired by ingesting soil which has been contaminated, usually by dogs' faeces. Young children are particular susceptible to toxocariasis because of their habit of eating dirt, and of handling soiled fur of puppies and then putting their fingers in their mouths. The severity of the disease depends upon the numbers of worms that have invaded the body and the duration of infection. It has been shown that puppies are more infected than adult dogs and that the incidence among bitches is lower at all ages. It is possible that nematode larvae other than *Toxocara* may be involved in visceral larva migrans. Viral encephalitis due to larval migration has been reported and the transmission of poliomyelitis virus by larvae of *Toxocara* has been suspected.

Laboratory diagnosis

A high, stable persistent eosinophilia reaching levels of 60 per cent is a prominent feature. *Toxocara* larvae can be identified in biopsy material and provide the most certain means of making a definite diagnosis. The fluorescent antibody test has also been used.

Control

Elimination of infection in puppies and dogs is the most effective way of controlling the disease. Puppies used as household pets should be regularly examined and treated. Children should be instructed in habits of personal hygiene. Treatment of pets can be effectively carried out with one of the piperazine compounds.

Toxocariasis—Summary

1 *Occurrence*—World-wide
2 *Organisms*—*T. canis* and *T. catis*
3 *Reservoir of infection*—Dogs and cats
4 *Mode of transmission*—Handling infected household pets
5 *Control*— (i) Treatment of household pets
        (ii) Personal hygiene

Trichuriasis

This infection is due to the whipworm *Trichuris trichiura* and it is often symptomless. Heavy infections of over 1000 worms, however, may cause bloody diarrhoea with anaemia and prolapse of the rectum.

Medical geography

Trichuriasis occurs throughout the world but is more prevalent in the warm humid tropics.

Applied biology

The sexually mature worms, which are about 5 cm long, have a whiplike shape and live in the caecum and upper colon of man. After fertilisation the eggs are passed in the faeces within 4 weeks of infection and embryonic development takes place in the soil. Under favourable conditions of moisture and temperature the larvae develop inside the eggs within 2–5 weeks. The embryonated eggs are infective.

When the eggs are ingested by man the larvae escape into the upper small intestine and migrate directly to the caecum, where they become adults within 1–3 months.

Epidemiology

Man is the reservoir of infection. Soil pollution is the determining factor in the prevalence and intensity of infection in a community, and clay soils are more favourable than sandy soils. Transmission occurs through the insanitary habit of promiscuous defaecation; and infection usually results from the ingestion of infective ova from contaminated hands, food or drink. Although *Trichuris* infection of domestic and other animals occurs, it is unlikely that animal reservoirs play a part in the epidemiology of human infection. Coprophagous animals can transport *Trichuris* eggs to locations other than human defaecation sites, since the eggs are passed unaltered through their intestine. The higher prevalence in children is probably due to greater exposure to infection.

Laboratory diagnosis

Direct smear examination of faeces will reveal the characteristic lemon-shaped ova. An egg count on an ordinary wet faecal smear (containing about 2 mg of faeces) of more than 100 ova is indicative of a heavy infection. Concentration and quantitative techniques can be applied.

Eosinophilia (10–20 per cent) is usually present, especially in massive infections. An associated microcytic hypochromic anaemia may be seen and the mucoid sticky stools may contain a preponderance of eosinophil cells and Charcot-Leyden crystals.

Control

1 Sanitary disposal of faeces
2 Personal hygiene.

Enterobiasis

This infection is due to the pinworm *Enterobius vermicularis* and is prevalent throughout the world and is probably less common in the tropics than in countries of the temperate zone. The infection may be symptomless or there may be mild gastro-intestinal discomfort and pruritus ani.

Applied biology

The female worm is about 8–13 mm long while the male worm—which is rarely seen—is only 2–5 mm. They both live in the caecum, where copulation takes place. The gravid females then migrate to the colon and rectum and at night pass through the anus to deposit their eggs on the perianal skin and genitocrural folds. Within a few hours larvae develop within the eggs, which are now infective. Upon ingestion by man, the larvae hatch in the duodenum and mature in the caecum. The life cycle from egg to adult lasts 3–7 weeks. The survival of the ova depends upon temperature and humidity; viability being greatest in cool, moist surroundings.

Epidemiology

Man is the reservoir of infection. The highest incidence of enterobiasis is in school-children from 5 to 15 years. It is very prevalent in crowded districts with faulty hygiene, in institutional groups, and among members of the same family.

The ova from the perianal region are transferred to night clothes, towels and bedding, and infection may follow when these are handled. Infective ova may be present in the dust and infection can therefore take place by inhalation. The intense pruritus around the perianal regions results in scratching and the hands, especially beneath the finger nails, become contaminated and ova are transferred directly to the mouth or indirectly through food and other objects which have been handled. Occasionally the larvae, after hatching in the perianal regions, re-enter the anus and migrate to the caecum, where they mature (retroinfection). There may be a racial susceptibility to infection, thus Puerto Rican children living in crowded conditions in New York had a lower incidence of infection than white, non-Puerto Rican children.

Laboratory diagnosis

Adult female worms may be found in the faeces or perianal skin. The method of choice making for a diagnosis is the Scotch adhesive tape swab applied to the perianal region in the morning before bathing or defaecation. Ova are identified by their asymmetrical shape and well-developed embryo when the tape is mounted on a slide for examination. The Scotch tape can be also applied to that part of the person's clothing which has been in contact with the perianal region. At least three examinations should be carried out before a negative diagnosis is made. Enterobiasis is very infectious and if one person is infected in a household all other members of the family should be suspect.

Control

Because enterobiasis is a family or institution infection, all members should be examined and those positive treated simultaneously. Scrupulous cleanliness, frequent washing of the anal region, the hands and the nails, especially after defaecating, controls the infection. Cotton drawers and gloves should be worn at night and boiled daily. The drug treatment of choice is Viprynium (Vanquin) in a single dose of 5 ml– 30 ml.

Dracontiasis

The guinea-worm *Dracunculus medinensis* has been known since ancient times. It results in the formation of ulcers with extrusion of embryos on contact with water.

Medical geography
In occurs in local distributions in Africa, the Middle East, India, Pakistan, the Caribbean islands, Guyana and Brazil.

Applied biology
The sexually mature female is up to 1 m long and 2 mm in diameter; the uterus, which occupies most of the body, contains millions of embryos. The male is small and its fate after copulation is not known.

When the gravid female is ready to discharge the larvae, the cephalic end of the worm approaches the skin and secretes a substance which causes a blister to form. When the surface of the blister comes in contact with water, the anterior end of the vagina protrudes and the uterus expels the embryos into the water until the supply is exhausted. The female worm then shrivels and dies.

The larvae liberated in water must be taken up by suitable species of *Cyclops*, in which they develop into infective forms in about 3 weeks. Man becomes infected by drinking water containing infected *Cyclops*. These are digested by the gastric juices and the freed larvae penetrate the wall of the digestive tract and eventually migrate to the subcutaneous tissues. The female worm requires about 1 year before it is ready to discharge her embryos.

Epidemiology
Contamination of water with larvae from infected persons takes place when such persons draw drinking water from shallow ponds or wells. The water in these ponds, being stagnant with a high organic content, favours the presence of the vector species of *Cyclops*. In the dry season in some areas these ponds are much frequented since they often provide the only readily accessible source of water, thus creating a high *Cyclops*/man contact ratio. In other places, transmission may occur during the rains when surface pools exist which disappear in the dry season. Infection can also be contracted when drinking water while bathing in contaminated pools or during ritual washing of the mouth in the performance of religious ablutions.

It has been suggested that gastric acidity may be responsible for resistance to infection in some exposed persons, but this hypothesis has been repudiated.

Laboratory diagnosis

A microscopical diagnosis can be made by placing a few drops of water on the guinea-worm blister. This stimulates the discharge of embryos which can be seen on examination of the water under a $\frac{2}{3}$-inch objective.

Control

Transmission can be interrupted by the provision of a piped water supply, providing wells with a sanitary well-head, straining or boiling all water for human consumption. DDT at 1 part per million, chloride of lime or 'Abate' (Cyanamid) will achieve immediate though temporary control of infected waters by killing the cyclops intermediate host. Treatment of individual infections with niridazole or thiabendazole has given excellent results. This economically important water-borne disease could be eliminated in extensive areas during the 'Water Decade'. The elimination of guinea-worm would be a visible, measurable and rapid result of the Water Decade's planned activities. Within affected countries guinea worm endemic foci should be given priority for the construction of safe water supplies.

Trichinosis

Trichinosis is a disease caused by encysted larvae of *Trichinella spiralis*. This parasite is more prevalent in temperate than in tropical countries and is mainly confined to those countries where pork is eaten.

Applied biology

The adult worms are found in the small intestine of a number of carnivorous animals including the pig, bush-pig, rats, hyenas and other hosts. Their life span in the intestine is approximately 8 weeks.

After fertilisation, the female worms bury themselves in intestinal mucosa and each produces about 1500 larvae. The larvae migrate via the intestinal lymphatics to the thoracic duct and into the blood-stream, whence they are distributed to the muscles. Here they develop and become encysted between the muscle fibres in 5–7 weeks. Calcification occurs in about 18 months but the encysted larvae remain alive for many years. When food containing encysted larvae is ingested by a suitable host the larvae are released by the action of digestive juices on the capsule and the cycle is repeated in the new host. In susceptible animals the larvae grow into sexually differentiated adults which on mating produce larvae which then invade striated muscle. In man, infection terminates at the cystic stage.

Epidemiology

Pigs are the chief reservoir of infection. Trichinosis in man results from eating raw or inadequately cooked pork or pork products, e.g. sausage meat. In Kenya, the bush-pig is a common source of infection. Pigs become infected chiefly from eating uncooked slaughter-house refuse containing infected meat scraps; occasionally rats, which have a high natural infection rate of trichinosis, can be a source of infection when they are eaten by pigs.

Serological tests have shown that in many communities the incidence of infection is apparently higher than the number of clinically diagnosed cases, and it is obvious that many light infections pass unnoticed. In recent years small and large epidemics have occurred. Congenital trichinosis has been reported.

Laboratory diagnosis
One of the most constant, single, diagnostic aids in trichinosis is a rising eosinophilia of 10–40 per cent. Parasitological diagnosis is based on the finding of the encysted larval worms in a thin piece of muscle biopsy compressed between two glass slides and examined under a low magnification of the microscope. In light infections, when direct examination is negative, the biopsy specimen should be incubated overnight in an acid-pepsin mixture and the centrifuged deposit examined for larvae.

Recently, intradermal and serological tests have been widely used. They include:
  (i) complement fixation
  (ii) bentonite agglutination
  (iii) latex agglutination
  (iv) cholesterol agglutination
  (v) fluorescent antibody.
The CFT can provide a diagnosis in the first week of the disease—the specificity of the test is high. The bentonite, latex, cholesterol agglutination tests are excellent tests for diagnosing recent infections, but are unreliable in chronic infections.

Control

Adequate cooking of pork meat will essentially protect the individual. Legislation compelling all pig food containing meat to be cooked virtually stops transmission of trichinosis to the pig.

Angiostrongyliasis

Eosinophilic meningitis due to the nematode worm *Angiostrongylus cantonensis* occurs sporadically and occasionally in small epidemics in certain Pacific Islands, including Tahiti and Hawaii, and in South-East Asia including Vietnam and Thailand.

Applied biology
A. cantonensis is essentially a parasite of rats and only occasionally infects man. The eggs hatch in the faeces of the rat in which they are expelled, and the infective larvae invade certain snails or slugs. These are later eaten by rats, which thereby become infected. The life cycle in man

is unknown, but young adult worms have been found in the cerebro-spinal fluid and the brain where they measured 8–12 mm in length.

Epidemiology
Human infection results from the accidental ingestion of infected snails, slugs and land planarians (worm-like creatures) found on unwashed vegetables, such as lettuce. Freshwater prawns may become infected from snails and slugs washed into rivers and estuaries during rainy weather. This was thought to be the main source of local, human infection in Tahiti. Eating raw or pickled snails of the genus *Pila* is considered the mode of infection in Thailand; the percentage of positive snails for *A. cantonensis* infections varying from 1.8 to 72 per cent. The peak incidence of eosinophilic meningitis occurs in the cooler, rainy months between July and November, during this period lettuces and strawberries are most consumed, and when unwashed lead to infection. In Thailand males are affected twice as frequently as females, the highest attack rate occurring in the second and third decade. It has been suggested that *A. cantonensis* originated in the islands of the Indian Ocean—Madagascar, Mauritius, Ceylon—and then spread eastwards to South-East Asia and so to the Pacific area, and the giant African snail *Achatina fulica* might have been instrumental in the spread of the parasite. In Malaysia, the shelled slug *M. malayanus* has been shown to shed infective third-stage larvae, but no human cases have yet been reported.

Laboratory diagnosis
Examination of the cerebrospinal fluid reveals increase in protein and a strikingly high eosinophilia (60–80 per cent)—larval worms are some-times found in the CSF and can be identified as *A. cantonensis*.

Control

The infection is prevented by not eating unwashed vegetables and strawberries and uncooked snails, slugs and prawns infected with larvae. Efficient rat control will reduce the reservoir of infection.

Gnathostomiasis

Gnathostoma infection may present as 'creeping eruption', transitory swellings or eosinophilic meningitis.

Medical geography
The normal hosts for *Gnathostoma spinigerum* are domestic and wild felines, dogs and foxes. Human infections have, however, been reported from Israel, the Sudan, India and the Far East. The majority of human cases to date have occurred in Thailand. One per cent of dogs in Bangkok are infected with gnathostomiasis.

Applied biology

The life cycle in the definitive animal hosts is well known, and involves two intermediate hosts—a *Cyclops* and a fish or an amphibian. Man is an unnatural host and the immature worms may locate either in the internal organs or near the surface of the body, but as the larvae rarely develop into adults the life cycle in man is not known. Adults have, however, been reported in the intestine and ova passed in human faeces.

Epidemiology

Gnathostoma infection in human beings is not uncommon in Thailand and a substantial animal reservoir of *G. spinigerum* has been reported. The parasite has been isolated from cats, dogs, domestic pigs, freshwater fish, eels, snakes, frogs, leopards, chickens and fish-eating birds. Human infection usually results from eating fermented fish, which is a Thai delicacy much liked by women. The dish known as *Somfak* is made up of raw freshwater fish, cooked rice, curry, salt and pepper and then wrapped in banana leaves. Recently it has been shown experimentally that penetration of the skin by the 3rd stage infective larva can occur. There is a possibility therefore that in addition to *ingestion*, human infection is possible during the preparation of raw fish dishes or raw chicken dishes by the 3rd stage larva penetrating the bare skin of the hands of individuals preparing these meals. Other ways for man to acquire the infection is by eating other forms of raw fish, frogs, and possibly snakes infected with encysted larvae.

Human infection has occasionally been attributed to *G. hispidum*, the definitive host in this instance is the pig.

Laboratory diagnosis

Diagnosis in human infections depends on finding the immature worms and identifying them. Cutaneous tests with antigens from larval or adult worms as well as precipitin test have been used for diagnosis. Eosinophilia is present.

Control

The infection is prevented by not eating uncooked fish and meats of other animals infected with encysted larvae. Ancylol (disophenol) kills both the larval and adult forms of *Gnathostoma* in dogs and cats. Unfortunately the compound is too toxic for man.

Taeniasis

Taeniasis occurs in all countries where beef or pork are eaten. The larval stage of *T. solium* produces cysticercosis.

Medical geography

The beef tapeworm *Taenia saginata* has a cosmopolitan distribution and is particularly common in the Middle East, Kenya and Ethiopia. The pork tapeworm *T. solium* is also widely distributed and its larval stage, *Cysticercus cellulosae*, produces cysticercosis in man.

Applied biology

The life cycle and pathogenesis of *T. saginata* and *T. solium* are similar, with the exception of the classical intermediate hosts which are cattle and pigs respectively.

The adult worms live in the small intestine of man only. The respective intermediate hosts become infected by swallowing eggs or mature segments passed in the faeces. The embryos hatch, penetrate the intestinal wall and are carried by the bloodstream to the skeletal muscles, as well as to the tongue, diaphragm and liver. The sites of predilection appear to vary in different areas, and in these sites the larvae invaginate, grow and encyst to become the infective *C. bovis* and *C. cellulosae* in about 10 weeks.

The encysted bladder-like larval forms are pearly-white in colour and contain the invaginated heads of the future adult worms. The cysts of *C. bovis* live for about 9 months, while those of *C. cellulosae* remain viable for 3–6 years.

When infected beef or pork is ingested by man, the cysts are dissolved by the gastric juices; the worms pass to the small intestine, and the heads evaginate and attach themselves to the intestinal wall, where they develop into adult worms and within 2–3 months gravid segments are discharged.

The adult *T. saginata* is from 4 to 10 m long, the head contains four suckers but no hooks, and the uterus has 20 to 25 compound lateral branches on each side; while *T. solium* is only 2–8 m long, the head contains four suckers as well as a double crown of large and small hooks, and the uterus has only 7 to 12 lateral branches on each side. Each mature segment of either worm contains a set of male and female reproductive organs. The ova of *T. saginata* and *T. solium* are indistinguishable from each other morphologically.

Epidemiology

Man is the only reservoir of infection.

The world incidence of *T. saginata* is much higher than that of *T. solium* and it is estimated that in some parts of Kenya infection rates of taeniasis in man may approach 100 per cent and that 30 per cent of cattle may harbour cysticerci.

T. saginata is uncommon in young children and the incidence increases with age. The sexes are equally susceptible—man acquires infection by eating raw or partially cooked beef, while cattle are infected while grazing on pastures, fertilised by human faeces, which are flooded with sewage-laden water. The role of birds in the transmission of the disease is not clear.

T. solium is spread by the insanitary disposal of faeces, thus providing the pigs with a ready opportunity for infection when they ingest human excreta. Man is infected when eating uncooked or insufficiently cooked pork.

Laboratory diagnosis

'Direct smear' examination of the faeces occasionally reveals the typical *Taenia* ova. The intact segments which usually are passed can be compressed between two glass slides and the branches of the uterus at their origin from the main uterine stem can be counted and a differentiation easily made between *T. saginata* (20 to 35) and *T. solium* (7 to 12). The haemagglutination test is positive in about 50 per cent of patients.

Cysticercosis

The adult *T. solium* is a parasite of man alone and the worm lives in the small intestine while the larval worm encysts in pork flesh as *Cysticercus cellulosae*. The pig acts as the classical intermediate host. Man can, however, become infected with the larval worm, and this condition is known as cysticercosis.

Epidemiology

Direct infection of man by larval worms of *T. solium* can occur by ingestion of water and food contaminated by faeces or flies or by unclean hands transferring eggs from the adult worm carrier. Moreover, auto-infection can occur by a person carrying eggs from the anus to the mouth on the fingers, or by massive regurgitation of ova from the small intestine into the stomach.

The liberated larvae penetrate the intestinal mucosa and are then carried by the bloodstream to various parts of the body where they encyst, the commonest sites being the subcutaneous tissues, skeletal muscles and the brain. The cysticercus takes about 4 months to develop and becomes enveloped in a fibrous capsule, which eventually calcifies and may be seen radiologically. *C. cellulosae* are small, oval or spherical, whitish bodies with an opalescent transparency and denser spot on one side where the scolex (tapeworm head) is invaginated. The life span of the cysticercus varies from a few months to 35 years. The geographical distribution of cysticercosis is necessarily similar to that of *T. solium*.

Control

Transmission of taeniasis and cysticercosis can be controlled by the sanitary disposal of human faeces, the thorough cooking of meat and raising the standards of personal hygiene.

(a) The individual

All persons suffering from taeniasis should be dewormed with niclos-amide given in a single dose of 2 g or dichlorophen (6 g) on each of two successive days. The thorough cooking of all beef and pork meat affords personal protection and health education should be carried on to raise the standards of personal hygiene, especially among persons harbouring *T. solium*.

(b) *The community*

Sanitary disposal of human excreta is essential. Untreated human faeces should not be used as fertilisers and if possible human faeces should be avoided altogether as a means of manuring crops.

Strict abattoir supervision resulting in adequate inspection of carcasses and condemnation of infected meat should be carried out. If meat containing cysticerci has to be consumed it should be thoroughly cooked under the close supervision of a health officer.

Taeniasis—Summary

1 *Occurrence*—World-wide
2 *Organisms*—*Taenia solium, T. saginata, Cysticercus bovis*
3 *Reservoir of infection*—Man
4 *Modes of transmission*—Uncooked meat, auto-human infection
5 *Control*— (i) Sanitary disposal of faeces
　　　　　　 (ii) Thorough cooking of meat
　　　　　　 (iii) Personal hygiene
　　　　　　 (iv) Individual specific treatment

Diphyllobothriasis

Infection by the fish tapeworm *Diphyllobothrium latum* is characterised by a megaloblastic anaemia due to vitamin B_{12} deficiency.

Medical geography

Diphyllobothriasis is more common in the temperate zones than in the tropics, where it has only been reported from the Philippines, Madagascar, Botswana, Uganda and southern Chile.

Applied biology

The adult, which may be 10 m long, lives in the ileum of man or of other mammals, and may have as many as 4000 segments. The gravid segments disintegrate and the ova are passed in the faeces. On reaching water the ciliated embryo escapes and is swallowed by the first intermediate host—a freshwater crustacean (*Cyclops* or *Diaptomus* species)—in which it develops as a *procercoid*. When the infected crustaceans are swallowed by various freshwater fishes (salmon, pike, etc.) further development takes place in the musculature of these second intermediate hosts to form *plerocercoids*. When man and other animals eat raw fish the plerocercoid is liberated and attaches itself to the small intestine, where it grows into an adult in about 6 weeks.

Epidemiology

Man and a number of fish-eating mammals, e.g. dog, cat, fox, pig, bear, seal, etc., are the reservoir of infection. Man is infected by eating raw or insufficiently cooked fish; the latter having acquired their infections in waters contaminated by faeces containing ova of *D. latum*. As with the other tapeworms, the adult fish tapeworm is long lived. The export of raw fish may cause infection outside the endemic areas.

Laboratory diagnosis
If segments are passed in the faeces or vomitus, diagnosis can be made by seeing the typical rosette-shaped uterus when the segment is crushed between two glass slides. More commonly, however, 'direct smear' examination of the faeces will reveal the characteristic operculate ova.

Control

Thorough cooking of fish affords personal protection and all infected persons should be treated with niclosamide (Yomesan) or dichlorophen (Antiphen) in the same dosage as for taeniasis. Control of export of smoked fish should be exercised. Sanitary disposal of the human faeces will reduce infection of fish, and fishing should be forbidden in infected waters.

Hymenolepiasis

Three dwarf tapeworm infections can occur in man due to *Hymenolepis nana, H. diminuta* and *Drepanidotaemia lanceolata* respectively. They all occur in the tropics and subtropis.

Applied biology
The adult *H. nana* measures about 20 mm in length and contains 100– 200 segments; it lives in the upper ileum attached to the intestinal mucosa by its globular head. The gravid segments rupture in the intestine and the eggs containing an infective embryo are passed in the faeces. When ingested by man, the embryo penetrates a villus and develops into a cysticercoid larva. On maturity it ruptures the villus, returns to the intestine and attaches itself to the mucosa, giving rise to segments. About a month is required from the time of infection to the first appearance of ova in the faeces.

The adult of *H. diminuta* also inhabits the small intestine and is larger than *H. nana*. The ova containing the embryo are passed in the faeces and it undergoes a cycle of development in rat fleas and other insects. When man ingests food contaminated with these insects, the liberated larva attaches itself to the intestine.

D. lanceolata is an infection of birds and man has only very rarely been accidentally infected.

Epidemiology
H. nana is a common tapeworm of man in the south-eastern United States, parts of South America, and India. Man becomes infected by ingesting the ova in food or water that has been contaminated by human

or rat faeces. The infection can also be transmitted directly from hand to mouth. Owing to the unhygienic habits of children, *H. nana* is more prevalent in them, with the highest incidence occurring between 4 and 9 years. Although rats and mice are commonly infected, man is the chief source of human infections, infection being spread directly from patient to patient without utilising an intermediate host.

H. diminuta is an infection of rats and mice, man being an incidental host. The principal source of infection is food contaminated by rat and mice droppings on which the intermediate insect hosts also thrive. When man eats food containing these insect vectors he gets accidentally infected. Human infection is chiefly in children who ingest rat fleas.

Laboratory diagnosis
A moderate eosinophilia (4–16 per cent) occurs in both *H. nana* and *H. diminuta* infections. Diagnosis is made by finding the characteristic ova in the faeces.

Control

Personal hygiene, sanitary disposal of faeces and food hygiene will control these infections with dwarf tapeworms. The treatment of the individual is as for taeniasis, but it is advisable to repeat the dose after an interval of 3 weeks to kill any further tapeworms which may have emerged from their larval state in the intestinal villi.

Hydatid Disease

This disease can be caused by any one of three species of the genus *Echinococcus*—*Echinococcus granulosus, E. multilocularis* and *E. oligaettas*. Since the epidemiological and pathological features of these three tapeworms are very similar, a detailed description of only *E. granulosus* is given here.

Medical geography
Hydatid disease—caused by the larval form of *E. granulosus*—has a cosmopolitan distribution, being particularly prevalent in the sheep- and cattle-raising areas of the world.

Applied biology
The adult *Echinococcus* is a small tapeworm about 5 mm in length which inhabits chiefly the upper part of the small intestine of canines, especially dogs and wolves.

When the ova, which are passed in the faeces, are swallowed by man or other intermediate hosts (e.g. sheep, cattle, horses, etc.) the enclosed embryo is liberated in the duodenum. It penetrates the intestinal mucosa, reaches the portal circulation, and is usually held up in the liver within 12 hours to develop into a hydatid cyst. If the embryo passes the liver filter, it enters the general circulation, and thus reaches the lungs and other parts of the body. It then develops into a hydatid cyst wherever it eventually comes to rest. Two main varieties of cysts occur— the unilocular and the multilocular. The unilocular hydatid cyst develops a wall with two layers, the outer layer is thick, laminated and elastic, while the inner layer is made up of a protoplasmic matrix containing many nuclei. Around the cyst there is a connective-tissue capsule formed by the tissues of the host. From the inner or germinal layer bulb-like processes arise which are termed brood capsules. By a process of localised proliferation and invagination of the wall of the brood capsules numerous scolices (tapeworm heads) are produced. Each scolex is borne on a pedicle and has suckers and two rows of hooklets. Some of the brood capsules separate from the walls and settle to the bottom of the cyst as a fine granular sediment, 'hydatid sand'. As the hydatid cyst enlarges invaginations of the wall may give rise to daughter cysts and from them granddaughter cysts may arise in a similar manner.

In some cases in which no effective encapsulation occurs the daughter cysts develop as a result of evagination of the cyst wall producing the *multilocular* or *alveolar* hydatid cyst. This variety of hydatid cyst is due to *E. multilocularis*. When the hydatid is eaten by definitive hosts—dogs, foxes, wolves and certain other carnivorous animals—the numerous larvae develop into sexually mature worms in a few weeks. Dogs are usually infected when they eat the infected viscera of sheep or cattle.

Epidemiology

Dogs are the main reservoir of human infection. Infected ova may live for weeks in shady environments but they are quickly destroyed by sunlight and high temperatures. Man acquires hydatid disease when he swallows infected ova as a result of his close association with dogs, and the insanitary habit of not washing his hands before ingesting food. Although infection is usually acquired in childhood, clinical symptoms do not appear until adult life. The dog faeces contaminating fleeces of sheep can also be an indirect source of human infection. It has been shown that in Kenya hydatid cysts are present in more than 30 per cent of cattle, sheep and goats, though the disease in man occurs infrequently, except in the areas of Turkana. Canines are heavily infected while light infections have been recorded in wild carnivores, e.g. jackals and hyenas. The main cycle of transmission in Kenya is between dogs and domestic livestock. Turkana tribesmen are the most heavily infected people in Kenya because of the intimate contact between children and the large number of infected canines in the area—here dogs are used to clean the face and anal regions of babies.

Laboratory diagnosis

If the hydatid cysts rupture, its contents—hooklets, scolices, etc.— may be found in the faeces, sputum or urine. Eosinophilia is present but is usually moderate in degree (300–2000 per mm^3) and there may be hypergammaglobulinaemia.

Intradermal and serological tests, and radiology are used in diagnosis.

Control

This depends on raising the standards of personal hygiene, deworming of infected dogs (with arecoline hydrobromide) and adequate supervision of abattoirs. Infected offal and meat should be destroyed, dogs excluded from slaughterhouses, and infected carcasses deeply buried or incinerated.

(a) *The individual*
People must be warned of the danger of handling dogs or sheep and the importance of washing their hands immediately afterwards.

(b) *The community*
Deworming of all infected dogs, if possible, is the best means of getting rid of the main reservoir of infection. The most suitable drug for this purpose is praziquantel (Droncit). In addition, all meat or offal containing hydatid cysts should be disposed of and thus be made inaccessible to dogs. Abattoir supervision and hygiene will exclude dogs from the premises and infected carcasses should be incinerated. In sheep-rearing areas burial or incineration of dead sheep should be carried out.

Hydatid Disease—Summary

1 *Occurrence*—World-wide
2 *Organism*—Genus *Echinococcus*
3 *Reservoir of infection*—Dogs
4 *Mode of transmission*—Ingestion of infected ova
5 *Control*— (i) Personal hygiene
              (ii) Deworming of dogs
              (iii) Abattoir hygiene

Paragonimiasis

This infection is characterised by cough, expectoration of bloody sputum and, later, signs of bronchiectasis or lung abscess.

Medical geography
Paragonimiasis is due to the lung fluke *Paragonimus westermani*, which has a wide geographical distribution. It occurs focally throughout the Far East, South-East Asia, the Pacific Islands, West Africa and parts of South America. A new species, *P. africanus*, which is considered to be the local causative agent of paragonimiasis, has been described from the Cameroons. Other species responsible for human infections are *P. siamensis* and *P. heterotremus*.

Applied biology

The adult worm is a reddish-brown, oval fluke (about 10 mm long and 5 mm wide) which lives mainly in cavities in the lungs. From these pulmonary pockets the ova escape through the bronchioles and are discharged in the sputum or in the faeces if the sputum is swallowed. In other anatomical sites the ova reach the outside world only when abscesses are formed and rupture.

The contained miracidia hatch in water and enter a suitable species of snail (e.g. *Melania* spp.) in which they develop into cercariae. The cercariae emerge from the snail and penetrate the flesh of certain freshwater crabs and crayfish, where they encyst. Man and susceptible animals are infected by eating these raw or partially cooked crustaceans.

After ingestion, the larvae encyst and penetrate the wall of the jejunum into the peritoneal cavity. They can pass through the diaphragm into the pleural cavity and finally burrow into the lungs where, enclosed in a cystic cavity, they grow to adult worms 5–6 weeks after ingestion.

Epidemiology

Man is the reservoir of infection. Although a considerable domestic and wild animal reservoir of *Paragonimus* infection exists, the part it plays in the epidemiology of human disease has yet to be fully determined.

Transmission is maintained by faecal and sputum pollution of water in which the appropriate snails and vector crustaceans live, and by the custom of eating uncooked crabs and crayfish soaked in alcohol, vinegar, brine or wine. Infection can also occur during the preparation of such food, when encysted cercariae can be left on the knife or other utensils.

Although in most areas infection is higher in males than in females, in the Cameroons women are infected three times as often as men. The peak age of incidence is between 11 and 35 years of age. It has been reported that during a measles epidemic in Korea 80 per cent of *Paragonimus* infections were produced by the administration of the fluid extract of crushed crabs given medicinally to the patients. The infection may persist for many years after leaving endemic areas.

Laboratory diagnosis

The infected sputum is characteristically sticky and bloody, usually of a dark, brownish-red colour. The characteristically shaped eggs are usually found in the sputum or in the faeces on 'direct smear' examination or by concentration techniques. In the first year of infection eggs are seldom found but there is usually an eosinophilia of about 20–30 per cent.

Precipitin reactions with crude and fractionated antigens, intradermal tests and complement-fixation tests have all been used for diagnostic and epidemiological purposes. Cross reactions with other trematodes limit the usefulness of these tests, although the weal is larger and more closely defined with the homologous antigen.

Control

Crabs and crayfish should be cooked before eating. Faecal pollution of water should be prevented. Elevation of standard of personal and public hygiene and the provision of latrines will reduce transmission.

Clonorchiasis

This infection is caused by the oriental liver fluke *Clonorchis sinensis* and may be symptomless or result in severe liver damage with the possibility of malignant change.

Medical geography

Clonorchiasis is mainly found in the Far East. Endemic foci occur in Japan, South Korea, South Eastern China, Taiwan and Vietnam.

Applied biology

The adult *C. sinensis* is a flat, transparent fluke which inhabits the bile ducts and sometimes the pancreatic ducts of man and other fish-eating mammals. It is from 10 to 25 mm long and 3 to 5 mm in breadth.

Self-fertilisation is the common means of fecundation and the ova are carried down the common bile duct to the duodenum and are passed in the faeces. On reaching water the ova are ingested by a suitable snail (e.g. genus *Bithynia*) and hatch in the snail's digestive tract. The enclosed miracidia develop in the snail host into sporocysts and rediae within which cercariae develop. These eventually break out of the mother redia and escape into the water.

The cercariae with unforked tails penetrate the scales of one of several freshwater fishes (e.g. Cyprinoid) and encyst in their flesh, skin, and gills. Here they develop into numerous encysted metacercariae which are the infective forms, and which remain viable for 2 months after the death of the fish.

When ingested by man the metacercariae are freed by the action of the gastric and duodenal juices, and the larvae migrate to the common bile duct and then into the smaller biliary radicles where they mature into adults.

Epidemiology

Man is the reservoir of infection. As with paragonimiasis many animals harbour. *C. sinensis*, but their importance in the epidemiology of the human disease has yet to be fully assessed.

Man and other mammals are infected by eating raw or undercooked fish containing metacercariae. Fish ponds fertilised with fresh human faeces are a common source of infection. Infected fish exported to other countries can result in the spread of the disease to areas where the parasite is not normally found.

Clonorchiasis is rare in infants under 1 year of age, it begins, however, at abour 2 years, rising to 65 per cent in those aged 21–30 years and to a peak of 80 per cent in those dying between the ages 51 and 60 years. Males are more frequently infected than females, but there are no social differences in the prevalence of the disease because of the universal custom of eating raw fish. The life span of the worm is 25–30 years.

Laboratory diagnosis

A definitive diagnosis is made by finding the typical operculated ova by 'direct smear' examination of the faeces or duodenal aspirate.

There is usually a leucocytosis (23 000–48 200) with eosinophilia. In severe cases with secondary infection of the bile ducts there may be severe hypoglycaemia with blood sugars of 22–45 mg per cent; bilirubin levels of 3–10 mg per cent and a raised alkaline phosphatase.

Control

Fish should not be eaten raw and the use of human faeces in fish ponds should be avoided. Sanitary disposal of faeces and raising the standards of personal and community hygiene will reduce transmission.

Opisthorchiasis

This infection is very similar to clonorchiasis, resulting in enlargement of the liver and eventually malignant change.

Medical geography

This disease is due to two parasitic trematodes—*Opisthorchis felineus* and *O. viverrini*. In the tropics the former is prevalent in the Philippines, India, Japan and Vietnam, while the latter has been reported from north and north-east Thailand and Laos.

Applied biology

The life cycle and pathogenesis of these two human hepatic trematodes are similar to that of *C. sinensis*. The adults inhabit the distal bile ducts and the ova are passed out in the faeces. After ingestion by the appropriate snails (e.g. *Bithynia*) the miracidia develop into cercariae, which in turn penetrate the flesh of suitable species of freshwater fishes (e.g. Cyprinoid family) in which they encyst and develop into metacercariae. When the metacercariae are ingested by a suitable host—man, domestic, wild and fur-bearing animals—they encyst in the duodenum and migrate to the distal bile ducts particularly those of the left lobe of the liver. The entire life cycle takes about 4 months.

Epidemiology

Man, domestic, wild and fur-bearing animals are the reservoir of infection. The chief reservoir of *O. felineus* is the cat. Man and the reservoir hosts are infected by the consumption of raw or insufficienty cooked fish. Snails and fish are infected by faeces deposited on the sandy shores and washed into the streams.

In north-east Thailand 90 per cent of people over the age of 10 are infected with *O. viverrini* and it is estimated that over 3.5 million persons in Thailand harbour the parasite. The source of infection is a popular dish called 'Keompla', consisting of raw fish, roasted rice, and vegetables seasoned with garlic, lemon juice, fish sauce and pepper. Chinese residents of Thailand who do not eat raw fish are free from infection. The largest number of human infections occur during the latter portion of the rainy season and the first part of the dry season, i.e. from September to February.

Laboratory diagnosis
This is made by finding the ova on 'direct smear' examination of faeces or duodenal aspirate.

Control

(i) Raw fish should be avoided; fish should be eaten only if cooked.
(ii) Sanitary disposal of faeces and a raised standard of personal and public hygiene will reduce transmission.

Fascioliasis

This infection may be silent or may present with symptoms of chronic liver disease and portal hypertension. Praziquantel is effective against liver and lung fluke infections.

Medical geography
Fascioliasis is caued by the trematode *Fasciola hepatica* (sheep-liver fluke), which has a world-wide distribution in ruminants, being especially prevalent in the sheep-rearing areas of the world. In some areas, e.g. Hawaii, the causative agent of fascioliasis is *F. gigantica*.

Applied biology
The adult worm, which is large (30 mm long and 13 mm broad), flat and leaf-shaped, lives in the bile ducts of liver parenchyma of sheep, cattle, goats and other animals, and man. The eggs are passed in the faeces and hatch in a moist environment. The released miracidia then enter the appropriate species of snails (*Limnaea*), and develop successively into sporocytes, rediae and cercariae. The cercariae then leave their snail host and encyst on various grasses and water plants. When this water vegetation is ingested by the appropriate hosts, the larvae excyst in the intestine, penetrate the mucosa, enter the liver through the portal circulation, and eventually reach the bile ducts, where they mature in about 3 months. *F. hepatica* obtains its nourishment from the biliary secretions and can absorb simple carbohydrates.

Epidemiology
The reservoir of infection is ruminants especially sheep. Man usually contracts infection by eating lettuce or water cress contaminated by sheep or other animals' faeces. The highest incidence of infection occurs

in low, damp pastures where the grasses and the water are infected with encysted cercariae.

Laboratory diagnosis

The finding of the typical operculated eggs in faeces (150×90 μm) is diagnostic, but unfortunately these do not appear till about 3 months after infection. Duodenal intubation may reveal the ova in biliary secretions at an earlier stage of the disease. There may be a leucocytosis ($12\,000$–$40\,000$ per mm^3) and an eosinophilia of 40–$85\,\%$.

Intracutaneous and serological tests are useful but not specific or sensitive enough, the haemagglutination test is reputed to be the most sensitive.

Control

Lettuce or water cress should be sterilised by momentary immersion in boiling water, this will destroy the encysted cercariae.

Fasciolopsiasis

This infection is often symptomless, but with heavy infections abdominal pain with alternating diarrhoea and constipation may occur.

Medical geography

Fasciolopsiasis is caused by the large, fleshy fluke—*Fasciolopsis buski*—which is found mainly in China, but also in India, Indo-China, Thailand, Malaysia, Indonesia, Taiwan and Europe.

Parasitology

F. buski is normally an intestinal parasite of the pig and of man and inhabits the small intestine. The eggs are passed in the faeces and the miracidium is released and swims in water until it penetrates a suitable mollusc host of the genus *Segmentina*—where it develops into a sporocyst, redia and cercariae. When the cercariae leave the snail they encyst on aquatic plants. When the encysted cercariae are ingested by man, the cyst wall is dissolved in the duodenum and the liberated larvae attach themselves to the mucosa, where they develop into adult worms whose nourishment is derived from the duodenal secretions. The egg output per worm is very high, averaging $25\,000$ eggs per day.

Epidemiology

Man, who is a source of infection, is infected when he eats raw waterplants contaminated with encysted cercariae. Pigs are also an important animal reservoir, infecting the stagnant ponds in which edible water plants grow. The commonest source of infected edible water plants are the water caltrops and water chestnuts which are often cultivated in ponds fertilised by human faeces. In China, these tubers are eaten raw and fresh from July to September and, as they are peeled with the teeth, an easy entry of the cercariae to the mouth is provided.

Laboratory diagnosis

The diagnosis can be made by finding the characteristic operculated ova in the faeces, there may be a leucocytosis and eosinophilia. Occasionally, adult flukes are vomited or found in the faeces.

Control

This consists in adequate cooking of the potentially infected foods and prevention of faecal pollution of water in which they grow. Provision of latrines and the raising of standards of personal and public hygiene by health education helps to reduce transmission.

Heterophyiasis and Metagonimiasis

These conditions are due to infection by two very minute flukes— *Heterophyes heterophyes* and *Metagonimus yokogawai*. In the tropics the former is found in Egypt, Tunisia, South China, India and Philippines, while the latter occurs in the Far East and Indonesia.

The **life cycle** and **epidemiology** of both flukes is similar. The adults live in the upper part of the small intestine embedded in mucus or in the mucosal folds. The eggs containing miracidia are passed in the faeces and, on ingestion by suitable snails, develop into sporocysts, rediae and cercariae. The cercariae then leave the snails and enter the appropriate fish, in which they encyst into infective metacercariae. When the fish are eaten raw or partially cooked the metacercariae are liberated and the larvae develop into adult worms in the small intestine.

The first snail intermediate hosts for *H. heterophyes* are brackish water snails (e.g. *Pirinella conica*), while the second intermediate hosts are mullets; for *M. yokogawai* the hosts are snails of the *Semisulcospira* species and salmonoid and cyprinoid fishes.

The pathogenicity of these parasitic infections is very low, unless aberrant ova enter the circulation when the spinal cord may be affected.

In addition to man, other mammals are also infected and, like clonorchis infection, heterophiasis is acquired by eating raw or partially cooked infected fish.

Diagnosis is made by finding the characteristic ova in the faeces. There may be eosinophilia.

Control

Control depends on avoiding eating raw and partially cooked infected fish and raising the standards of personal and community hygiene. *Food hygiene.* See p. 318. *Disinfection.* See p. 318.

The Control of Diarrhoeal Disease

Diarrhoeal diseases as a group remain a major cause of death in developing countries especially in children. Programmes for the reduction of morbidity and mortality include three main elements:

(a) *Oral rehydration*
This measure is most valuable in lowering mortality. The community, especially the mothers of young children, should be taught how to produce the fluids most easily from ready made packets of glucose and salt.

(b) *Infant feeding*
Breast feeding should be encouraged in babies. Mothers should be taught how to produce infant weening foods in a hygienic manner from locally available ingredients.

(c) *Improvement of sanitation*
The provision of adequate and safe water supplies and the general improvement of environmental sanitation should be emphasised.

FURTHER READING

WHO CDD. Ser. 80.1: *Guidelines for the trainers of community Health workers on the treatment and prevention of acute diarrhoea.*
WHO CDD. Ser. 80.2: *A manual for the treatment of acute diarrhoea.*
WHO CDD. Ser. 80.3: *Guidelines for the production of oral rehydration salts.*
WHO CDD. Ser. 80.4: *Guidelines for cholera control.*
EURO Reports and Studies No. 44: *Surveillance and control of acute diarrhoeal diseases.*
EURO Reports and Studies No. 63: *Oral enteric vaccines.*
FEACHEM R. G. (1981). *Environmental aspects of cholera epidemiology.* Part I. Trop. Dis. Bull. No. 8. p. 675.
FEACHEM R. G. *et. al.* (1981). Ibid. Part 2. Trop. Dis. Bull. No. 10. p. 865.
FEACHEM R. G. (1982). Ibid. Part 3. Trop. Dis. Bull. No. 1. p. 1.

CHAPTER 5

INFECTIONS THROUGH SKIN AND MUCOUS MEMBRANES

In one group, transmission of infection occurs by contact with contaminated persons or objects. In the other groups, infection may be acquired by exposure to infected soil (hookworm), water (schistosomiasis, leptospirosis), by the bites of animals (rabies) or through wounds (tetanus).

CONTACT INFECTIONS

Table 5.1 gives examples of disease which are spread by contact.

Table 5.1 Examples of infections acquired through skin and mucous membranes

Viruses	Bacteria	Fungi	Protozoa	Helminths	Arthropods
Smallpox	Gonorrhoea*	Superficial fungal infection e.g. ringworm	Trichomonas vaginalis	Schistosomiasis	Scabies
				Hookworm	
Chicken-pox	Syphilis*				
Trachoma	Yaws				
Inclusion conjunctivities	Endemic treponematoses				
Lymphogranuloma venereum*	Leprosy				
	Tetanus				

* Venereal diseases.

The Infective Agents

The infective agents include viruses, bacteria, fungi and arthropods.

Physical and biological characteristics
Some of the agents which are transmitted by direct person-to-person contact are notably delicate organisms which do not survive long

outside the human host and cannot become established in any part of the environment, neither in an alternate host nor in an inanimate object such as soil or water. The venereally transmitted diseases such as gonorrhoea and syphilis are the best examples of this group; the usual mode of infection is therefore through intimate contact, mucous membrane to mucous membrane, or skin to skin. Some of the other infective agents which can survive in the environment for relatively longer periods, may be spread indirectly through the contamination of inanimate objects.

In most of these infections man is the sole reservoir of infection, although some of the superficial fungal infections may be acquired from lower animals.

Mode of transmission

This may be by *direct contact* from touching an infected person; also through kissing and sexual intercourse, especially in the case of venereally transmitted diseases.

It may be by *indirect contact* through the handling of contaminated objects such as toys, handkerchiefs, soiled clothing, bedding or dressings.

Environmental factors which aid the transmission of these infections include high population densitiy as in urban areas, overcrowding and poor environmental and personal hygiene.

Epidemiological features of contact infections

A contact infection would tend to spread from an infected source to susceptible persons in the same household and to others who make contact with him at work and in other places. There is therefore a tendency for cases of contact infections to occur in clusters among household contacts, and within groups of persons who have close contacts, e.g. children's play groups, schools and factories.

In the case of venereal diseases, the clustering occurs in relation to those who are in sexual contact.

Host Factors

The behaviour of the human host is an important factor in the occurrence of certain contact infections. For example, a high level of personal cleanliness discourages the spread of some superficial infections. Age is another important factor, as for example in infections such as scabies and tinea capitis to which children are generally more susceptible than adults. The occurrence of venereal diseases is largely determined by the sexual behaviour of the host.

In some of the infections, e.g. measles, one attack confers lasting immunity but this is not a general rule for all the contact infections. Thus, repeated attacks of gonorrhoea may occur. The herd immunity that is derived from the high frequency of an endemic treponemal infection such as yaws may protect the community, though not the individual, from venereal syphilis.

Control of Contact Infections

1 *Infective agent*
   (a) Elimination of the reservoir by case finding, selective or mass treatment.
2 *The route of transmission*
   (b) Improvement of personal hygiene.
   (c) Elimination of overcrowding.
   (d) Avoidance of sexual promiscuity.
3 *The host*
   (e) Specific immunisation, e.g. smallpox.
   (f) Chemotherapy and chemoprophylaxis, e.g. yaws.

SMALLPOX

In May 1980, the eradication of smallpox from the world was formally declared at the World Health Assembly in Geneva. This unique achievement was the result of a global campaign, initiated and co-ordinated by the World Health Organisation (WHO) in collaboration with the national health authorities and governments. The final certification of eradication was based on a stage by stage, country by country, region by region examination of evidence which led to the final conclusion that the transmission of smallpox is no longer occurring in the world. Following this declaration, a number of questions are being asked:

(i) *Is it possible that smallpox is still being transmitted in some hidden foci?*
Some people have wondered whether the disease is still occurring in remote areas which were not reached by the global campaign. An examination of the process employed in the search for cases even in the most remote communities is very reassuring. Eradication was proclaimed after no naturally transmitted case had been found for over two years. It is most unlikely that such a focus could exist without causing outbreaks in more accessible areas. Each passing day without the detection of a case further strengthens the conviction that transmission has ceased.

(ii) *How about the possibility of an animal reservoir?*
Although a certain number of pox viruses occurring in animals occasionally affect man, e.g. monkey pox, there is no evidence of a natural reservoir of smallpox in animals.

(iii) *Could any of these poxes mutate to produce a fresh strain of smallpox?*
Such speculation cannot be completely ruled out but it is extremely unlikely.

(iv) *Can transmission occur from variola viruses lying dormant but viable in nature?*
For example, it has been suggested that the virus could remain viable in corpses and that fresh transmission could occur if the graves of former victims are disturbed. Variola virus can survive in dried scabs but the viability of the material declines month by month and becomes non-infectious within a year.

(v) *What are the implications of smallpox eradication for public health authorities?*
(a) LABORATORY STOCKS OF VARIOLA VIRUS   By international agreement, four centres which provide adequate security against accidental infection have been designated for holding stocks of variola virus. According to the agreement reached among the nations, other stocks should have been destroyed or transferred to the four centres.
(b) VACCINATION POLICY   It is now generally agreed that it is no longer desirable to vaccinate populations routinely against smallpox nor is it necessary for governments to require certificate of smallpox from international travellers. Most governments have adopted this policy.
(c) VACCINE STOCKS   Even though most people are firmly convinced that smallpox has been eradicated, stocks of vaccine are still being held. This is a wise precaution in support of the policy of suspending routine vaccination.

(vi) *What lessons can be learnt from the eradication of smallpox?*
First and foremost, this successful campaign illustrates the value of international collaboration. Governments throughout the world contributed to the success through generous donations in cash and kind, through various forms of technical cooperation including the free exchange of information and through the coordinating function of WHO.
Technical improvements in the vaccine (freezedrying) and in vaccination (the bifurcated needle), aided the eradication of smallpox. More important than the technical advances was the development of a revised strategy for the application of these tools. At first, smallpox campaigns were largely based on repeated rounds of immunisation of the population. In the course of the eradication programme, the importance of epidemiological surveillance was recognised. The systematic tracing of foci of infection through surveillance techniques proved to be a powerful measure in the campaign. The value of epidemiological surveillance is a most important lesson which should be applied in the control of other communicable diseases.

CHICKENPOX

Chickenpox is an acute febrile illness with a characteristic skin rash. The *incubation period* is usually from 2 to 3 weeks.

The main importance of chickenpox lies in its differentiation from smallpox. The typical clinical features of chickenpox and smallpox are compared in Table 5.2 The clinical diagnosis should be confirmed by laboratory tests if these are available. In any case, public health measures should be carried out and precautions maintained until the diagnosis of smallpox can be firmly excluded.

Table 5.2 Clinical features of smallpox and chickenpox compared

	Smallpox	*Chickenpox*
PRODROMAL SYMPTOMS	Fever, headache, severe prostration for 2 to 4 days before rash appears	Mild or no marked constitutional signs until just before rash appears
SKIN RASH Pattern of appearance	Only one crop, all lesions appearing within 1 to 2 days	Lesions appear in crops over several days to one week
	Lesions are at the same stage of development	Many stages of the lesions from vesicles to scabs are seen together on same part of the body
Distribution	*Centrifugal*—most numerous on the face and the distal parts of arms and legs	*Centripetal*—more numerous on the body than on the limbs
	Involves the palms and soles	Palms and soles not often involved
Individual lesions	Axilla usually spared	Axilla usually involved
	Evolution from macule to scab takes at least one week	Lesions evolve more rapidly—scabs appear within 3 to 4 days
	Circular	Oval
	Deep set	Superficial
	Vesicles are multilocular	Vesicles are unilocular
	Become umbilicated with rupture of central lobes	Vesicles collapse and become flat with rupture of vesicle
SCAR	Depressed	Superficial

Medical geography
Chickenpox is a common infection all over the world.

Virology
The aetiological agent is the varicella-zoster virus.

Epidemiology

Man is the reservoir of infection. Transmission is from person to person, either directly through contact with infectious secretions from the upper respiratory tract and through droplet infection or indirectly through contact with freshly soiled articles. The patient remains infectious for about 1 week from the onset of the illness.

Host factors play an important part in determining the clinical manifestations of this infection. In most cases, it is a mild, self-limiting disease. It tends to be more severe in adults than in children. The overall case fatality rate is low, but it is high in cases complicated with primary viral pneumonia. Fulminating infection with haemorrhagic bullae may occur in patients on corticosteroid therapy.

One attack of chickenpox usually confers lifelong immunity; the patient may subsequently exhibit a recrudescence of infection in the form of herpes zoster from latent infection.

Laboratory diagnosis

The organism may be isolated from the early skin lesions or from throat washings. A rising titre of complement-fixing antibodies in acute and convalescent sera is also diagnostic.

Control

The disease is usually notifiable, the main interest being in investigating cases and outbreaks to exclude smallpox. No specific immunisation against chickenpox is available. Infected persons may be isolated from other susceptibles, rigid isolation being enforced until the differentiation from smallpox is established.

Chickenpox—Summary

1 *Occurrence*—World-wide
2 *Organism*—Varicella-zoster virus
3 *Reservoir of infection*—Man
4 *Modes of transmission*—Contact, droplets, fomites
5 *Control*—Exclude smallpox

TRACHOMA

Trachoma is a major cause of blindness in the tropics and is characterised by a mucopurulent discharge initially progressing to a chronic kerato-conjunctivitis, with the formation of follicles, with hyperplasia, vascular invasion of the cornea and, in the late stage, gross scarring with deformity of the eyelids. Vision may be impaired, and in severe cases it may lead to blindness. The *incubation period* is from 4 to 12 days.

Medical geography

The occurrence of the infection is world-wide, including tropical, subtropical, temperate and cold climates, but the distribution of disease is uneven, being mostly in the Middle East, Mediterranean coast, parts of tropical Africa, Asia and South America. In the United States of America, it selectively affects certain groups such as American Indians and Mexican immigrants. It is estimated that throughout the world 400 million persons are infected with trachoma and 20 million are blind.

Virology

The organism responsible for trachoma is termed TRIC agent (trachoma inclusion conjunctivitis agent). It belongs to the PLT (psittacosis, lymphogranuloma venereum, trachoma) group of atypical viruses which are midway between true viruses and bacteria—*Chlamydia trachomatis*. The causal agent was first isolated with certainty in Peking and confirmed in the Gambia.

Epidemiology

Man is the reservoir of infection and the three serotypes of *Chlamydia trachomatis* (*a*, *b* and *c*) affect 200–300 million people in the world, mostly in Africa, the Middle East and Asia, despite good progress in the global control of the disease. *C. trachomatis* (serotypes d to k) are a common cause of urethritis and can also be responsible for ophthalmia neonatorum.

The common mode of transmission is mechanical from eye to eye by contaminated fingers, cloths, towels, bed clothes and flies (particularly *Musca sorbers*). Infected nasal discharge and tears can also be agents of transmission. The severer the infection the greater is the degree of virus shedding, which in most areas of the world occurs in children under 10 years of age. Infection is particularly common where there is poor personal hygiene; exposure to sun, wind and sand may aggravate the clinical manifestations.

Immunity to trachoma is only partial and non-protective. Cell mediated immunity develops eventually, leading to hypersensitivity which is responsible for the blinding complications of trachoma. The disease traces a variable course with spontaneous healing in some cases or progressive damage in others. In countries with a high incidence of bacterial conjunctivitis, particularly of the seasonal epidemic variety, the severity of the trachoma is enhanced and disabling complications are more frequent. In other areas, e.g. the Gambia, the disease is mild, and serious sequelae uncommon.

Laboratory diagnosis

Intracytoplasmic inclusion bodies 0.25–0.4 μm in diameter, staining purple with Giemsa or reddish-brown by iodine, may be seen in conjunctival scrapings. These elementary particles have been termed Halberstaedter-Prowazek bodies and are the principal microscopic diagnostic feature in trachoma but are also seen in inclusion conjunctivitis of the newborn. The number of inclusions tends to be proportional to the intensity of the infection and are most numerous in scrapings from the upper lid.

In early lesions neutrophils may be abundant. In later lesions plasma cells, lymphoblasts and macrophages containing necrotic debris (Leber cells) may be seen.

The agent may be cultured in the yolk of the sac of the embryonated egg.

Control

Improvement of living standards and mass treatment campaigns are the most effective methods for the prevention of trachoma.

(a) *The individual*
Topical or systemic treatment with sulphonamides; erythromycin; tetracycline or doxycycline is very effective. Surgical treatment is required for the complications, such as entropion, etc.

Hygienic measures include improvement in personal cleanliness, and avoiding the sharing of handkerchiefs, towels and eye cosmetics. It involves health education and the provision of adequate water supply.

(b) *The Community*
The main objectives are: (a) to reduce shedding of virus and (b) to stop transmission.

Topical administration is effective but because the period of treatment is long (6 months) compliance falls off as does the persistence of health personnel. This regime is most effective in schools 'a captive population' where it has been successfully used both curatively and prophylactically. It is important to bear in mind, however, that in areas of high endemicity the main reservoir of infection is the preschool child and suitable mass campaigns against this particular age group are also vitally important. Active research on vaccination is making slow progress. It only provides partial protection, and on the whole, has so far proved disappointing.

Trachoma—Summary

1 *Occurrence*—World-wide, uneven distribution, mainly tropical and sub-tropical
2 *Organism*—*Chlamydia trachomatis.*
3 *Reservoir of infection*—Man
4 *Modes of transmission*—Contact, fomites, mechanically by flies
5 *Control*— (i) Improvement in personal hygiene
         (ii) Mass treatment with systemic or topical antibiotics or sulphonamides

INCLUSION CONJUNCTIVITIS

This infection manifests itself as an acute purulent conjunctivitis of neonates or as follicular conjunctivitis of adults. The *incubation period* is from 5 to 12 days.

Medical geography
The distribution of infection is probably world-wide but the frequency of the infection is not fully appreciated except in places where interested clinicians have adequate laboratory facilities.

Virology
The causative agent is a virus which is closely related to the trachoma virus, both being referred to jointly as the TRIC agents.

Epidemiology
Man is the reservoir of infection, the usual habitat of the organism being the genital tract in the female cervix or the epithelium of the male urethra. The genital infection is asymptomatic.

The newborn baby is infected from its mother's genital tract during delivery; the infection may also be transmitted mechanically from eye to eye, but adults often acquire the infection in the swimming pool.

Control

Topical treatment with tetracycline ointment is usually effective but sulphonamides may also be administered by the oral route. Routine eye toilet of newborn babies is of no apparent value. Chlorination of swimming pools is useful in preventing adult infections.

Inclusion Conjunctivitis—Summary

1 *Occurrence*—World-wide
2 *Organism*—A TRIC virus
3 *Reservoir of infection*—Man, mainly carriers with genital infection
4 *Modes of transmission*—Intrapartum, contact, swimming
5 *Control*— (i) Early treatment
           (ii) Chlorination of swimming pools

SEXUALLY TRANSMITTED DISEASES (STD)

These are infections which are specifically transmitted during sexual intercourse. Although various other infections may be transmitted during sexual intercourse, the commonly recognised venereal diseases are:
Syphilis
Gonorrhoea

Lymphogranuloma venereum
Granuloma inguinale (Donovanosis)
Soft Chancre
Non-gonococcal urethritis
Herpes genitalis.

Epidemiology of venereal diseases

The infective agents include viruses, bacteria and protozoa, but most of them share the characteristic of being delicate, being easily killed by drying or cooling below body temperature, with the reservoir exclusively in man. Hence, transmission is mainly through direct close contact but rarely indirectly through fomites.

Route of transmission

Lesions are generally present on the genitalia, and the infective agents in the secretions and discharges from the urethra and the vagina, but extragenital lesions may occur through haematogenetic dissemination as in syphilis or through inoculation of the infective agent at extragenital sites. Transmission occurs:

(a) mainly through genital contact
(b) through extragenital sexual contact such as kissing
(c) through non-sexual contact, e.g. congenital syphilis, gonococcal ophthalmia neonatorum, or accidental contact as when doctors, dentists or midwives handle tissues infected with syphilis
(d) through fomites, e.g. soiled moist clothing such as wet towels, may transmit vulvovaginitis to pre-pubescent girls.

It is not uncommon for patients to claim that they contracted the venereal infection through some indirect contact such as the lavatory seat; such mechanism is extremely unlikely and the patient will usually admit to sexual exposure once his confidence has been obtained.

Host

The most important host factor is sexual behaviour, the significant feature being sexual promiscuity. The transmission of a venereal disease almost always implies sexual activity involving at least three persons. For if A infects B, it implies that A has also had sexual contact with at least one other person X, who infected A. Thus, venereal diseases have the highest frequency in those who are most active sexually, particularly those who indulge in promiscuous sexual behaviour with frequent changes of partners. Thus, young adult males away from home (sailors, soldiers, migrant labourers, etc:) are often at high risk.

Cultural attitudes to sex also play an important role. In some communities sexual matters are treated on a system of double standards in that whilst young unmarried girls are expected to remain chaste, young men are permitted or even encouraged to indulge in promiscuous sexual activities often with a small group of notorious women including prostitutes. Even after marriage, similar standards may apply; married women may be veiled, confined to special quarters in the household, or chaperoned on outings but with little or no restrictions on the extramarital sexual activities of the male. A more permissive attitude to sexual relations has developed in some communities which now tend to take a liberal view of all forms of sexual relations regardless of the sex or the marital status of the partners.

Promiscuity before marriage and infidelity after marriage represent the major behavioural factors underlying the transmission of venereal disease, whilst sexual abstinence and marital fidelity are protective.

Sexual behaviour

The pattern of sexual behaviour is undergoing major changes in developing countries as they evolve from rural traditional societies to modern urban industrial communities. There is also greater mobility from one community to the other, and easier communication through books, the cinema and television. The overall effect of these changes is to challenge and destabilise traditional values and customs especially with regard to sexual behaviour. On the one hand those who fear and respect sexual mores dictated by religious beliefs, by strict parents, by public opinion and by the law, are less likely to indulge in promiscuous sexual behaviour than those who are no longer bound by these considerations. The risk of unwanted pregnancy and of contracting sexually transmitted diseases also discourage sexual promiscuity. Self release through masturbation also avoids these two risks. On the positive side, interest in work and absorbing leisure pursuits also tend to diminish promiscuity. The use of sex for gain encourages sexual promiscuity and increases the risk of spread of these infections.

Control

The general guide-lines for the control of venereal diseases are as follows:

A Infective Agent

(1) Eliminate the reservoir of infection

The reservoir is exclusively human; it includes untreated sick patients but inapparent infection especially in women represents the most important part of the reservoir. The identification and treatment of the promiscuous female pool is of great importance. Regular medical examination and treatment of known prostitutes, inhabitants of brothels, and other places where promiscuous sexual behaviour is known to occur. Such medical supervision of prostitutes cannot entirely eliminate the risk of infection.

B Route of Transmission

2 *Discourage sexual promiscuity*
Through sex education, make the community aware of the dangers of sexual promiscuity. One objective would be to influence young persons before their sexual habits become established.

Encourage stable family life by providing married quarters in work camps, etc.

3 *Local prophylaxis*
The use of rubber condoms diminishes but does not eliminate the risk of infection of the male.

Careful toilet of the genitals with soap and antiseptic creams immediately after exposure also gives partial protection.

C Host

4 *Specific prophylaxis*
Specific immunisation is not available against any of the venereal diseases. Although a measure of protection can be obtained by using antibiotic chemoprophylaxis, this approach can be dangerous for the individual and the community. Chemoprophylaxis may suppress the acute clinical manifestations but the disease may remain latent and progress silently to late complications. The widespread use of a particular antibiotic in sub-curative doses may encourage the emergence and dissemination of drug-resistant strains.

5 *Early diagnosis and treatment*
Patients—This is one of the most important measures for the control of venereal diseases. Facilities for the diagnosis and treatment of those diseases must be freely accessible to all infected persons. Experience has shown that in order to reach the whole community everyone must have access to a free and confidential service.

Contacts—In addition to treating the patient, his sexual contacts must be investigated and treated. In hightly promiscuous groups where sexual activities occur in association with the use of alcohol or drugs, the details of the chain of transmission may be difficult to unravel. In such cases, one may use the technique of 'cluster tracing'. Apart from seeking a list of sexual exposures with dates, the patient is asked to name friends of both sexes whom he feels may profit from investigation for venereal diseases.

LYMPHOGRANULOMA VENEREUM

This is a chronic infection of the genitals which spreads to involve regional lymph nodes, and the rectum. Typically it produces ulcerative lesions on the genitalia with induration of the regional lymph nodes ('climatic bubo'). Anal and genital stricture may occur at a late stage; so also may elephantiasis of the vulva. Extragenital lesions and general dissemination occasionally occur.

Medical geography
The infection is endemic in many parts of the tropics and subtropics.

Virology
The causative agent is a large virus of the psittacosis group.

Laboratory diagnosis
Stained smears of pus and other pathological material may show virus particles. The organism can be identified on culture in the yolk sacs of embryonated eggs. The complement fixation test becomes positive some 2 to 4 weeks after the onset of the illness. A skin test, the Frei test, is available, but cross-reactions with other viral infections of the psittacosis group may occur depending on the purity of the antigen. It tends to remain positive for long periods.

Epidemiology
Man is the reservoir of infection, the source being the open lesions in patients with active disease. Transmission is mainly by sexual contact but also by indirect contact through contaminated clothing and other fomites.

As with other venereal diseases, the sexual behaviour of the host is a major factor determining the distribution and spread of this infection. Recovery from a clinical attack does not confer immunity.

Control

The main principles are as for other venereal diseases. The early stages of infection respond to sulphadiazine, but tetracyclines are the drugs of choice especially for the severe or advanced cases.

Lymphogranuloma Venereum—Summary

1 *Distribution*—Tropics and subtropics mainly
2 *Organism*—Lymphogranuloma venereum virus
3 *Reservoir*—Man
4 *Transmission*—Genital sexual contact—indirect contact
5 *Control*—As for other venereal diseases; the organism is sensitive to sulphonamides and broad-spectrum antibiotics

SOFT CHANCRE

This is an acute venereal infection which typically presents as a ragged painful ulcer on the genitalia; the inguinal lymph nodes become enlarged and may suppurate. Extragenital lesions may be found on the abdomen, fingers or other sites.

The *incubation period* is usually from 3 to 5 days but it may be very short (24 hours) where the lesion affects mucous membranes.

Medical geography

The infection occurs in many parts of the world, especially in tropical seaports.

Bacteriology

The causative agent is *Haemophilus ducrei*, a Gram-negative non-sporing bacillus.

Epidemiology

Man is the reservoir of infection. The open lesions are the most important source of infection although it has been suggested that the carrier state may exist in women.

Sexual contact is the usual mode of transmission but extragenital lesions may occur from non-sexual infection of children or accidental infection of doctors, nurses or other medical personnel who come into contact with infected lesions.

Laboratory diagnosis

Microscopy of the stained smear of the exudate from ulcers or pus from the regional lymph nodes may show a mixed flora including Gram-negative bacilli. The organism can be isolated on culture of pus from the ulcer or bubo. An intradermal skin test is available but it does not differentiate active infections from previous attacks.

Biopsy of the regional lymph nodes may also provide useful information.

Control

The general measures for the control of venereal diseases apply to the problem of chancroid. Active infections usually respond to treatment with sulphonamides but in resistant cases, antibiotics such as strepto-mycin, tetracycline, or chloromycetin may be used.

Soft Chancre—Summary

1 *Occurrence*—Tropics, especially seaports
2 *Organism*—Haemophilus ducrei
3 *Reservoir of infection*—Man
4 *Mode of transmission*—Sexual contact, accidental infection through non-sexual contact
5 *Control*—As for other venereal diseases

GRANULOMA INGUINALE

This is a chronic infection which presents with granulomatous lesions of the genitalia; regional lymph nodes may be affected and metastatic lesions occur.

The *incubation period* is 1 week to 3 months.

Medical geography
The infection occurs in various parts of the tropics and subtropics, particularly in poorer communities.

Organism
The aetiological agent is *Donovania granulomatis.*

Epidemiology
Man is the reservoir of infection. Transmission may be by sexual contact, but non-sexual contact may also be importnat.

Laboratory diagnosis
Stained smears from active lesion show the typical Donovan bodies. A skin test is available and the complement fixation test can also be used in diagnosis.

Control

General hygienic measures are important. Known cases should be treated with antibiotics (streptomycin, tetracycline, chloramphenicol or erythromycin). Contacts should be examined and treated if indicated.

Granuloma Inguinale—Summary

1 *Distribution*—Tropics and subtropics
2 *Organism*—*Donovania granulomatis*
3 *Reservoir of infection*—Man
4 *Transmission*—Contact, including sexual contact
5 *Control*—General hygienic measures—as for other venereal diseases

GONORRHOEA

This disease is caused by infection with *Neisseria gonorrhoeae.* In the male, it usually presents as an acute purulent urethritis with spread in some cases to involve the epididymis and testis. Late complications include urethral stricture, urethral sinuses and sub-fertility. A high proportion (80–90 per cent) of infected females are unaware of the infection; the others present with symptoms of urethritis and urethal or vaginal discharge. Complications in the female include Bartholinitis, salpingitis, pyosalpinx and pelvic inflammatory disease. Late complications include sub-fertility resulting from tubal obstruction. The *incubation period* is usually between 2 and 5 days, occasionally shorter (1 day), but may be as long as 2 weeks. It is usually notifiable nationally.

Geographical distribution
The distribution is world-wide with particular concentrations at seaports, and in areas having a high concentration of migrant labour or military personnel.

Bacteriology
N. gonorrhoea is a Gram-negative diplococcus, with a characteristic bean shape. It dies rapidly outside the human body, being susceptible to drying and heat.

Epidemiology
Man is the reservoir of infection; the most important part is the female pool with asymptomatic infection.

Transmission of the infection is mostly by:
(a) *Sexual genital contact*
(b) *Indirect contamination.* This may produce infection in prepubertal females. Vulvo-vaginitis may occur in a young girl who is infected by sharing towels or other clothing with an infected older relative. Post-pubertal girls do not become infected in this way; some cases of vulvo-vaginitis in young girls are the result of sexual contact with infected males.
(c) *Ophthalmia neonatorum.* This infection occurs in the course of delivering the baby of an infected mother.

All persons are susceptible. There is no lasting immunity after recovery; repeated infections are common. As with other venereal diseases, the most important host factor is sexual behaviour.

Laboratory diagnosis
Clinical diagnosis can be confirmed by bacteriological examination of stained smears of urethral discharge, cervical discharge or other infected material; the characteristic diplococci, some within pus cells, can be seen. The organisms can also be cultured on chocolate agar as a form of enrichment medium or on selective media such as the Thayer-Martin medium which contains antibiotics which suppress the growth of other organisms. Fluorescent antibody techniques are also available for diagnosis.

Control

The control of gonorrhoea is posing a difficult problem in most parts of the world. Various factors have contributed to this difficulty:
(a) Revolutionary change in sexual mores
(b) Replacement of the condom by effective contraceptive techniques which do not provide a mechanical barrier to infection

(c) Emergence of drug resistant strains

The control of gonorrhoea is based on the principles set out in the section on venereal diseases.

Gonococcal ophthalmitis can be prevented by treating all infected pregnant women and by toilet to the eyes of all newborn babies. The latter consists of instilling one drop of 1 per cent silver nitrate into the eyes of every newborn baby.

Gonorrhoea—Summary

1 *Occurrence*—World-wide
2 *Organism*—*Neisseria gonorrhoeae*
3 *Reservoir of infection*—Man
4 *Modes of Transmission*—Sexual contact. Rarely through fomites.
           Eye infection during delivery
5 *Control*— (i) As for other venereal diseases
     (ii) Toilet to the eyes of newborn babies

TREPONEMATOSES

The treponematoses are diseases caused by spirochaetes which belong to the genus *Treponemata*. The most important diseases in this group are:
(a) Venereal syphilis (*Treponema pallidum*)
(b) Yaws (*T. pertenue*)
(c) Pinta (*T. carateum*)
(d) Non-venereal syphilis (*T. pallidum*)

There has been much speculation about the origin and differentiation of these organisms. One view regards the organisms as being virtually identical but apparent differences in clinical manifestations result from epidemiological factors; the other view regards the organisms as separate but related entities. In practical terms, the pattern of treponemal diseases is still evolving with the eradication of the non-venereal treponematoses from endemic areas and with the rise in the frequency of venereal syphilis in some areas where the disease was previously not recognised as an important public health problem.

VENEREAL SYPHILIS

This is a chronic infection which is characterised clinically by a localised primary lesion, a generalised secondary eruption involving the skin and mucous membranes, and a later tertiary stage with involvement of skin, bone, abdominal viscera, cardiovascular and central nervous systems. The *incubation period* is usually 2 to 4 weeks but may be from 9 to 90 days. The primary lesion is usually a painless sore associated with firm enlarged regional lymph nodes. The initial lesion tends to heal spontaneously after a few weeks. Six weeks to 6 months or even a year later, secondary lesions appear usually as generalised non-itchy, painless and non-tender rash, shallow ulcers on the oral mucosa, widespread lymphodenopathy and mild systemic disturbance, including fever. These manifestations regress spontaneously, and the infection enters a latent phase which may last for 10 years or more before the tertiary lesions appear, although spontaneous healing may occur during the latent stage.

Although venereal syphilis was previously unknown or was not recognised in some parts of the world, the distribution of the venereal infection is now virtually world-wide.

Bacteriology

T. pallidum is a spirochaetal organism, a thin organism, 1–15 μm long with tapering ends; there are about 5–20 spirals. It is a motile organism, fresh preparations under dark-ground illumination show characteristic movements.

The organism is delicate, being rapidly killed by drying, at high temperature (50°C), disinfectants such as phenolic compounds, and by soap and water. It may survive in refrigerated blood for 3 days. The organism may remain viable for several years if frozen at −78°C.

Epidemiology

Man is the reservoir of infection, the sources of infection being moist lesions on the skin and mucosae, and also tissue fluids and secretions such as saliva, semen, vaginal discharge and blood.

Transmission is mainly venereal through genital or extragenital contact, but it may be non-venereal.

(i) VENEREAL TRANSMISSION   Genital contact may lead to infection with the organisms penetrating normal skin and mucous membranes. In the male, the infection may be quite obvious in the form of a primary chancre on the penis but the infective female may be unaware of a similar lesion on her cervix. Inapparent infection in the female, especially the promiscuous female, is an important source of infection.

Infection may also be transmitted during sexual play from extra-genital sites such as the mouth during kissing; the infected partner may develop primary lesions on the lips, tongue or breast.

(ii) NON-VENEREAL TRANSMISSION   This may be accidental, through touching infected tissues as in the case of dentists or midwives.

Congenital infection may occur in a child who is born to an infected mother, even though the mother is at a latent phase. Intra-uterine syphilitic infection may be associated with repeated abortions, still-births, or congenital infection in a live child, who may show lesions at birth, but more commonly clinical signs appear later.

The most important host factor in the epidemiology of syphilis is sexual behaviour, a high frequency of infection being associated with sexual promiscuity. A current infection with syphilis may provide some immunity, but if super-infection occurs, the clinical manifestations may be modified. There is some degree of cross-immunity to syphilis in persons infected with the other non-venereal treponematoses but such immunity is not absolute.

Laboratory diagnosis

1 DARK-FIELD MICROSCOPY of exudates of primary and secondary lesions usually reveal the spirochaete.

2 SEROLOGICAL TESTS on blood and cerebrospinal fluid. A variety of serological tests for syphilis are in use, but they fall into two main groups:

(a) *Non-treponemal antigen* These tests are based on the presence of the antibody complex—reagin, in syphilitic infections. This complex may be detected by using a flocculation test, e.g. VDRL slide test, Kahn test, Mazzine cardiolipin, or Kline cardiolipin. Alternatively, a complement-fixation test may be used, e.g. Kolmer test.

(b) *Treponemal antigen tests* These include the Treponema Pallidum Immobilisation test (TPT), Fluorescent Treponemal Antibody (FTA) and the Reiter Protein Complement-Fixation test (RPCFT).

The serological tests usually become positive 1–2 weeks after the appearance of the primary lesions, and are almost invariably positive during the secondary stage of the illness but may later become negative spontaneously or after successful chemotherapy at any stage.

False positive reactions

Using non-treponemal antigens false positive serum reactions are encountered in some persons who have not been infected with syphilis or other treponemal organism. Such *biological false positive* reactions are particularly associated with certain infections: protozoal (malaria, trypanosomiasis), spirochaetal (leptospirosis, relapsing fever), bacterial (leprosy, tuberculosis) and viral (atypical pneumonia, glandular fever, lymphogranuloma venereum). It has also been noted in cases of collagen vascular disease and following vaccination against smallpox or yellow fever.

Tests based on treponemal antigens, being more specific, are less liable to give such biological false positive reactions. Neither type of test can, however, differentiate syphilis from other treponemal infections.

A positive serological test therefore indicates the probable presence of a specific treponemal infection, the nature of which can be determined on clinical and circumstantial evidence.

Control

The general principles for the control of venereal diseases apply to the control of syphilis:

(1) *General health promotion*

Through health and sex education make the population aware of the danger of promiscuous sexual activity. Young persons especially should be encouraged to take up diversional activities in the form of games, interesting hobbies and other absorbing interests. Although the provision of good recreational facilities is highly desirable, it cannot however, by itself, make a significant change in sexual habits.

(2) *Control of prostitution and promiscuous sexual behaviour*

There are conflicting views about the best way to deal with the problem of prostitution in relation to venereal disease. At the one end it is suggested that prostitution being a social evil should be totally abolished, if necessary, by imposing severe penalties. An alternative view holds that whilst it may be desirable to abolish prostitution, it is not feasible to do so, and that harsh laws merely drive the practice underground and discourage the prostitutes and their partners from seeking appropriate medical treatment. In place of clandestine prostitution, licensed brothels are allowed to operate under the close supervision of the health authorities. Neither method provides a satisfactory solution.

The role of prostitutes in the transmission of syphilis varies from community to community. In some societies, professional prostitutes make a major contribution but, in others, much of the transmission results from promiscuous behaviour not involving immediate financial gain.

(3) *Early diagnosis and treatment*

Serology plays an important role in the detection of cases of syphilis, especially in the latent phase. Whenever feasible, there should be routine serological screening of pregnant women, blood donors, those who are about to get married, immigrants, hospital patients, prisoners and other groups.

Where there is a high probability that a person has been infected, such as the contact of a patient with open lesions, 'epidemiological treatment', i.e. treatment on the basis of presumptive diagnosis, should be given. Penicillin is the drug of choice; given early and in appropriate doses, syphilitic infection can be eradicated. Other antibiotics, e.g. tetracyclines, may be used if the patient is allergic to penicillin. There is as yet no effective artificial immunisation against syphilis.

Syphilis—Summary

1 *Occurrence*—World-wide
2 *Organism*—*Treponema pallidum*
3 *Reservoir of infection*—Man
4 *Modes of transmission*—sexual contact, non-sexual contact, transplacental

5 *Control*— (i) Control of sexual promiscuity
         (ii) Early detection and treatment of infected persons, including serological screening

NON-VENEREAL TREPONEMATOSES

YAWS

This non-venereal treponemal infection mainly affects skin and bones, rarely if ever affecting the cardiovascular or the nervous system. The skin lesions may be granulomatous, ulcerative or hypertrophic; destructive lesions of bone and hypertrophic changes are late lesions of bone. The *incubation period* is usually about 1 month, varying from 2 weeks to 3 months.

The disease was highly endemic in many parts of the tropics and subtropical zones of Africa, South-East Asia, the Pacific, the Caribbean and Central and South America. There has been a marked fall in the incidence of the disease, but constant surveillance is required to detect resurgence and institute prompt and energetic treatment. Several thousand cases were reported from Ghana in 1979.

Bacteriology
The infective agent, *Treponema pertenue*, cannot be distinguished from *T. pallidum* on microscopy (light, phase contrast or electron).

Epidemiology
Man is the reservoir of infection, the source of infection being the often moist skin lesions in the early phase of the disease. Transmission is mainly by direct contact, but flies, especially *Hippelates pallipes*, may carry the infection from a skin lesion to a susceptible host.

Most early cases are seen in children under 15 years. The disease occurs predominantly in rural communities where there is the combination of poverty, low level of personal hygiene, warm humid climate, and where children especially usually wear little clothing. Transplacental transmission does not occur.

Laboratory diagnosis
1 *Dark field microscopy* of the exudates from moist lesions will reveal the spirochaete.
2 *Serological tests* of blood become positive at an early stage of the infection, but tend to become negative when the disease has been latent for several years. None of the serological tests can differentiate syphilis from other treponemal infections.

Control

Yaws has been successfully controlled and virtually eradicated from some parts of the world where it had been highly endemic. The successful programme was backed by the World Health Organisation and it consisted of:

(a) *Epidemiological survey* by clinical examination of the entire population.

(b) *Mass chemotherapy with penicillin* of patients, including those with latent infection, and contacts. Specific treatment is with a single intramuscular injection of long acting penicillin in oil with 2 per cent aluminium monostearate (PAM).

(c) *Surveillance* through periodic clinical and serological surveys.

Apart from such specific campaigns, general improvement in personal hygiene and in level of living standards has contributed greatly to the disappearance of the disease.

Yaws—Summary

1 *Occurrence*—Tropics and subtropics of Africa, South-East Asia, Philippines, Pacific Islands, Caribbean, Central and South America. Mainly rural. Now well controlled in or eradicated from most areas

2 *Organism*—*Treponema pertenue*

3 *Reservoir of infection*—Man

4 *Mode of transmission*—Direct contact

5 *Control*— (i) Mass survey and chemotherapy
        (ii) Improvement of personal hygiene

PINTA

This is a spirochaetal infection which initially presents as a superficial non-ulcerating papule. Later flat hyperpigmented skin lesions develop, and these may become depigmented and hyperkeratotic. The *incubation period* is from 7 to 20 days.

Medical geography
It occurs predominantly in the dark-skinned people of Mexico, Central and South America, North Africa, Middle East, India, the Philippines and some areas in the Pacific.

Bacteriology
The infective agent is *Treponema carateum* a spirochaete which is morphologically indistinguishable from *T. pallidum*.

Epidemiology
Man is the reservoir of infection; the patients with early active lesions are the sources of infection.

Transmission is mainly from direct non-venereal contact, or through indirect contact. It has been suggested that certain biting insects play a role but this is not proven.

Infection is commoner in children than in adults. The relatively high frequency of cases in negroid persons may be related to socio-economic factors and personal habit, rather than to genetic factors. There is some cross-immunity with syphilis and other treponemal infections but protection is partial and syphilis may co-exist with pinta.

Pinta—Summary

1 *Occurrence*—Tropics and subtropics—America, Africa, Middle East, India, Philippines
2 *Organism—Treponema carateum*
3 *Reservoir of Infection*—Man
4 *Mode of transmission*—Direct and indirect contact
5 *Control*—As for yaws

ENDEMIC (NON-VENEREAL) SYPHILIS

This refers to a manifestation of infection with *Treponema pallidum* in an epidemiological situation in which the infection is highly endemic with non-venereal transmission occurring predominantly in young persons. A primary chancre is not commonly encountered and it is mainly extragenital. In the secondary stage, mucosal lesions (mucous patches) occur in the mouth, tongue, larynx and nostrils. Condylomata lata are also found in the moist areas: ano-genital area, groins, axillae, below the breast and the angles of the mouth. A variety of other skin lesions may also be present at this stage. Late lesions include skin gummata, nasopharyngeal ulceration, and bone lesions (osteitis, gummata). Cardiovascular and neurological involvement may occur but are apparently rare. Congenital infection is also rare.

The *incubation period* is 2 weeks to 3 months.

Medical geography
The infection is found in remote rural areas in parts of tropical Africa, the Middle and Near East, and southern Europe. It has virtually been eliminated from most of these areas where it was formerly endemic.

Bacteriology
The causative organism, *T. pallidum*, is indistinguishable from the aetiological agent of venereal syphilis.

Epidemiology
The distribution of the disease is associated with poverty, overcrowding and poor personal hygiene. Early infections occur predominantly in childhood.

Man is the reservoir of infection. Transmission is by close person-to-person contact; indirect transmission may occur through indirect contact from sharing pipes, cups and other utensils.

With improvement in social conditions, the endemic syphilis recedes, few children become infected but adults acquire venereally transmitted syphilis.

Laboratory diagnosis
The organism can be seen under dark-field microscopy from wet lesions such as mucous patches and condylomata. Serology becomes positive by the time that secondary lesions occur.

Endemic Syphilis—Summary

1 *Distribution*—Tropical Africa, Middle and Near East, Southern Europe
2 *Organism*—*Treponema pallidum*
3 *Reservoir of infection*—Man
4 *Mode of transmission*—Direct and indirect contact
5 *Control*— (i) Mass survey and chemotherapy with penicillin
     (ii) Improvement in personal hygiene

LEPROSY*

This is an infection due to the specific micro-organism, *Mycobacterium leprae*, which is of low invasive power and pathogenicity. The four main clinical forms described are: indeterminate leprosy; tuberculoid leprosy; borderline leprosy (probably the commonest form) and lepromatous leprosy.

Medical geography
This disease is common in the Indian subcontinent, tropical Africa, South-East Asia and South America. Small foci of infection exist in southern Europe and in the countries bordering the Mediterranean Leprosy has been introduced by immigrants into countries that have been free of indigenous cases for many years, e.g. the United Kingdom. It is estimated that the total number of cases throughout the world may well exceed 12 million.

Bacteriology
M. leprae is a slender rod-like organism which is both acid and alcohol fast and Gram-positive. It is found singly or in masses (globi). The bacilli are scanty in some clinical forms of leprosy (indeterminate and tuberculoid), while they are very numerous in the lesions of lepromatous leprosy. The organism has never been consistently cultured on artificial media. *M. leprae* has been successfully inoculated into the footpads of

* We are grateful to Dr S. Browne for the liberal use of his writings in the preparation of this section.

mice; it thrives in the armadillo and the hedgehog. The viable organism stains deeply and uniformly; irregular staining or beading indicates non-viability.

Epidemiology

The incubation period of leprosy is long and indefinite. Man is the only source of infection. The infectiousness of leprosy is not high, and repeated skin to skin contact seems to be necessary. The mechanism of contagion probably consists of the transfer of living *M. leprae* from skin to skin, and the introduction of the bacilli into the corium by some slight and unremembered trauma. The discovery of the viability of the large numbers of bacilli emerging from the nasal mucosa of patients with lepromatous leprosy is very important. *M. leprae* may also be shed by such patients from lepromatous skin ulcers, in the milk of lactating mothers and in much smaller numbers from the skin appendages. There is no positive evidence for the existence of an extrahuman reservoir of leprosy bacilli; nor for different strains. The role of fomites contaminated by skin squames or by nasal secretions is not clear. Conjugal infections are usually 5 per cent or less.

While prolonged and intimate contact is still classically considered to be necessary for infection to develop, there are well-authenticated cases of patients acquiring the infection after a brief passing contact with a person suffering from leprosy. Studies have shown that immunological conversion has taken place in a large proportion of leprosy contacts. These observations provide a firmer basis for placing leprosy in the group of infectious diseases (e.g., tuberculosis, and poliomyelitis) in which the rate of transmission of the infecting agent is very significantly higher than the disease attack rate. It is quite rare, for example, for workers in leprosaria to contract leprosy. Although leprosy is commonest in moist and humid lands, climatic factors *per se* are probably not important. Children and adolescents are commonly held to be more susceptible than adults, as are males more than females, but these generalisations are not as definite as they are sometimes made out to be. Hormonal influences may play a part, since there seems to be an increased incidence at puberty in both sexes, and clinical exacerbation of the disease may occur during pregnancy and particularly after parturition. Racial and genetic susceptibility affect the pattern of the disease from Central Africa since, as one moves eastwards or westwards from this central point, the ratio of lepromatous to tuberculoid patients increases.

The natural history of leprosy can conveniently be represented as in Fig. 5.1.

All persons exposed to repeated contact with open cases of leprosy do not contract the disease, and, moreover, a variable proportion of those who do develop leprosy, suffer from a self-healing form. Many persons infected with leprosy manifest a vigorous response to the organism,

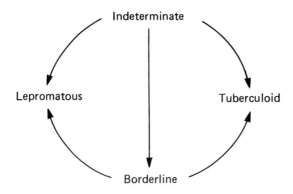

Fig. 5.1 Natural history of leprosy

while a variable proportion develop the severe progressive form of the disease characterised by minimal response (lepromatous).

Recent work has emphasised the complex nature of the immune response in leprosy. Both immunoglobulins and lymphocyte-mediated immune mechanisms are involved. Patients whose resistance is impaired lack cell-mediated immunity.

Secondary and primary dapsone resistance have become a major problem in many countries. Primary dapsone resistance is now estimated to be as high as 37 % in South India, and 38 % in Mali. Moreover, there is emerging the relatively new problem of persistence of leprosy bacilli. In this situation the majority of *M. leprae* are killed but some of the bacilli survive and are able to multiply after a period of quiescence—'persisters'.

The lepromin test
The antigens used for the lepromin test are prepared by the maceration of tissue containing great numbers of bacilli, such as a nodule obtained from a patient suffering from active lepromatous leprosy. The organisms are killed by heat or by other means. A refined lepromin is obtained by treating the tissue with chloroform and ether, and then centrifuging at high speed. The deposit is suspended in carbol-saline. The test is performed by injecting 0.1 ml of antigen intradermally; the site of injection is inspected after 24 hours, and daily thereafter. There are other methods of preparing a suitable antigen from bacillus-containing material and sundry modifications of the test.

There are two types of cutaneous response to the lepromin test. The early reaction of *Fernandez* consists of an erythematous infiltrated area which appears 24–72 hours after injection, while the *Mitsuda* reaction is nodular in form and most intense 21–30 days after injection. The early reaction is now interpreted as a response to soluble substances of the bacillus, and the late reaction as resistance to the bacillus excited by insoluble substances. Variation of the intensity of the lepromin test occurs among leprosy patients as well as among contacts. The best site for the inoculation is the anterior aspect of the forearm.

The Mitsuda reaction is negative in pure lepromatous leprosy, strongly positive in major tuberculoid leprosy, and variably positive in intermediate forms. BCG vaccination may result in conversion of a negative lepromin reaction to positive, this conversion occurring in a variable proportion of subjects to a variable degree.

Neither an early nor a late lepromin reaction proves immunity. The lepromin test is essentially an allergic reaction, though many leprologists believe that the reaction tests both allergy and immunity to leprosy bacilli. The proportion of persons in endemic areas giving positive Mitsuda reactions increases with age from nil at birth up to 80 per cent in adults. It has been speculated that an intrinsic natural factor exists—which is called factor N (N for natural)—that gives an individual the capacity to react specifically to *M. leprae*. Thus about 20 per cent of the population, for no apparent reason, will not become lepromin-positive however strong the natural or artificial extrinsic stimuli may be, this minor group probably lacks intrinsic factor N.

Laboratory diagnosis

The cardinal point in diagnosis is the demonstration of *M. leprae* in a smear of clinical lesion stained by the Ziehl-Neelson method. The best sites for taking smears are the following:
1 the active edge of the most active lesion
2 the ear lobes
3 the mucosa of the nasal septum.
Biopsy of typical macules, nodules, infiltrations or enlarged nerves is often used. Bacterial assessment of patients with leprosy is made by counts on skin smears or biopsy specimens, from which two indices can be derived—(*a*) the *Morphological Index* (M.I.), and (*b*) the *Bacteriological Index* (B.I.).

The *morphological index* is the average percentage of morphologically normal and viable (i.e. solid-staining or deeply staining) bacilli in smears from the various sites.

The *bacteriological index*, expressed by various notations (0 to 4 or 5 or 6), is a measure of the average concentration of recognisable bacillary forms in smears from various sites on the skin (and possibly nasal mucosa).

Control

Where determined and sustained efforts can be made, leprosy can be cured in the individual and controlled in the community.

(a) The individual

Primary and secondary dapsone resistance has become increasingly common throughout the world occurring in lepromatous (LL) and borderline (BL) cases. Triple drug therapy is mandatory if resistance is to be minimised using (1) rifampicin, (2) dapsone, and either prothionamide, clofazimine or ethionamide as the third drug. Various regimens are on trial to determine the best combinations for both multibacillary as well as paucibacillary leprosy. Limiting the duration of treatment is one of the objectives of these trials.

(b) The community

The threshold below which leprosy ceases to be a public health problem depends on a number of factors and probably varies from country to country.

Although the factors that determine the persistence or disappearance of leprosy in a community are still unknown, the general principles of control of a slightly contagious bacillary disease can be applied to leprosy, namely:

(i) reduction of contagious sources by chemotherapy to a level at which there is little danger of spread

(ii) control of the frequency and duration of potentially infective contacts

(iii) tracing and supervision of all persons exposed to infection.

Methods of control depend on the incidence of leprosy in the community, the state of the existing medical services and the willingness of the authorities to accord leprosy control the place its importance deserves.

In lands where leprosy is more highly endemic (namely most of the tropics and subtropics) its control is a most difficult problem. All the adverse factors are present in some degree, namely:

(i) overcrowding and low standards of hygiene

(ii) lack of medical services

(iii) limited financial resources

(iv) ignorance and prejudice

(v) the existence of diseases that kill (malaria) or are more prevalent (schistosomiasis, onchocerciasis), more contagious (tuberculosis, cholera) or more amenable to control measures (poliomyelitis, water-borne diseases, trachoma).

The essence of leprosy control is survey, education and treatment. *Survey* may mean a whole-population survey, a pilot or sampling operation, or be limited to certain readily available groups such as schoolchildren, schoolteachers, workmen and their families, or army and police recruits. When the prevalence is high, regular whole-population surveys conducted annually by teams of auxiliaries working under a doctor are essential. Clinical examination of stripped subjects, conducted with due regard to privacy and social habits, is the rule.

Doubtful lesions are examined by the doctor in charge, smears are taken and either stained on the spot or fixed for subsequent staining at the central laboratory. If possible, contacts of known leprosy patients are seen even more frequently. Treatment is instituted at once for all patients in whom active leprosy has been diagnosed. Advantage is taken of the presence of relatives and fellow-villagers to establish good public relations and to embark on a suitable scheme of education. From the beginning, leprosy should be integrated into the comprehensive medical service for the control of transmissible diseases and treatment provided for leprosy patients suffering from other diseases as well. This also fosters good public relations, for duplication of services is avoided and the health of the whole community is improved.

The mainstay of the anti-leprosy campaign in an urban or rural area in the developing countries is the all-purpose dispensary in charge of a competent paramedical worker. After being instructed in the rudiments of leprosy diagnosis and treatment, the latter is able to recognise early leprosy, ensure regularity of treatment of all patients and participate in health education, simple physiotherapy, etc.

Leprosy patients are treated either at *static dispensaries* or in *mobile clinics*. The choice will be determined largely by local conditions, such as the status of the public health service, distribution of the population, the prevalence of leprosy, local communications, etc. The drugs used should be restricted to a few (the fewer the better) and they should be given according to a simple codified regime. The great majority of patients, whatever the form or stage of leprosy and whatever their age and sex, may be safely and satisfactorily treated in this fashion, and the risk of untoward side-effects is minimal.

The mobile clinic—whether for leprosy only or an all-purpose type—has proved its worth in Francophone Africa. The itinerary is planned so that regular visits are paid every so often along a certain route. Patients foregather at set points from surrounding villages and hamlets to receive a supply of drugs sufficient to last until the next visit. Paramedical workers travel on bicycles where the truck cannot go, rejoining it further along the route. The essential features of the service are diagnosis, examination of contacts and the taking of slit-smears. While the drawbacks and shortcomings of this system are obvious, it is the only way of tackling the leprosy problem in a scattered population with primitive and precarious communications. One real disadvantage of rural control schemes is that patients no longer suffering from active disease may have to walk long distances to receive a supply of anti-leprosy tablets that have no effect on their burnt-out disease, but with possible worsening of the ulcers on their anaesthetic feet. The campaign will inevitably suffer as a result.

In some circumstances, the *segregation village* has been advocated. When arable land is available and the patients can support themselves by farming, the temporary expedient of the segregation village has much in its favour, provided the goodwill of tribal chiefs and populace has been assured. Sometimes the local authorities themselves take the initiative. The village should fall within the purview of a resident medical auxiliary who may also have either a small ward for in-patients or access to beds in a local hospital. If such villages can be properly supervised and patients can return home when this is deemed advisable they may play a useful part in the leprosy campaign. However, they may also perpetuate false notions about leprosy; the inmates stay on and acquire a landed and vested interest in the village, perhaps holding the local population to ransom by begging. In some countries (for instance Korea) these communities, which include cured patients, raise enormous problems. Their upkeep makes heavy financial demands on the government, and special schools have to be set up for the children, thus strengthening the fears of the healthy population that leprosy sufferers transmit a taint. The segregation village is now in general out of favour.

The *central hospital* forms an essential element in a leprosy control scheme. At any one time about 1 per cent of the patients will be inpatients. Facilities for reconstructive surgery should be available, as also for pre- and post-operative physiotherapy, for training in the use of anaesthetic limbs, for occupational therapy or vocational training, and for the provision of prostheses.

In no other disease do social and psychological factors loom so large as in leprosy. Since no specific psychological changes can be attributed to leprosy *per se*, the factors determining the psychological changes that occur are rather the outcome of the patient's attitude to his disease and the attitude of society. In the patient, traditional beliefs as well as guilt feelings may result in either apathy and resignation or a resentful aggressiveness towards society. Leprosy in the present 'incarnation' may be regarded as retribution for misdeeds in a previous one, so that nothing can or should be done to ameliorate it. When seen as punishment for a sexual misdemeanour, leprosy may lead to such intense feelings of remorse and recrimination that suicide is contemplated or even committed. On the other hand, the person with leprosy may be led to believe that his only hope of cure is to deflower a virgin and thus pass on his disease to someone else.

Tolerance by society is the exception rather than the rule. As a result the patient tries to conceal his trouble for as long as possible, for the consequences may be compulsory segregation or shunning of the whole family by the community. Apparently healthy relatives are regarded as 'tainted' and may find it impossible to secure marriage partners, or those already married may be forced into divorce. Concealment of early (and treatable) leprosy lesions not only allows the disease to progress to irreversible deformity but also perpetuates an endemic situation.

BCG vaccination has given conflicting results. Current research is focused on the possibilities of developing a vaccine based on killed *M. leprae*.

Chemoprophylaxis with dapsone to children under 15 years of age who were contacts of lepromatous and other bacteriologically positive index cases, has given encouraging results in India but has been less convincing in the Philippines.

Leprosy—Summary

1 *Occurrence*—Indian subcontinent, tropical Africa, South-East Asia, South America
2 *Organisms*—*Mycobacterium leprae*
3 *Reservoir of infection*—Man
4 *Mode of transmission*—Intimate contact
5 *Control*— (i) Individual treatment with triple drug therapy
      (ii) Survey
     (iii) Static dispensaries or mobile clinics
     (iv) Education of society
      (v) BCG and/or prophylactic dapsone

SUPERFICIAL FUNGAL INFECTIONS

A wide variety of fungi infect skin, hair and nails, without deeper penetration of the host tissues. The various clinical manifestations include favus, ringworm of the scalp, body, feet ('athlete's foot') and nails; some produce dyspigmentation, e.g. Tinea versicolor. The lesions are mostly disfiguring but apart from the aesthetic aspect some are disabling, e.g. athlete's foot could lead to splitting of the skin and secondary bacterial infection.

Medical geography
These infections have a world-wide distribution but some of the clinical manifestations such as ringworm of the feet tend to be more severe in the moist tropics. There are geographical variations in the incidence of various species, e.g. the predominant cause of tinea capitis in North America is *M. audouini* but it is *T. tonsurans* in South America.

The infective agents include species of *Epidermophyton, Trichophyton, Microsporon* and *Mallassezia furfur* (causative agent of Tinea versicolor).

Epidemiology
Man and animals represent the main reservoir of many of these infections but some of the fungi are also found in the soil. Domestic pets play an important role for some infections, e.g. *M. canis* which is transmitted from dogs and cats.

Transmission may be from direct contact but also indirectly through contact with contaminated floors, barber's instruments, clothing, combs and other personal articles.

All age and racial groups are susceptible to these infections but some of the infections show variation with age and sex, e.g. ringworm of the scalp due to *Microsporon audouini* is most prevalent in pre-pubertal children. Subclinical infections occur; some of these organisms can be cultured from persons who do not show clinical signs.

Laboratory diagnosis
Specimens for examination include scrapings from the skin and nails, and also infected hairs. The organisms may be demonstrated on microscopy of skin scrapings which can be cleared with a solution of 10 per cent potassium hydroxide. Some of the organisms can be cultured on selective media such as Sabouraud's glucose agar at 20°C. Some of the fungal lesions in hairy areas display fluorescence when examined under ultraviolet light ('Wood's light') and this serves as a useful screening test.

Control

Prompt identification and treatment of infected persons will help to reduce the reservoir of infection, but the existence of subclinical infections may limit the value of this measure.

General hygienic measures in homes, schools and public places such as baths and swimming pools can help reduce the hazard of infection. The sharing of towels and other personal toilet articles should be discouraged. The handling of animals including domestic pets is also an avoidable risk.

Fungal Infections—Summary

1 *Occurrence*—World-wide, but certain manifestations, e.g. clefts, are more severe in the tropics
2 *Organisms*—Various species of *Epidermophyton, Trichophyton,* and *Microsporon*; also *Malassezia furfur*
3 *Reservoir of infection*—Man, animals and soil
4 *Transmission*—Direct contact, indirect contanct with contaminated articles
5 *Control*— (i) Personal hygiene
         (ii) Sanitation in baths and pools

CANDIDIASIS

This is a mycotic infection which usually affects the superficial layers of the oral cavity (thrush), female genitalia, and other mucous membranes; lesions of the skin especially in the moist folds, may occur; involvement of nails may present as chronic paronychia; and rarely the organism becomes disseminated systemically in debilitated persons, e.g. leukaemia and other neoplasms especially under treatment with corticosteroids, and broad-spectrum antibiotics.

The *incubation period* varies widely, but in children, it may be of order of 2 to 6 days.

Medical geography
It has a world-wide distribution.

Mycology
Candida albicans is the main pathogenic organism producing these lesions, rarely other organisms such as *Saccharomyces* may produce a similar oral lesion.

Epidemiology
Man is the reservoir of infection. Transmission is by contact with infected persons, both patients and carriers.

The carrier state is very common, the organism being found as part of the oral and intestinal flora. The occurrence of disease is therefore largely determined by host susceptibility. Newborn babies and infants, debilitated persons such as diabetics, cachectic patients with advanced cancer, and patients with advanced tuberculosis.

Ill-fitting dentures, tuberculous cavities and similar local factors may predispose to lesions of candidiasis. Treatment with broad-spectrum antibiotics may so alter the normal flora as to promote the overgrowth of these yeasts with consequent pathological manifestations. House-wives, cleaners and bartenders who soak their hands in water for long periods are liable to chronic paronychia due to candidiasis.

Transmission is by contact. The newborn infant may be infected by her mother during childbirth.

Control

This includes prompt treatment of infections using mycostatin, in severe cases. Genital infections should be treated in late pregnancy. Prolonged use of broad-spectrum antibiotics should be avoided.

Candidiasis—Summary

1 *Occurrence*—World-wide
2 *Organism*—Candida albicans
3 *Reservoir of infection*—Man
4 *Transmission*—Contact, during parturition
5 *Control*— (i) Careful use of broad-spectrum antibiotics
       (ii) Elimination of local predisposing factors
      (iii) Treatment of pregnant women

TRICHOMONIASIS

This is a chronic infection of the genital tract of both sexes. In the female, it presents with vaginitis accompanied by copious discharge; and with urethritis in the male.

The *incubation period* is from 1 to 3 weeks.

Medical geography
It has a world-wide distribution

Parasitology
The causative agent is *Trichomonas vaginalis*, a protozoan flagellate.

Laboratory diagnosis
Microscopy of wet film preparation of vaginal or urethral discharge may show the motile organism. The organism can also be identified in stained smears.

Epidemiology
Man is the reservoir of infection, the infected genital discharges being the source of infection. Transmission is by sexual intercourse or by indirect contact through contaminated clothing and other articles. Clinical manisfestations occur more frequently in males than in females.

Control

Although the general principles for the control of venereal diseases apply, the main approach is the treatment of infected persons and their sexual partners. Improvement in personal hygiene is also important.

Trichomoniasis—Summary

1 *Occurrence*—World-wide
2 *Organism*—*Trichomonas vaginalis*
3 *Reservoir of infection*—Man
4 *Transmission*—Sexual contact, indirect contact through fomites
5 *Control*— (i) As for other venereal diseases
            (ii) Improvement in general hygiene

SCABIES

This is an infection of the skin by the mite, *Sarcoptes scabiei*. The skin rash typically consists of small papules, vesicles and pustules, characterised by intense pruritus. Another typical feature is the presence of burrows which are superficial tunnels made by the adult mite. Secondary bacterial infection is common. Lesions occur most frequently in the moist areas of skin, e.g. web of the fingers.

The *incubation period* ranges from a few days to several weeks.

Medical geography
The distribution of the disease is widespread in the tropics with particular concentration in poor overcrowded areas; it is also found in the temperate zones, especially in slums and where disasters such as wars have led to crowding and insanitary conditions.

Causative agent

The infective agent is the mite *Sarcoptes scabiei*. The female mite which is larger than the male, measures 0.3 to 0.4 mm. The gravid female lays its eggs in superficial tunnels. Within 3–5 days, the eggs hatch to larvae and nymphs which pass through four stages and finally moult after 3 weeks to become sexually mature adults. The adults pair and mate on the skin surface.

Epidemiology

Man is the reservoir of infection. There is a related species of mite in animals—*Sarcoptes mange*; man may acquire this infection on contact with infected dogs, but this mite cannot reproduce on human skin.

Transmission of scabies is by direct contact with an infected person or indirectly through contaminated clothing. Infection may be acquired during sexual intercourse.

All persons are apparently susceptible but infection is particularly common in children; several cases are commonly found within the same household.

Laboratory diagnosis

The adult mite can be seen using a hand lens, and identified under the microscope; the female mite can be brought to the surface by teasing the burrows with a sharp pointed needle.

Control

A high standard of personal hygiene must be maintained, with particular emphasis on regular baths with soap and water, frequent laundering of clothes, and the avoidance of overcrowding also help to prevent the spread of infection.

Infected persons should be treated by the application of benzyl benzoate emulsion or tetraethylthiuram monosulphide following a thorough bath. Other affected members of the family should be treated at the same time to prevent re-infection. Mass treatment may be useful in large institutions such as work camps.

Scabies—Summary

1 *Occurrence*—World-wide, overcrowded poor areas
2 *Organism*—Sarcoptes scabiei
3 *Reservoir of infection*—Man
4 *Mode of transmission*—Direct contact; or indirectly through contaminated clothing
5 *Control*— (i) Improvement in personal hygiene
         (ii) Treatment of affected persons

OTHER INFECTIONS ACQUIRED THROUGH SKIN AND MUCOUS MEMBRANES

Apart from infections transmitted by contact with infected persons, some infections are acquired through skin by exposure to infected soil (tetanus, hookworm), to water (schistosomiasis, leptospirosis) or animal bites (rabies).

HOOKWORM

This is an important intestinal parasite which occurs commonly in warm climates especially in communities with poor environmental sanitation. Anaemia secondary to blood loss is the most important clinical feature of hookworm infection. Although light to moderate loads of infection may be well tolerated in well-nourished persons who have an adequate intake of iron, heavy infection usually leads to iron-deficiency anaemia and occasionally to severe protein depletion. Thus, the occurrence of diseases in hookworm infection depends on the interaction of the load of infection, the state of the iron stores and the diet of the host.

Medical geography
The infection is endemic in the tropics and subtropics; it is receding from the more developed areas being most highly prevalent in the rural areas of the moist tropics. It occurs in various parts of tropical Africa, south-eastern USA, Mediterranean countries, Asia and the Caribbean. In parts of West Africa, *N. Americanus* is the predominant species, whereas *A. duodenale* is found in the Mediterranean area; in most other areas, in Asia, Central and South America, mixed infections occur. During the past decades both parasites have become widely distributed throughout the tropics and subtropics, and rigid demarcations are no longer tenable.

Parasitology
The two main species which infect man are *Ankylostoma duodenale* and *Necator americanus*. The adult worms living in the intestine, are attached to the intestinal wall from which they suck blood; they migrate from site to site. The eggs are passed in faeces, and after hatching the larvae mature in the soil. The infective larvae may survive in the soil for many weeks. Man is infected on contact with soil, the infective larvae penetrating the unbroken skin and this may give rise to a pruritic rash (ground 'itch'). The larvae migrate to the lungs and ascend the trachea to be swallowed and carried to the intestine where the adult worms become established.

The hookworms of cats and dogs, *Ankylostoma braziliense* and *A. caninum*, fail to achieve full maturity in man but may cause a serpiginous skin rash—cutaneous larva migrans.

Laboratory diagnosis

Hookworm infection is diagnosed by the identification of the eggs in stool; concentration methods are used for detecting light infections. Quantitative assessment of the load can be made by using a dilution method, e.g. the Stoll technique. The larvae can be cultured from stool on moist filter paper at room temperature, 25°C; the species of the worm can be identified from the larval stage or from expelled adults.

Epidemiology

Although man is the only important source of human hookworm infection, the epidemiology of the disease is dependent upon the interaction of three factors—the suitability of the environment for the eggs or larvae; the mode and extent of faecal pollution of the soil; and the mode and extent of contact between infected soil and skin.

Thus survival of hookworm larvae is favoured in a damp, sandy, or friable soil with decaying vegetation, and a temperature of 24°–32°C. Larvae move very little horizontally but can migrate upwards as much as 1 metre. *A. duodenale* eggs resist dessication more than those of *Necator*, while the development of hookworm larvae in the eggs and subsequent hatching can be retarded in the absence of oxygen. Insanitary disposal of faeces or the use of human faeces as soil fertiliser are the chief sources of human infection in countries where individuals are bare-footed. Thus, it is to be expected that hookworm infection will have a higher prevalence in agricultural than in town workers—and that in many tropical countries it is an occupational disease of the farming community. Experiments have shown that although *Necator* infection is acquired almost exclusively by the percutaneous route, *Ankylostoma* infection may be contracted either percutaneously or orally—the latter mode of entry gives special point to the reports of contamination of vegetables by these larvae.

Contrary to the general belief, it has been shown that larvae of *A. duodenale* do not always develop directly to adulthood upon invasion of man. Thus, in West Bengal, India, arrested development appears to be a seasonal phenomenon which results in (a) reduction of egg output wasted in seeding an inhospitable environment and (b) a marked increase in eggs entering the environment just before the monsoon begins. The relationship of some key behavioural and social factors to the levels of hookworm infection by studying the defaecation behaviour of a population can have direct implications for control.

Provided people are equally exposed to hookworm infection, both sexes and all ages are susceptible. In communities in which the parasite has long been endemic, the inhabitants develop a host/parasite balance in which the worm load is limited, thus although the infection rate in some rural areas of the tropics may be 100 % only a small proportion develop hookworm anaemia. It is not known whether these heavy infections resulting in anaemia are dependent upon repeated exposure to a high intensity of infection, or whether they represent a failure of immunity. There is little direct evidence about the effects of host immunity on hookworm in man.

Control

Control of hookworm infection involves four approaches: (1) the sanitary disposal of faeces, (2) health education, (3) chemotherapy, and (4) correction of the anaemia.

The provision of latrines and *education* in their proper usage are crucial to the control of hookworm infections. If fresh human faeces is used as fertiliser, it should be treated in order to kill the larvae either by composting before usage or by the addition of chemicals such as sodium nitrate, calcium superphosphate or ammonium sulphate. The wearing of protective footwear is a useful complementary measure.

Anthelminthics

The approach to treatment requires orientation in the context of intensity of infection, probability of reinfection and economic consider-ations. Thus, whereas in non-endemic areas it is justifiable to treat all infections however light, in endemic areas where reinfection is likely to occur only heavy or moderate infections are worth treating *unless simultaneous attempts* are also made to improve environment hygiene. In the tropics, therefore, the main aim of anthelmintic treatment should be to reduce the load of infection below the level of clinical significance; complete parasitological cure is unnecessary except within the context mentioned above. Nevertheless, in patients who are severely ill from other causes such as protein-energy malnutrition, marasmus, tubercu-losis, or sickle-cell anaemia, worm infections, however light, should be treated even though reinfection is certain to occur.

In the past, laxatives were routinely given before and after treatment; they are now usually considered unnecessary except in the presence of constipation. In many countries of the tropical world *economic* con-siderations must determine the choice of drug that is given.

The recommended anthelminthics are relatively non-toxic and in most instances can be given straight away even to debilitated patients. When the anaemia is very severe (less than 5 g per 100 ml) some practitioners prefer to raise the haemoglobin level to about 7–8 g per 100 ml before dealing with the worm infection specifically. Patients with severe hypoalbuminaemia should be adequately and quickly dewormed.

Several drugs are available for treating hookworm infections; their efficacy varies according to the species in question. Repeated treatments are usually necessary except in light infections, and this generalisation is valid for all the drugs mentioned below.

For *A. duodenale* infections treatment may be given with pyrantel embonate, bephenium hydroxynaphthoate, mebendazole or bitos-canate. For *N. americanus* treatment with tetrachlorethylene, pyrantel embonate, mebendazole or bitoscanate is available. Drugs that have a better effect on one species usually also have some effect on the other species.

Broad-Spectrum Anthelminthics

Multiple intestinal helminth infections are common in the rural tropics. In these cases anthelmintics that are effective against more than one parasite may be useful. Even so, their activity against one species may be selectively lower than against another. Mebendazole, pyrantel embonate, oxantel-pamoate, oxantel-pamoate/pyrantel pamoate suspensions, and thiabendazole are good examples of broad-spectrum anthelmintics that have been used both for individual and mass treatment. When the multiple infections are generally light, the convenience, range and economic advantages of using such compounds are well worth considering. With heavy infections, however, selective treatment for the appropriate species of helmintic infection is preferable.

Anaemia

The response to iron therapy is usually rapid. A cheap and very effective treatment is ferrous sulphate, 200 mg tds given by mouth and continued for three months after the haemoglobin concentration has risen to 12 g per 100 ml. Even without deworming, this regime will rectify the anaemia and a rise in haemoglobin of 1 g per 100 ml per week occurs; unless the worms have been removed, however, the haemoglobin will drop as soon as iron therapy is discontinued and anthelminthics are therefore mandatory in heavy infections. When indicated, e.g. if regular oral administration cannot be guaranteed, intramuscular or intravenous iron preparations are given.

Hookworm—Summary

1 *Distribution*—Tropics and subtropical area of Africa, South America and Asia
2 *Organisms*—*Necator americanus*; *Ankylostoma duodenale*
3 *Reservoir of infection*—Man
4 *Transmission*—Contact with contaminated soil
5 *Control*— (i) Sanitary disposal of faeces
             (ii) Wearing of shoes

TETANUS

This is an acute disease caused by the action produced by *Clostridium tetani*. The disease is characterised by an increase in muscle tone, and spasms, fever and a high mortality in untreated cases. Usually the hypertonia and the spasms are generalised, but in some mild cases, the muscle rigidity may be confined to a local area, e.g. a limb, and spasms may also be localised to the laryngeal muscles. Trismus is usually an early symptom. A peculiar grimace 'risus sardonicus' is often noted in these patients. In tetanus neonatorum, the first symptom is failure to suck in a baby who had sucked normally for the first few days after delivery.

The incubation is usually between 3 days and 3 weeks. The interval between the first symptom of stiffness and the appearance of spasms is known as the period of onset.

Medical geography
This is world-wide with a high concentration in some parts of the tropics. Farmers and others living in areas are usually more frequently affected than urban dwellers. With routine immunisation of children and prophylactic care of wounds, the disease is now rare in the developed countries.

Bacteriology
Clostridium tetani is a Gram-positive rod, an obligate anaerobe, which forms terminal spores giving it a characteristic drumstick shape. The spores are highly resistant to drying and to high temperatures; they may withstand boiling for short periods.

Epidemiology
The reservoir of infection is the soil and the faeces of various animals including man. The organism gains entry into the host through wounds; any wound may serve as the portal of entry for tetanus:

(a) POST-TRAUMATIC   Deep penetrating wounds especially when associated with tissue necrosis, and particularly when contaminated with earth, dung or foreign organic material. Superficial wounds including burns may also cause tetanus. The umbilical wound is the usual portal of neonatal tetanus.

(b) POST-PUERPERAL AND POST-ABORTAL   These arise from the use of contaminated instruments and dressings.

(c) POST-SURGICAL   These may also be from instruments and dressings, but the infection may be endogenous, from the presence of the organism in the host's bowel or in his wounds.

(d) CHRONIC ULCERS AND DISCHARGING SINUSES   Chronic ulcers, guinea-worm infections, chronic otitis media, infected tuberculous sinuses may serve as portals of entry.

(e) CRYPTOGENIC   In a high proportion of cases, no focus is found, presumably some of these are due to minor injuries which have healed. All non-immune persons in all age-groups are susceptible. Infection does not confer immunity; repeated attacks occur.

Laboratory diagnosis
The diagnosis can be firmly made without laboratory tests. The isolation of the organism from the wound is of little value since it may be recovered from the wounds of persons who show no sign of tetanus.

Control

There are three main lines of prevention:

(1) Antibacterial measures

These include the protection of wounds from contamination, adequate cleansing of wounds and careful débridement. Antibiotics especially long-acting penicillin can also be given to suppress the multiplication of *Clostridium tetani*. If the wound is old, i.e. more than twelve hours, tetanus may occur despite an adequate dose of penicillin.

(2) Passive immunisation

Tetanus antitoxin (ATS) in the form of horse serum is used. 1500 units are given in the average case although a larger dose may be required for patients who present with heavily contaminated wounds. Repeated doses of ATS will lead to sensitisation of the patient creating the hazard of allergic reactions. These later doses are also rapidly eliminated from the body and therefore are less effective for prevention and treatment. Efforts have been made to replace serum antitoxin with human immunoglobulin containing tetanus antitoxin.

(3) Active immunisation

Active immunisation with tetanus toxoid is the most satisfactory method of preventing tetanus. Ideally everyone should be given a course of active immunisation. Booster doses can then be given periodically, e.g. every 5 years or whenever the person is injured. Special preparations are available for combined active-passive immunisation. Active immunisation of the pregnant woman will protect the infant from neonatal tetanus. The persistence of clinical cases of tetanus in any community is a direct indictment of the health authorities of the country concerned because tetanus toxoid is simple to administer, safe, effective and cheap. With the stimulus of the WHO expanded programme of immunisation and the slogan of health care for all by the year 2000, tetanus should be one disease *at least* that should become rare in the developing world.

The goal of the Expanded Programme on Immunisation (EPI) is to reduce morbidity and mortality by providing immunization against the target diseases of diphtheria, pertussis, tetanus, measles, poliomyelitis and tuberculosis for every child in the world by 1990.

Tetanus—Summary

1 *Occurrence*—World-wide, but very low incidence in developed countries as a result of immunisation programme
2 *Organism*—*Clostridium tetani*
3 *Reservoir of infection*—Man
4 *Mode of transmission*—Through wounds
5 *Control*— (i) Active immunisation with tetanus toxoid
    (ii) Toilet of wounds
    (iii) Penicillin prophylaxis
    (iv) Passive immunisation with antitetanus serum

MYCOBACTERIUM ULCERANS INFECTION
(Buruli ulcer)

Mycobacterium ulcerans which results in the formation of chronic necrotising ulcers of the skin and subcutaneous tissues is being recognised as a common problem in many parts of the world. The predominance of lesions occur in the extremities.

Medical geography

The infection has been recognised in Australia, Uganda, Zaire, West Africa, Malaysia, Mexico and Papua New Guinea. The condition is probably more widespread in the tropics than is generally reported, being confused with tropical ulcer.

Bacteriology

M. ulcerans grows preferentially at a temperature of 32–33°C. It belongs to the group of slow-growing mycobacteria requiring 4–18 weeks to grow from initial isolation.

Epidemiology

The prevalence of Buruli disease varies considerably in the various reported areas. A careful recent study of the epidemiology of Buruli disease was carried out in Uganda, where the outstanding geographic feature was the distribution of Buruli lesions near the Nile. Thus, the section of the Kinyara refugee settlement closest to the Nile had the highest incidence of the disease. In these parts, more than 25 per cent of refugee children under 15 years of age developed Buruli lesions. The disease apparently is more common in sparsely settled areas, and may be related to the cultivation of previously undisturbed areas.

Buruli disease occurs from infancy to old age, but the highest incidence is in children from 5 to 14 years. Among adults it is more common among women than men. Two factors are mainly responsible for the age and sex distribution: immunity to the disease and exposure to the agent. People with a naturally positive tuberculin reaction are partially protected from Buruli disease. The most important reasons for the age, sex distribution and differences in anatomic sites are probably attributable to differential exposure. The method of transmission is unknown and the disease has only been tentatively included in this section until conclusive evidence of its mode of spread has been obtained. Atypical mycobacteria have been isolated from grasses in areas of high endemicity in Uganda. The usual *incubation period* is about 4 to 10 weeks. There is a peak seasonal incidence between September to November each year.

Laboratory diagnosis

Classically, histological examination of the lesions, reveals complete necrosis of subcutaneous tissue with numerous organisms in subcutaneous fibrous septa. There is a notable absence of inflammatory cells.

Control

(a) *The individual*
The first principle of surgical treatment is excision of all involved tissue; the second is early covering of the denuded area with skin.

(b) *The community*
BCG vaccination has given promising results. Health education emphasising to the communities the significance of the early lesion—a small nodule—has resulted in Uganda in an overall reduction in total hospitalisation and operative time, as well as the elimination of crippling deformities.

SCHISTOSOMIASIS

This remains one of the most important parasitic infections in the tropics. Human infection, due mainly to *Schistosoma haematobium, S. mansoni* and *S. japonicum*, causes chronic inflammatory changes with progressive damage to various organs. The localisation of the worms varies from species to species. At first the lesions are granulomatous with damage to parenchymatous host cells; later fibrotic changes take place. Even after the worms have been eliminated, residual sequelae may persist. Four clinical stages are identified (Table 5.3). Local dermatitis occurs at the site of penetration ('cercarial dermatitis'), fever and malaise may occur after the appearance of the skin lesions. Later during the migratory phase, more systemic manifestations may occur, fever, transient skin rashes, cough with radiological evidence of pulmonary infiltration and eosinophilia. These early manifestations of schistosomiasis are usually missed, and diagnosis is made only at the stage of established infection. *S. haematobium* mainly affects the urogenital system and classically presents with haematuria; later frequency and dysuria may occur.

The late effects of *S. haematobium* include contraction of the bladder, obstructive uropathy from involvement of the ureter and secondary bacterial infection; cancer of the bladder is associated with chronic vesical schistosomiasis.

Established infection due to *S. mansoni* and *S. japonicum* mainly affect the bowel with secondary changes in the liver. Initially, the patient may present with weakness, tiredness, loss of weight, anorexia, dysenteric symptoms, abdominal tenderness and hepatosplenomegaly. Late effects include progressive fibrosis of the liver and secondary portal hypertension. Infection with *S. japonicum* has been associated with cancer of the bowel. Ectopic lesions occasionally occur in the skin, brain, spinal cord and other sites. Pulmonary arteritis may lead to cor pulmonale in severe long-standing schistosomiasis.

Table 5.3 A classification of the course of Bilharziasis—based on para-sitological, clinical and pathological aspects

Stage	Parasitological	Clinical	Pathological
Stage of invasion	Migration and beginning of maturation	Incubation period, including cercarial dermatitis, if present	Slight inflammatory reactions in skin, lungs and liver
Stage of maturation	Completion of maturation and early oviposition	Toxaemic stage of the disease (or acute febrile stage) not always recognised or present	Allergic reactions, generalised and local to products of eggs and/or young schistosomes
Stage of established infection	Intensive oviposition accompanied by a corresponding egg discharge	Stage of early chronic disease, characterised for instance by haematuria, or intestinal and other digestive manifestations possibly with cardiopulmonary or other complications	Local inflammatory reactions due to ova, resulting mainly in granuloma formation. Fibrosis is not a predominant feature
Stage of late effects	Prolonged infection (usually with reduced or discontinued egg extrusion)	Stage of late chronic disease, due to irreversible effects, and/or sequelae or complications	Progressing formation of fibrous tissue, with its consequences according to the organs involved intensity of infection and possibly other factors

Medical geography

It has been estimated that a total of about 200 million persons are affected in various parts of the world.

S. *haematobium* occurs in many parts of Africa, North, West, Central and East Africa, parts of the Middle East and a few foci in Southern Europe (Portugal).

S. *mansoni* is found in the Nile delta, West, East and Central Africa, South America and the Caribbean.

S. *japonicum* occurs in China, Japan, the Philippines and other foci in the Far East.

Parasitology

These worms are trematodes with the peculiar morphological feature in that the body of the male is folded to form a gynaecophoric canal in which the female is carried. The adult worms are found in the veins; *S. haematobium* are predominantly in the vesical plexus, *S. mansoni* in the inferior mesenteric veins and *S. japonicum* predominantly in the superior mesenteric veins.

Other schistosomes which infect man include *S. bovis, S. mattheei,* and *S. intercalatum.*

Life Cycle of the Schistosomes

The female lays eggs which pass through the bladder or bowel into urine and faeces respectively. A proportion of eggs are retained in the tissues and some are carried to the liver, lungs and other organs. If an excreted egg lands in water, it hatches and produces a free living form, the miracidium, which swims about with the aid of its cilia. It next invades an intermediate host, a snail of the appropriate species. Within the snail it undergoes a process of asexual multiplication, passing through intermediate stages to become the mature cercaria. The cercaria, which is the infective larval stage for man, emerges from the snail and swims being propelled by its forked tail. On contact with man, the cercaria penetrates the skin, sheds its tail and becomes a schistosomule. The latter migrates to the usual site for mature adults of the species.

Intermediate hosts

All the intermediate hosts of schistosomes are snails belonging to the Gastropoda class in the orders Pulmonata and Prosobronchiata. Various species of *Bulinus* snails are the vectors of *S. haematobium,* whilst *Planorbid* snails, species of *Biomphallaria,* are the intermediate hosts of *S. mansoni.* Both *Bulinus* and *Biomphallaria* are aquatic snails which breed in ponds, lakes, streams, marshes, swamps, drains, dams, and irrigation canals. *Oncomelania* species, the intermediate host of *S. japonicum,* are amphibious snails, living in moist vegetation. These snail hosts are affected by physical factors such as temeprature; and by chemical factors, pH and oxygen tension. The snails are hermaphrodite but not self fertilising; they lay eggs usually on vegetation; these hatch and grow to mature adult forms.

During the dry season, the aquatic snails aestivate in the drying mud, with the openings on the shells covered with dried mucus. Although snails with immature infections may survive the dry season, those with mature infections usually die. *Oncomelania,* being an operculated snail, survives drying much better than the non-operculated snails.

Laboratory diagnosis

Parasitological and immunological methods are used in the diagnosis of schistosomiasis. Eggs of *S. haematobium* are usually found in urine and occasionally in faeces. The optimal time for urine collection is around midday. For a quantitative assessment of the load of infection, a 24-hour collection of urine can be examined, or timed collection around midday (e.g. 11 a.m. to 1 p.m.) when egg count is highest, may be used. For *S. mansoni* and *S. japonicum* infection, examination of faeces may reveal the eggs; concentration techniques may be required for light infections; quantitative techniques are available and are useful in determining both pathogenicity as well as the effects of intervention. Eggs of *S. mansoni* are occasionally found in urine. Rectal biopsy ('rectal snip') is useful in diagnosing infections, particularly those due to *S. mansoni* and *S. japonicum* but it is also positive in some cases of *S. haematobium*; the specimen is easily obtained by curetting the superficial layers of the rectal mucosa and examining the material fresh between two glass slides; it can later be fixed and stained.

Other diagnostic techniques include cystoscopy, pyelography, liver biopsy, biochemical tests of hepatic and renal function. These are mainly used for the detailed assessment of individual patients but some have been adapted for field survey.

Immunological tests include a skin test in which antigen is injected intradermally and the size of the test weal from the antigen is compared with a control.

A variety of serological tests, e.g. circumoval precipitin (COP), Cercariahüllen, fluorescent antibody tests (ELISA) are used for the diagnosis of schistosomiasis; the tests are group specific and so cannot identify the particular infecting species. Some of the tests (e.g. COP) become negative after treatment or spontaneous cure, but others, e.g. the skin test, remain positive for indefinitely long periods. False positive results may occur in persons who have been exposed to avian and other non-human schistosomes.

Epidemiology

Man is the main reservoir of *S. haematobium* but naturally acquired infection with *S. mansoni* has been found in various animals including primates. *S. japonicum* is widely distributed in various mammals—cats, dogs, cattle, pigs and rats—and they constitute a significant part of the reservoir. Other schistosomes, e.g. *S. bovis* and *S. intercalatum*, are basically infections of animals with occasional infection in man.

Man acquires the infection by wading, swimming, bathing or washing clothes and utensils in the polluted streams. Certain occupational groups, e.g. farmers and fishermen, may be exposed to a high risk.

The age and sex distribution of schistosomiasis varies from area to area. One fairly common pattern is of high prevalence rates of active infection in children, who excrete relatively large quantities of eggs, and a lower prevalence rate of active infection among adults; the latter show late manifestations and sequelae. Epidemiological studies indicate that the load of infection is an important factor in determining the severity of pathological lesions and clinical manifestations. Epidemiological evidence also suggests that some degree of immunity to all schistosomal infections occurs in man. Considerable interest exists in mathematical models of schistosome transmission and their relevance to control strategy.

MAN-MADE WATER RESOURCES   In the past decade water resource development programmes were undertaken in endemic areas of the world, and during this period an increase has been observed in the transmission of schistosomiasis in the areas around man-made lakes and irrigation schemes. Real economic returns could well be seriously jeopardised unless provision for human welfare is made at the planning stage.

Control

The control of schistosomiasis depends on a profound understanding of the epidemiology of the disease complex, and in particular of the biology, ecology, and distribution of the parasites, their snail intermediate hosts and mammalian reservoir hosts. A sound knowledge of the role of man and his behaviour in maintaining the infection is crucial. Moreover, the ultimate success of any control programme is dependent upon a full understanding of the local socio-economic conditions and upon the appreciation by the health authorities as well as by the community of the benefits of the proposed measures.

There are six basic approaches to the control of schistosomiasis:
(a) *Elimination of the reservoir*
(b) *Avoidance of pollution of surface water*
(c) *Elimination of the vector*
(d) *Prevention of human contact with infected water*
(e) *Health education*
(f) *Community participation*

(a) *Elimination of the reservoir*
The use of *chemotherapy* in control requires a clear definition of aims, selection of the appropriate chemotherapeutic agent, and decisions on the dosage and frequency of administration to be followed as well as on the organization of the delivery system.

While other means of schistosome control merely reduce transmission without any direct effects on human worm load, chemotherapy reduces the output of live eggs from the patient's body and, in doing so, diminishes transmission. Moreover by killing worms in the treated individual it not only reduces the risk of morbidity and mortality due to the disease, but also enables the patient to recover from reversible lesions. It is important to distinguish between these two beneficial effects. The second benefits only those who are treated, while the first helps the whole community. Even when the reduction in transmission is incomplete, the fall in disease risk may still be considerable. Chemotherapy is thus a tool for both primary and secondary control of schistosomiasis.

The object of primary control is clearly to end egg output, especially in those most likely to pollute transmission sites. In situations where egg output cannot be reduced to zero, it is not known at what level persisting egg excretion ceases to be a public health problem. Some epidemiological models suggest that egg production is so great relative to what is needed for continued transmission that even a small residual percentage of egg output will be sufficient to maintain transmission at a considerable level; however, data are not yet available to test this hypothesis. Nor is it possible to say whether a few people with high egg excretion rates are epidemiologically more or less of a problem than a large number of people with a low egg output. It follows that the goal of primary control should be to reduce the egg output of as large a part of the population as possible to as near zero as can be obtained within the constraints of drug toxicity, cost, and possible effects on immunity.

The severity of schistosomiasis increases with rising egg output and intensity of infection. An appreciable proportion of patients with low egg excretion rates also show severe lesions, though it is not clear whether these lesions are due to a previous heavy infection or greater susceptibility to pathological consequences. It is therefore desirable to treat *all* infected individuals to achieve maximum secondary control—selective population chemotherapy—; in situations where there are operational constraints priority must be given to the heavily infected or to other high-risk groups such as schoolchildren—targeted population chemotherapy.

The drugs available for the control of schistosomiasis are metrifonate, oxamniquine and praziquantel.

With the exception of metrifonate, the antischistosomal drugs are expensive in relation to the health budgets of many developing countries. Both the drug costs and the expenses of administering a multiple-dose regime may be reduced by shortening the course of treatment or decreasing the dose. The consequences of such reductions in parasitological terms must be assessed for each proposed regimen.

It is clear that the lower toxicity and simpler dosage regimens of the drugs now available will enable chemotherapy to play an increasing part in control programmes. Already over one million persons have been treated for *S. mansoni* infection in the Brazilian control programme, while hundreds of thousands have received metrifonate in the Egyptian *S. haematobium* control measures.

When the prevalence is high in a community and mass treatment is required, two main approaches are possible. In one, the whole population is examined and those found infected are treated. In this case the treatment is on an individual risk basis and the efficiency and cost of the examination will have to be considered before opting for this approach. In the alternative approach, high-risk groups with high prevalence of infection are identified and treatment is given to all members of those groups regardless of whether each individual is infected or not. This may be called a group risk approach.

Several factors must be considered in deciding between the two approaches. The safety of the treatment is the overriding consideration, since it is not wise to give a hazardous drug to an uninfected person. However, in economic terms, the cost of identifying infected persons must be balanced against the cost of chemotherapy given unnecessarily and this has to be worked out individually for each programme. Both these costs will rise as prevalence falls. For some drugs the cost is relatively low compared with that of case detection; but, since the drugs have to be imported into most endemic areas, the use of shadow pricing, in which such items as foreign exchange and local labour are differentially weighed, may alter this balance.

Most schistosomiasis control programmes use diagnosis based on the examination of excreta and apply treatment on the basis of individual risk. This is true, for example, of the large Egyptian programme, which uses an inexpensive drug distributed through the national primary health care facilities. However, in the extensive Brazilian programme, treatment of the whole community is undertaken at defined prevalences of *S. mansoni*.

(b) *Avoidance of pollution of surface water*
This can be achieved by providing suitable sanitary facilities for the disposal of excreta and teaching people how to use them appropriately. It is important for the programme to include children since they usually have relatively high outputs of viable eggs. Unless the programme is highly successful, little benefit will be derived from these measures because infected communities usually produce many more eggs than are required to maintain infection in the snails.

(c) *Elimination of the vector*
Physical alteration of the habitat, e.g. drainage of swamps, may solve the problem by eliminating the breeding sites of the snails. Where such radical cure is not feasible, the situation can be improved by rendering the environment hostile to the snails, e.g. removal of aquatic vegetation, altering the flow rate of the streams, or building concrete linings to the walls of the drains.

Chemical measures are very useful now that more effective and safer molluscicides have been devised. The older chemicals, copper sulphate and sodium pentachlorophenate are being replaced by niclosamide ('Bayluscide') and N-trityl morpholine ('Frescon'); the latter two are safer and more effective. Molluscicides must be applied under the direction of those who have expert knowledge and experience to assure effective action against the snails and minimal risk to man and other living things. For the amphibian snail vectors of *S. japonicum*, calcium cyanamide or yuramin are very effective molluscicides. Endod (*Phytolacca dodecandra*) remains the most thoroughly studied example of a molluscicide of plant origin. Molluscicides can be applied locally or area-wide depending on specific situations.

Biological control has been attempted by the use of predatory fishes, e.g. *Astatoreochronics albiacide*. The most successful biological method has been through the use of the *Marissa cornuarietis* snail which feeds voraciously, thereby competing with *Biomphallaria glabrata*, and also it consumes their egg masses and their young. Great care needs to be applied in the use of this method lest the predator becomes a more serious menace.

(d) *Prevention of human contact with infected water*
This requires the provision of alternative supplies of safe water, thereby eliminating the risk of exposure to infected streams coupled with health education. Where contact with such waters is unavoidable, protective clothing such as rubber boots should be worn; this may prove impractical for peasant farmers or subsistence fishermen.

(e) *Health education*
Human attitudes towards water and waterborne disease transmission frequently need to be modified, particularly in areas with endemic schistosomiasis.

Health education should be the responsibility of all health workers and should be based on a clear understanding of the people's perception of disease and its relation to the environment. Efforts should be directed towards those groups that are at greatest risk and most involved in transmission—usually young children. It is recommended that, whenever possible, efforts be positive rather than negative in orientation. In other words, it is better to encourage children to refrain from initially polluting water sources than to try to prevent water contact. Infection is likely to be associated with certain types of water-contact behaviour which will vary in different transmission situations. If a link is established between specific activities and schistosomiasis transmission, then these activities should be discouraged.

An effective health education programme should promote active community participation. Such participation may range from a community installing its own water supply to a community simply cooperating with the health authorities in reducing contact with unsafe water bodies.

(f) *Community participation*
Community participation must be considered as an essential element of any schistosomiasis control programme.

National interest should be promoted once the schistosomiasis problem is considered to be a serious public health problem. Governments or communities implementing schistosomiasis control programmes have the responsibility of organising national or local efforts through mechanisms acceptable to the communities concerned.

Recognition of the problem by the local population and its awareness of the risks and possible consequences of infection must be the basis of its cooperation. To this end, the advice should be prepared in a clear, simple and convincing form, and presented in the most suitable style. Simple, inexpensive, and appropriate technology must be carefully selected and transmitted to those members of the community most involved in schistosomiasis control.

Community participation must be organised as an integral part of basic health care activities and the primary health workers must be prepared to assume their responsibilities at the local level.

Schistosomiasis—Summary

1 *Distribution*—*S. haematobium*—tropical Africa, Middle East
    S. mansoni—tropical Africa and South America
    S. japonicum—China, Japan and other areas in Far East
2 *Organisms*—*S. haematobium, S. mansoni* and *S. japonicum*; also animal schistosomes including *S. mattheei, S. bovis*, and *S. intercalatum*
3 *Reservoir of infection*—*S. haematobium*—man. *S. mansoni*—man, some primates and rodents, *S. japonicum*—man, various domestic and wild animals.

LEPTOSPIROSIS

This is an acute febrile illness usually accompanied by malaise, vomiting, conjunctival injection and meningeal irritation; in severe cases, jaundice, renal involvement and haemorrhage may occur. The *incubation period* is from 3 days to 3 weeks.

Medical geography
Various pathogenic species of leptospira are present in most parts of the world. The occurrence of human disease is determined by the distribution of the organisms in animal reservoirs.

Bacteriology
Leptospira are thin spirochaetal organisms, which can remain viable in water for several weeks. Many different serotypes have been identified, some of the common ones being *Leptospira icterohaemorrhagica* (the agent of Weil's disease), *L. canicola* (canicola fever), *L. pomona*, and *L. bovis*

Laboratory diagnosis
The organisms may be seen on microscopy of blood or centrifuged specimen of urine using dark ground illumination, or of a thick blood film stained with Giesma's technique. The organism can be isolated on culture or by inoculation of blood intraperitoneally into hamsters or

guinea-pigs. The serotype is identified by serological tests. Agglutinating and complement fixing antibodies can be detected in infected patients.

Epidemiology
The reservoir of infection is in various vertebrates; both wild and domestic animals are involved—cattle, dogs, pigs, rats and other rodents, and reptiles. Urine is the source of infection.

The infection may be acquired by contact with infected water, the organism penetrating the skin, or by ingestion of contaminated water or food. Certain occupations carry the risk of exposure to leptospirosis, e.g. fish workers, persons working in sewers, rice paddies, or other collections of surface water, and soldiers who may have to wade across streams.

Control

Domestic animals should be segregated as far as possible from water sources for human use. The reservoir in wild animals should also be eliminated, e.g. by the control of rodents.

Human contact with potentially contaminated water should be avoided, and where such contact is unavoidable protective clothing be worn.

Immunisation for persons at high risk has been suggested using the local strain of leptospira as antigen; similarly pet dogs can be vaccinated.

Leptospirosis—Summary

1 *Distribution*—World-wide
2 *Organisms*—Leptospira species—various serotypes
3 *Reservoir of infection*—Domestic and wild animals
4 *Transmission*—Contact with polluted water—ingestion
5 *Control*— (i) Limit animal contact with human sources of water
          (ii) Avoid contact with contaminated water
          (iii) Immunisation

RABIES

Rabies is a viral infection which produces fatal encephalitis in man. The clinical features include convulsions, dysphagia, nervousness and anxiety, muscular paralysis and a progressive coma. The painful spasms of the throat muscles make the patient apprehensive of swallowing fluids, even his own saliva ('hydrophobia'). Once clinical signs are established the infection is invariably fatal.

The *incubation period* is usually 4 to 6 weeks but it may be much longer, 6 months or more.

Medical geography

The infection is endemic in most parts of the world with the exception of Great Britain, Australia, New Zealand, Scandinavia, areas of the West Indies and the Pacific Islands. The disease is most commonly encountered in parts of South-East Asia, Africa and Europe. There has recently been a dramatic spread of animal rabies in Europe, foxes being the main reservoir of infection.

Virology

The causative agent is a myxovirus which can be isolated and propagated in chick embryo or tissue culture from mouse and chick-embryos. The freshly isolated virus ('street virus') in experimental infections has a long incubation period (1 to 12 weeks) and it invades both the central nervous system and the salivary glands. After serial passage in rabbit brain, the virus ('fixed virus') multiplies rapidly solely in brain with a short incubation period of four to six days after experimental inoculation.

Epidemiology

Rabies is basically a zoonotic infection of mammals, especially the wild carnivores in the forest (foxes, wolves, jackals). The urban reservoir includes stray and pet dogs, cats and other domestic mammals, and in a part of South America, vampire bats play an important role in spreading infection to fruit bats, cattle, and other animals including man.

The transmission of the infection is by the bite of the infected animal, the virus being present in the saliva. It can also presumably be transmitted by the infected animal licking open sores and wounds. Airborne infection has been demonstrated in some special circumstances, notably in caves heavily populated by bats.

Rabies in Animals

With the exception of the vampire bat which tolerates chronic rabies infection with little disturbance, other mammals rapidly succumb to this infection once clinical signs develop. At first, there may be a change in the behaviour of the animal: restlessness, excitability, unusual aggressiveness or friendliness. Later, there are signs of difficulty in swallowing fluids and food. Paralysis of the lower jaw gives the 'dropped jaw' appearance in dogs. Finally the animal may become comatose and paralysed ('dumb rabies') but even at the terminal stage running around, attacking indiscriminately ('furious rabies').

Laboratory diagnosis

Various laboratory tests are used to establish the diagnosis in suspected animals or in human cases. The rabies virus may be demonstrated in the brain tissue, saliva, spinal fluid and urine, but brain tissue is most commonly examined. Microscopic examination of the brain may show characteristic cytoplasmic inclusion bodies (Negri bodies) in the nerve cells especially those of the hippocampal gyrus. These may be demonstrated on microscopic sections of the brain or by staining smear impressions from fresh brain tissue. The organism can be demonstrated by inoculation of suspected material into mice (intracerebral) or into hamsters (intramuscular), infection being identified by the presence of Negri bodies in the brains of the animals which die, by the fluorescent antibody technique or by neutralisation tests using specific antibody.

Control

In urban areas, the problem is best tackled by the control of dogs and also the appropriate management of cases of dog bite; stray dogs should be impounded and destroyed if unclaimed. Pet dogs, and preferably also cats, should be vaccinated every 3 years. In rabies-free areas, the importing of dogs, cats and other mammalian pets should be strictly controlled, such animals being kept in quarantine for at least 6 months. Whenever a dog is found to be rabid, other animals that have been exposed to it should be traced so that they can be vaccinated, kept under observation or destroyed. The control of rabies in wildlife is much more difficult. The risk can be minimised by trapping and killing wild animals which serve as reservoir of rabies.

Post-exposure Treatment

(1) *Local treatment*
The wound should be cleaned thoroughly with soap or detergent; an antiseptic such as chlorine bleach should be applied.

(2) *Artificial immunisation*
Rabies can be prevented in persons who have been exposed to risk by the use of active immunisation alone or in combination with passive immunisation. The decision to use active immunisation should be based on a careful consideration of the risk in each case.

Broad guidelines are provided in Table 5.4, but three points need to be carefully considered:
(a) PREVALENCE OF RABIES IN THE AREA   Vaccine may not be indicated in areas which are consistently free of animal rabies.
(b) BITING ANIMAL: ITS SPECIES AND STATE OF HEALTH   Carnivores are particularly important in the spread of rabies.

In the case of a dog bite, the animal should be captured alive if possible, and kept under observation for 10 days. If the animal has been killed or if it dies during the period of observation, steps should be taken to find out if it was rabid; the animal should be decapitated and the head sent to the laboratory. In the case of a wild animal, it should be killed and the brain examined for rabies.

It must be assumed that there has been exposure to rabies in cases of unprovoked bites by wild animals, or if the biting animal has escaped or

Table 5.4 Post-exposure treatment for the prevention of rabies

| Biting Animal | | Treatment — Type of exposure | | |
Species	Status at time of exposure	None	Mild	Severe
Domestic: Dog Cat	Healthy	None	None Begin vaccine at first sign of rabies in biting animal	RIG or ARS Begin vaccine at first sign of rabies in biting animal
	Signs suggestive of rabies	None	Rabies vaccine Stop treatment if animal is normal on fifth day after exposure	RIG or ARS plus rabies vaccine Stop treatment if animal is normal 5 days after exposure
	Rabid	None	Rabies vaccine	RIG or ARS plus rabies vaccine
	Escaped, killed Unknown	None	Rabies vaccine	RIG or ARS plus rabies vaccine
Wild Animal	Regard as rabid if unprovoked attack	None	RIG or ARS plus rabies vaccine	RIG or ARS plus rabies vaccine

Abbreviations: Rabies immunoglobulin, human (RIG)
Antirabies serum, equine (ARS)
Human diploid cell rabies vaccine (HDCV) } Rabies vaccine
Duck embryo vaccine (DEV)

been destroyed without examination. A dog which has been adequately vaccinated is unlikely to be rabid.

(c) THE SITE AND EXTENT OF THE BITE *Severe exposure.* This includes cases of multiple or deep puncture wounds; bites on the head, neck, face, hands or fingers. After such a severe exposure, the incubation period tends to be very short.

Mild exposure. Single bites, scratches and lacerations away from the dangerous areas listed under severe exposure; also the licking of open wounds.

Vaccines

For post exposure treatment there are 3 types of rabies vaccine:

(1) *Human diploid cell rabies vaccine* (HDCV—the vaccine of choice). This is a freeze-dried suspension of rabies virus prepared in human diploid cell cultures and inactivated by beta-propriolactone or tri-n-butyl phosphate. 1 ml of vaccine is given intramuscularly on day 0, 3, 7, 14, 28 and 90.

(2) *The duck-embryo vaccine* (DEV)

(3) *Semple type rabbit brain vaccine*

Passive Immunisation

RIG (or ARS if RIG is not available) is given only once at the beginning of antirabies prophylaxis, to provide antibodies until the patient responds to vaccination. The recommended dose of RIG is 20 IU/kg, that of ARS is 40 IU/kg. RIG is the product of choice when available because it rarely causes adverse reactions.

Pre-exposure Treatment

Certain persons such as veterinarians, dog catchers and hunters who run a high risk of rabies can be protected by using HDCV. Three 1 ml injections are given intramuscularly on days 0, 7 and 21. DEV, e.g. two doses of 1.0 ml given subcutaneously 1 month apart, followed by a booster dose 6–7 months later is also effective if HDCV is not available.

Rabies—Summary

1 *Occurrence*—Endemic in most parts of the world except Great Britain, Australia, New Zealand, Scandinavia and parts of the West Indies and the Pacific Islands

2 *Organism*—Rabies virus

3 *Reservoir of infection*—Wild animals, strays and pets

4 *Modes of transmission*—Bite of infected animals. Airborne in restricted circumstances

5 *Control*— (i) Immunisation of pet dogs and control of stray dogs

    (ii) Passive and active immunisation after exposure

    (iii) Prophylactic immunisation of high-risk groups

ANTHRAX

This is an acute infection which may present as a localised necrotic lesion of the skin (malignant pustule) with regional lymphadenopathy; further dissemination will cause septicaemia. Pulmonary and gastro-intestinal forms of infection occur from inhalation or ingestion respectively of the infected material.

The *incubation period* is usually less than 1 week.

Medical geography

The infection is endemic in most agricultural areas both tropical and temperate.

Bacteriology

The causative agent, *Bacillus anthracis*, is an aerobic spore-bearing organism. The resistant spore survives drying, routine disinfection and other adverse environmental conditions; it remains viable for long periods on hides, skins and hairs.

Epidemiology

Anthrax is a zoonosis, the reservoir of infection being farm animals, cattle, sheep, goats horses and pigs. The animal products such as hides, skins and hair (e.g. brushes) are potential sources of infection.

Transmission may be by contact with these infected materials or animals. The organism may also be inhaled (wool sorter's disease) or swallowed, for example in contaminated milk.

Laboratory diagnosis

A smear of the skin lesion may show typical organisms as chains of large, Gram-positive rods. The organism can be isolated from skin, sputum or blood, by culture on blood agar. Virulence is tested by intraperitoneal injection into mice.

Control

Sick animals should be isolated. The carcasses of animals which die should be burnt or buried in lime, avoiding any contamination of soil. Animals and human beings at high risk can be immunised using a live attenuated vaccine. Animal products such as hides, bone meal, and brushes, should be disinfected usually by autoclaving where feasible. Protective clothing especially gloves should be worn when handling potentially infected material.

Anthrax—Summary

1 *Distribution*—Widespread in agricultural areas
2 *Organism*—Bacillus anthracis
3 *Reservoir of infection*—Farm animals
4 *Modes of transmission*—Contact with infected animals or their products. Inhalation. Ingestion

5 *Control*— (i) Isolation of sick animals
           (ii) Careful disposal of infected carcasses
           (iii) Disinfection of hides, skins and hairs
           (iv) Protective clothing, e.g. gloves

VIRAL HAEMORRHAGIC FEVERS

There are several viral haemorrhagic fevers that infect man, namely, (1) smallpox, (2) chikungunya fever, (3) dengue fever, (4) Rift Valley fever, (5) yellow fever, (6) Crimean haemorrhagic fever, (7) Kyasanur Forest disease, (8) Omsk haemorrhagic fever, (9) Argentinian haemorrhagic fever (Junin virus), (10) Bolivian haemorrhagic fever (Machupo virus), (11) Lassa fever, (12) Marburg virus disease, and (13) Ebola virus disease. Some of these are dealt with elsewhere in the book.

In this section we shall deal with three that have been recently discovered namely—*Lassa fever*; *Marburg virus disease*; and *Ebola virus disease*. The epidemiology of these diseases is far from clear but for transmission all seem to require intimate exposure to the patient or exposure to his or her blood or other bodily secretions.

LASSA FEVER

Lassa fever is an acute febrile disease caused by a virus belonging to the arenavirus group. Since it was first described in 1969, outbreaks of varying size and severity have occurred in Nigeria, Liberia and Sierra Leone. Lassa virus has been isolated from blood, pharyngeal secretions and urine.

The multimammate rat, *Mastomys natalensis*, is the possible reservoir host of Lassa fever. Once it has been successfully transmitted from its natural reservoir host to man, it is capable of adaptation to man-to-man transmission. No seasonal, yearly, sex or age pattern has been seen. The case fatality ratio in hospitalised cases is around 12%. Subclinical infections are, however, quite frequent and in some locations in Sierra Leone as many as 40% of the population had antibody to Lassa fever virus. Lassa fever does not appear to be a highly communicable disease. Airborne spread, mechanical transmission and accidental inoculation occur.

Control

Patients suspected of Lassa fever should be isolated. Collection of specimens must be done wearing a mask and protective clothing. High risk contacts should be identified and kept under active surveillance. Strict barrier nursing procedures must be observed.

MARBURG VIRUS DISEASE

The first documented outbreak of Marburg virus disease occurred in 1967 in Marburg, West Germany and Belgrade, Yugoslavia. Contact with the blood, organs and cell cultures of imported African green monkeys was responsible for the epidemic. A total of 31 people were affected and seven died; all secondary cases survived. The disease appeared again in a young Australian man who was admitted to a Johannesburg hospital in February 1975 after having toured Rhodesia and Zambia. His female travelling companion and one female attendant nurse were also infected. The index case died, the other two survived. Although in the 1967 epidemic the immediate source of infection was the African green monkey no reservoir-host-vector chain has yet been identified.

The incubation period is estimated to be between three and nine days. Two cases were reported from Kenya in 1980.

Control

This is as for Lassa fever above.

EBOLA VIRUS DISEASE

Two outbreaks of Ebola haemorrhagic fever occurred in the Southern Sudan and in Zaire in 1976. One of the outbreaks in the Sudan appeared to have originated in the workers of a cotton factory while the other was hospital based. A second epidemic occurred in the Southern Sudan in 1979.

Transmission of the disease requires close contact with an acute case such as the act of nursing a patient. The incubation period is 7–14 days. The fatality rate is high between 30–50 %, but subclinical infections do occur; thus 11 % of case contacts, in hospital and in the local community, had antibodies to Ebola virus. No animal reservoir has yet been identified, and the cycle of transmission is not known.

Control

This is as for Lassa fever.

FURTHER READING

WHO Public Health Papers, No. 65: *Social and Health Aspects of Sexually Transmitted Diseases.*

WHO Tech. Rep. Ser. No. 607: *Expert Committee on Leprosy.*

WHO Tech. Rep. Ser. No. 675: *Chemotherapy of Leprosy for Control Programmes.*

CHAPTER 6

ARTHROPOD-BORNE INFECTIONS

Arthropods play an important, and in some cases a determinant role, in the transmission of some infections. The epidemiology of these infections is closely related to the ecology of the arthropod vector, and hence the most effective measures for the control of these infections often relate to the control of the vector. The arthropod vector introduces a further dimension to the complex host-parasite interrelationship, and for some of these infections, a fourth factor is added when there is a non-vertebrate animal reservoir.

THE INFECTIVE AGENTS

These include a wide variety of organisms ranging from viruses to helminths. The viral infections are known under the collective term 'arbo viruses', a contraction of 'arthropod-borne viruses'. These arboviruses cause a variety of clinical syndromes:
  (i) Fever
 (ii) Aseptic meningitis
(iii) Encephalitis
 (iv) Haemorrhagic fever.

Vector-parasite Relationship

The vector may be specifically involved in the biological transmission of the infective agent, in which case, this is an essential phase in the life cycle of the agent. The phase within the vector which is often referred to as the *extrinsic incubation period* may involve (a) *morphological development* of the agent without multiplication, e.g. filiarial worms, (b) *Asexual multiplication*, e.g. arboviruses, plague, (c) *Sexual multiplication*, e.g. malaria. The extrinsic incubation period is important epidemiologically for only after its completion is the infection transmissible. Usually, the arthropod acquires the infection from an infected host but in a few specific instances the vector may acquire the infection congenitally by transovarian passage, e.g. mites in scrub typhus.

The vector may bring about a simple mechanical transfer of the agent from the source to the susceptible host. The housefly and other filth flies are important mechanical vectors of various infections especially gastro-intestinal infections, e.g. shigellosis, which rely on the faeco-oral route of transmission, and are dealt with in Chapter 4.

Mode of Transmission

In the case of mechanical transfer of infections, the vector may carry the infective agent on its body or limbs, or the infective agents may be ingested by the vector passing through its body unmodified and excreted in faeces.

In most cases, biological transmission takes place when the vector bites the host. In this process, the vector may acquire the infective agents from the blood or skin tissues of the infected host or, alternatively, the infected vector may inoculate the infective agents from its salivary secretions into a new host, e.g. malaria.

In other cases, the host becomes infected through contamination of his mucous membranes or skin by the infective faeces of the vector, e.g. Chagas' disease; or by the infective tissue fluids which are released when the vector is crushed, e.g. louse-borne relapsing fever. The host may acquire infection by ingesting the vector; the transmission of guinea-worm occurs by this unusual route, when man ingests the infected cyclops, the crustacean intermediate host of this worm (see p. 82).

Host Factors

Many of the arthropod vectors which bite mammals show marked host preferences. Some of them bite man preferentially, and these are said to be *anthropophilic*; whereas others which bite animals preferentially are *zoophilic*. There is some evidence that mosquitoes are attracted to and bite some persons more often than others, but the basis for this preference is not as yet clearly understood.

Acquired immunity plays an important role in the epidemiology of some of the arthropod-borne infections. For example, previous exposure to the yellow fever virus may confer lifelong immunity; some protection from yellow fever may also be derived from exposure to related viruses of the B group. In other cases, immunity is of short duration and is not absolute, e.g. plague.

Control of Arthropod Infections

1 Infective Agent

(a) Destruction of animal reservoir, e.g. rats in the control of plague.
(b) Isolation and treatment of infected persons, e.g. yellow fever patient is nursed in a mosquito-proof room or bed.

2 Route of Transmission

(a) *Control of vectors*
Preventing the vector from coming into contact with the human host.
 (i) *Biological barriers*, e.g. clearing an area to free it of breeding and

resting places for the vectors; siting houses away from known breeding places of mosquitoes.

(ii) *Mechanical barriers*, e.g. protective clothing, screening of houses, mosquito nets.

(b) *Destruction of the vectors*

(i) *Trapping, collection and destruction of the vectors.* Various mechanical devices are in use, e.g. sticky strips to which flies adhere.

(ii) *Chemical insecticides.* Some of these are active against the larval aquatic forms, others are directed against the adult vectors.

(iii) *Biological methods.* These include the alteration of the physical constitution of the environment, and alteration of the flora and fauna.

Alteration of physical environment includes such things as the drainage of ponds, drying up of lakes and alteration in speed and course of a river. Alteration of the fauna may affect the food supply and shelter of the vector, e.g. by driving away the 'big game' from an area, there is a reduction in the food supply of *Glossina morsitans*, the vector of *Trypanosoma rhodesiense*. Alteration in the predator or parasite fauna may also affect the vector.

Table 6.1 Some examples of arthropod-borne infections

Viruses	Rickettsiae	Bacteria	Protozoa	Helminths
Arthropod-borne (ARBO-) viruses causing various diseases: (i) Fever (ii) Aseptic meningitis (iii) Encephalitis (iv) Haemorrhagic fever	*R. prowazekii* var. *prowazekii* (louse-borne typhus) *R. mooseri* (murine typhus) *R. tsutsugamushi* (scrub typhus) *R. rickettsii* (tick-borne typhus) *Coxiella burnetii*	*Yersinia pestis* (Bubonic plague) *Borrelia recurrentis* *Bartonella bacilliformis*	Malaria *Trypanosoma gambiense* *T. rhodesiense* *T. cruzi* *Leishmania donovani* *L. tropica* *L. mexicana* *L. braziliensis*	*Wuchereria bancrofti* *Brugia malayi* *Onchocerca volvulus* *Dipetalonema perstans* *D. streptocerca* *Mansonella ozzardi* *Loa loa*

Alterations in the flora may also affect food supply and shelter for the vector, as for example the clearance of low-level foliage to control *Glossina tachinoides* or the clearance of the water lily, *Pistia*, in the control of mansonia larvae and pupae.

3 Host

Immunisation with an attenuated live virus gives protection against yellow fever, but specific immunisation is not generally available against other arboviruses. The use of specific chemoprophylaxis in the control of malaria and other arthropod borne infections is described in the section dealing with each infection.

THE ARBOVIRUSES

The arthropod-borne viruses (arboviruses) may cause various syndromes in man or, alternatively, may present as atypical or subclinical infections only recognisable by antibody studies. The majority are zoonoses, and about 70 out of the 200 different arboviruses identified are known to cause disease in man. The definitive diagnosis depends upon isolation of the virus from patients early in the infection, with demonstration of a rise in titre of antibodies to the particular agent in at least two sera taken during the acute and convalescent stages of the disease.

Three main groups of arboviruses have been serologically defined as groups A (alphaviruses), B (flaviviruses) and C (bunyaviruses), and the important viruses within these groups are listed in Table 6.2. The majority produce non-fatal infections. Control of the vector population where practicable will reduce the risk of infection. Steps can also be taken to avoid being bitten by vectors.

A number of arthropod-borne viruses infecting man, including sandfly fever and Colorado tick fever, do not fit into any of the groups so far described, which is indicative that other groups exist. Colorado tick fever is found in the United States, where small rodents are believed to be the normal hosts. Man, in whom it causes acute illness, becomes infected as the result of being bitten by the vector tick *Dermacentor andersoni*.

Because infection usually produces prolonged immunity, attack rates in all age-groups indicate the introduction of a new arbovirus, while disease confined to children implies reintroduction of virus or overflow from a continuous animal cycle to susceptible humans. Mosquitoes are the most common vectors of arboviruses, ticks the next most common, and *Phlebotomus* and *Culicoides* the least frequently involved.

ARBOVIRUSES: GROUP A (Alphaviruses)

All the viruses in this group (about seventeen) have a number of general properties common to each other and to the rest of the arboviruses. The natural vectors or suspected vectors for all the known Group A viruses

Table 6.2 Some clinically recognised arboviruses in the tropics.

Group A Alphaviruses	Group B Flaviviruses	Group C Bunyaviruses	Other
Chikungunya	Yellow fever	Apeu	Bunyamwera group
Mayaro	Dengue	Caraparu	
O,Nyong-Nyong	St Louis encephalitis	Itaqui	Bwamba group
Venezuelian equine encephalitis	Japanese B encephalitis	Marituba	Phlebotomus fever
	Murray Valley encephalitis	Oriboca	
Western equine encephalitis		Ossa	Simbum group— Oporonche
Eastern equine encephalitis	West Nile		Vesicular stomatitis group
	Ilheus		
	Spondweni		Colorado tick fever
	Uganda S-H336		
	Wesselsbron		Rift Valley fever
	Tick-borne encephalitis		California encephalitis complex
	Kyasanur Forest disease		Nairobi sheep disease

are mosquitoes. Clinically recognisable diseases of man have been described for:
  (i) *Chikungunya virus* which occurs in Africa, Thailand, Cambodia and India
 (ii) *Mayaro virus* which is found in Trinidad, Brazil and Bolivia
(iii) *O'Nyong-Nyong virus* which produced an explosive epidemic disease in East Africa
 (iv) *Venezuelan equine encephalitis virus*. This is an apizootic of horses which affects man, and human outbreaks with fatalities have occurred in Venezuela, Colombia and Panama.

ARBOVIRUSES: GROUP B (Flaviviruses)

The diseases most important to man result from infections with arboviruses of this group, most of which have mosquitoes as their vectors, with the exception of a subgroup which are tick-borne.

Antigenic cross-reactivity is marked in the group B viruses, so that in areas where there is a high endemicity, e.g. tropical Africa, serological diagnosis may be difficult, and most rapid and definitive diagnostic method of active infection is by virus isolation. Many infections are symptomless. Clinically recognisable disease has been described for the following viruses in this group:

(i) *Murray Valley encephalitis virus* which occurs in Australia and New Guinea producing a high attack rate in children

(ii) *West Nile virus* has been isolated in Africa, the Near East and India; it produces a dengue-like syndrome

(iii) *Ilheus virus* is found in South and Central America and Trinidad

(iv) *Spodnweni, Uganda S-H336* and *Wesselsbron* viruses respectively occur in South Africa and Nigeria, Uganda and South Africa and in South Africa and Portuguese East Africa

The most important diseases are (1) Yellow fever, (2) Dengue fever, (3) Japanese B encephalitis, (4) Kyasanur Forest disease.

Diseases caused by Group B Arboviruses (Flaviviruses)

1 Yellow Fever

Yellow fever is an acute infectious disease of sudden onset and variable severity caused by a virus transmitted by mosquitoes. It is characterised by fever, jaundice, haemorrhagic manifestations and albuminuria. The *incubation period* in man is 3–6 days.

Medical geography

Yellow fever is endemic in large areas of South America and tropical Africa. The endemic zone in Africa approximately covers that part of the continent which lies between latitudes 15°N and 10°S. In South America the endemic zone stretches from south of Honduras to the southern border of Bolivia and includes the western two-thirds of Brazil, Venezuela, Colombia, and those parts of Peru and Ecuador which lie east of the Andes. Certain towns are considered as not forming part of these zones provided they maintain continuously an *Aëdes* index not exceeding 1 per cent. This index represents the proportions of houses in a limited, well-defined area in which breeding places of *Aëdes aegypti* are found. Epidemics occur from time to time and have been described from the Sudan, Ethiopia, the Senegal, Nigeria, Ghana and the Gambia as recently as 1978/79. In the Gambia a serological survey indicated that 8000 cases occurred with about 1700 deaths.

Yellow fever does *not* occur in Asia or the Pacific region, though the urban vector is widespread (*vide* South-East Asian haemorrhagic fever). It is not clear whether this is because the disease has not been introduced or because of a peculiar racial immunity, in any case the risk of introduction must be avoided at all costs. (Yellow fever *receptive areas*.)

Applied biology
Unmodified yellow fever virus attacks the cells of all three embryonic layers (pantropic). All strains show some degree of neurotropism, but the severity of the illness is largely due to the degree of viscerotropism shown; i.e. the degree of affinity shown for the abdominal viscera, particularly the liver. The degree of virulence shown by the virus can be modified by serial passage through mouse brain, or by culture in chick embryos or in tissue culture. The virus actually multiplies in the mosquito host: after biting an infected person or monkey, the mosquito itself becomes infective after an interval of about 12 days (extrinsic incubation period) and remains infective for the rest of its life. Mosquitoes are the only insects able to transmit infection.

Epidemiology
There are two main epidemiological forms of yellow fever:
(i) URBAN TYPE The mosquito vector is *Aëdes aegypti*, which is primarily a domestic mosquito which breeds in or near houses, with the female preferring to lay her eggs in water collecting in artificial containers, such as old tins, etc.

The virus cycle is Man-Mosquito-Man; this method of spread requires large numbers of susceptible hosts, and hence tends to occur in large towns. Villages, with frequent passage of people from one village to another, will also be suitable for this type of spread. Urban-type yellow fever can effectively be controlled by anti-mosquito measures.
(ii) JUNGLE TYPE This may occur either in endemic or epizootic forms. In the endemic form, the disease, which is primarily one of monkeys, is almost constantly present, and sporadic cases of human infection occur from time to time. The primary spread of the virus is from monkey to monkey, via *A. africanus* in Africa (Fig. 6.1) and *Haemagogus* spp. in South America (Fig. 6.2): both these mosquitoes live in the tops of trees. *Haemagogus* species will occasionally bite man, for example when a tree is felled, and South American jungle yellow fever is thus maintained.

In Africa, however, there is another way in which jungle yellow fever virus can be transmitted from the monkey to man. Certain monkeys have the habit of raiding crops, particularly bananas. Another mosquito, *A. simpsoni*, occurs on the edges of forests, and becomes infected by biting infected raiding monkeys, and then later bites the farmer when he collects his crop. *A. simpsoni* thus acts as a so-called 'Link-host'. It is important to remember that, in endemic areas, many cases of yellow fever are mild illnesses resulting in subclinical infections leading to immunity among the indigenous population.

Laboratory diagnosis
Virus isolation from the blood up to the 4th day of the disease is the diagnostic procedure of choice. Isolation of virus is by intracerebral inoculation of mice. After the 3rd day the mouse protection test can be used. This test involves demonstrating whether or not mice are protected

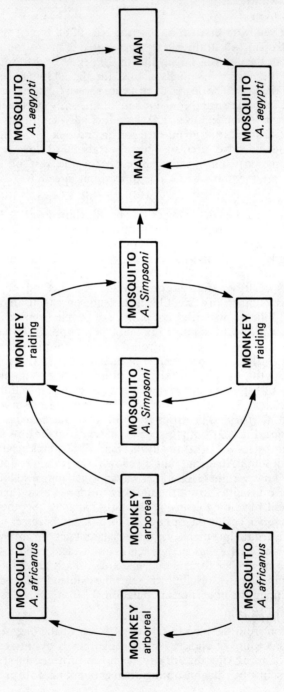

Fig. 6.1 Epidemiology of African yellow fever

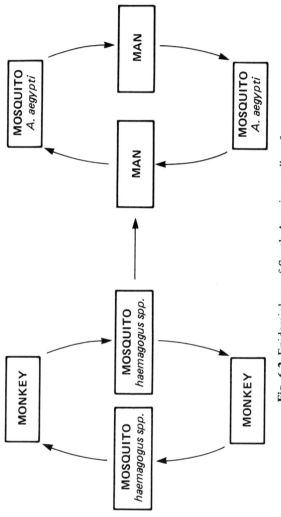

Fig. 6.2 Epidemiology of South American yellow fever

from a challenge dose of the virus by antibodies in the patient's serum. A second protection test should be made some 5 days later. A significant rise of titre in the second sample would confirm the diagnosis, while an unaltered titre would only indicate an immunity due to a past infection or vaccination. It must be borne in mind that there may be cross-reaction with other viruses of the group B arbovirus group. Neutralisation, complement fixation, or haemagglutination inhibition tests are also employed, depending on the particular circumstances and the likelihood of previous exposure to other group B viruses. Histology of the liver in fatal cases establishes the diagnosis. Occasionally virus can be isolated from this organ.

Control

(a) The individual
Since the virus circulates in the blood during the first few days of the disease, a suspected case must be isolated for the first 6 days in a screened room or under a mosquito net. Steps should be taken at once to obtain laboratory confirmation of the diagnosis, but institution of control measures should not await results from the laboratory. Domestic contacts also should be isolated under screened conditions for 6 days, and the patient's house and all premises within a radius of 55 m (60 yards) should be sprayed with a residual insecticide. The first cases of yellow fever in an epidemic are likely to be mistaken for other illnesses, especially infective hepatitis. It is therefore very important always to remember the possibility of yellow fever in endemic areas and when in doubt to take blood for serological examinations or specimens of the liver (if necessary with a viscerotome) from corpses. A life-long immunity follows recovery from the disease. There is evidence to suggest that the presence of extensive immunity to other group B viruses modifies the severity and spread of yellow fever.

(b) The vector
In densely populated areas elimination of vector breeding must be undertaken at once. *A. aegypti* is a peri-domestic mosquito and will breed in practically anything that will hold water. This includes water containers such as jars and cisterns, as well as innumerable objects which may hold rain-water: defective gutters, old tins, jars and coconut shells (often hidden in the grass), and the bottoms of small boats and canoes. These breeding foci should be reduced as far as possible by suitable measures; water containers covered or screened, tins and other rubbish buried, and so forth. This is unlikely to prevent all breeding, but it will simplify treatment of the remainder by regular oiling or by addition of insecticidal briquettes.

Residual spraying of the interiors of all houses and out-buildings or of all surfaces close to breeding places (peri-focal spraying) will reduce the

Aëdes population rapidly. Epidemic transmission will cease when the *Aëdes index* is reduced to below 5 per cent. To prevent introduction of an infected mosquito into countries where the disease is absent but conditions exist for transmission, aircraft coming from the endemic zone must be disinsecticised (by insecticidal aerosol) as specified by the World Health Organisation. This is particularly important in Asia, where vigorous antimosquito measures around airports should be carried out, international certificates of all persons coming from endemic zones scrupulously checked and adequate quarantine of animal reservoirs such as monkeys instituted. International notification provides health authorities with up-to-date information regarding the status of yellow fever throughout the world.

(c) *Immunisation*
Protection of scattered populations by vector control is, however, impracticable, and recourse must be had to vaccination of the whole community. This will afford protection for at least 10 years. Mass vaccination is advisable in epidemic conditions. Two vaccines are available: the 17D strain maintained by passage in chick embryo or in tissue culture and the Dakar strain maintained in mouse brain. This latter is prepared in a form which permits administration by scarification and is very suitable for use in scattered populations in rural areas; it is however associated with a higher incidence of meningoencephalic reactions than the 17D strain which is more generally recommended. Infants under 1 year of age should preferably not be vaccinated, since encephalitis follows vaccination in this age-group more frequently than in adults. Some countries do not require vaccination certificates in the case of infants.

The spread of the disease is controlled by requiring all persons entering or leaving an endemic area to be in possession of a valid certificate of vaccination. Those not in possession of such a certificate may, on arrival in a non-endemic area, be subjected to quarantine for a period of 6 days from the date of last exposure to infection or until the certificate becomes valid. A vaccination certificate becomes valid 10 days after vaccination and remains so for 10 years. A certificate of revaccination done not more than 10 years after a previous vaccination becomes valid on the day of vaccination. Vaccination is contraindicated in patients whose immune responses are suppressed by steroids or immunosuppressive drugs.

(2) Dengue Viruses

Dengue viruses produce, in general, a non-fatal, short, febrile illness, characterised by severe myalgia and joint pains. The occurrence of haemorrhagic phenomena with a significant mortality, especially in childhood, has been a feature of recent epidemics in South-East Asia. There are four main serotypes of Dengue viruses, numbers 1, 2, 3 and 4.

(a) 'Classical' Dengue fever

A. aegypti is the established mosquito vector of the dengue viruses responsible for dengue fever which is widely distributed throughout urban areas of the tropics and subtropics. A pandemic of 'Classical' dengue fever began in the Caribbean in 1977 and involved major outbreaks on many of the islands, including Puerto Rico. The virus circulates in the blood at the onset of symptoms and for a few days. The extrinsic incubation period of the virus in *A. aegypti* is about 2 weeks. Infection confers immunity to the homologous strain for about a year. Diagnosis must be based on the clinical findings, intracerebral inoculation of blood in suckling mice, and other virological and serological tests. The only practical preventive measures are control of the vectors in their aquatic or adult stages as described for yellow fever. The prevention of mosquito bites by screening or repellents provides further protection.

(b) South-East Asian haemorrhagic fever

In recent years, epidemics of dengue with haemorrhagic phenomena have been reported from widely spaced regions—in Calcutta, the Philippines, Thailand, Malaysia, Indonesia, Burma and Singapore, and, all types of dengue viruses have been isolated from *A. aegypti* during these epidemics. The epidemics have an urban distribution with cases clustered in the crowded, poorer, central districts of cities. Although uncontrolled urbanisation has been responsible for some of the epidemics that have occurred in Southeast Asia in recent years, the disease is now spreading to rural areas as well. The disease is usually seen in races of oriental origin; and haemorrhagic fatal manifestations are usually confined to persons under 15 years of age with a peak incidence in the 3–6 year group.

A fatal case of dengue haemorrhagic fever in an American child has recently been described from Thailand. Some outbreaks of haemorrhagic fever have been caused by the arbovirus *Chikungunya* (group A). On the whole the syndrome associated with chikungunya infection is milder than haemorrhagic dengue.

Control

Control of South-East Asian haemorrhagic fever is based on eradicating the urban vector mosquito *A. aegypti* as described for yellow fever.

3 Japanese B Encephalitis

The majority of infections are inapparent or mild. The disease occurs in China, Taiwan, Korea, Japan, Malaysia, Singapore and India. The most efficient vector is *Culex tritaeniohynchus*, and the preferred vertebrate hosts are birds and domestic animals, e.g. pigs; man being only an incidental host. The virus is spread from rural to urban areas by viraemic birds. The peak age specific prevalence in most areas is between 4–8 years of age. In 1977, there were 1699 cases of encephalitis with 415 deaths reported in Thailand. Here, the highest percentage of sero-positive cases was found in patients aged 10–19 years. Control of the vector mosquitoes is not practicable on a large scale. Isolation of pig sties from human habitats reduces the mosquito/man contact.

4 Kyasanur Forest Disease

The virus of Kyasanur Forest disease has to date been found only in Mysore State, India. The disease occurs more frequently in the dry season and in persons working in the forest. The principal vector is the tick *Haemaphysalis spinigera*. Human infection is often preceded by illness and death in forest-dwelling monkeys, which act as amplifiers of the virus which is maintained in small mammals. Personal protection against the vector tick is the only practicable method of control.

ARBOVIRUSES: GROUP C

The Group C viruses have only been isolated from Brazil, Trinidad, Panama and the USSR, while antibodies in man have been reported from Africa.

OTHER VIRUSES

Many other viruses, some grouped and others as yet ungrouped, are known to produce disease in man. The illness is usually mild and large segments of the population show neutralising antibodies to the various viruses resulting from subclinical infections.

(i) Bunyamwera Group

Bunyamwera virus was isolated from Uganda and neutralising anti-bodies have been detected from Uganda, Tanzania, Mozambique, Nigeria and other parts of Africa. No fatal cases have been reported.

(ii) Phlebotomus Fever Group

The diseases caused by viruses in this group are non-fatal. The vectors are various species of *Phlebotomus* and the distribution of the disease is limited between the latitudes 25° and 45°N. There are two types of viruses, the Sicilian and the Neapolitan. Sandfly fever appears epidemically over much of the tropics and subtropics, where it is transmitted by *Phlebotomus papatasii*. Recovery from the disease is followed by a long-lasting immunity to the homologous strain of virus. Sandfly breeding can be controlled to some extent by clearing piles of rubbish and mending cracked and dilapidated walls. The insects are particularly susceptible to DDT, and have been drastically reduced in many places by residual house spraying employed for the control of mosquitoes.

(iii) Simbum Group—Oporonche Virus

Oporonche virus disease occurs in Trinidad and Brazil.

(iv) Rift Valley Fever Virus

This virus usually causes a non-fatal disease in man, characterised by fever, myalgia, severe headache, epistaxis and occasionally ocular complications. It is a cause of severe disease in sheep and cattle in East and South Africa. Man is infected through handling sick animals or carcasses. More recently Rift Valley fever virus has caused disastrous epizooties in the Sudan and Egypt. In the Egyptian outbreak in 1977 there was around 20 000 human infections and at least 90 deaths. The natural reservoir is unknown, the vectors are mosquitoes of the Aedes and Culex groups.

Arbovirus Infections—Summary

	Yellow fever	Dengue fever	S.E. Asian haemorrhagic fever
1 *Occurrence*	South America, Tropical Africa	Widely in tropics	S.E. Asia
2 *Organisms*	Yellow fever virus	Dengue virus	Dengue virus
3 *Reservoir of Infection*	Man, monkeys	Man	Man
4 *Mode of transmission*	*Aëdes* spp. bites	*Aëdes* spp.	*Aëdes* spp.
5 *Control*	(i) Isolation of individual (ii) Vector control (iii) Immunisation	(i) Vector control	(i) Vector control

THE RICKETTSIAL DISEASES

The typhus fevers are caused by rickettsiae which are intracellular organisms living and multiplying in arthropod tissues such as those of the lice, fleas, ticks and mites. The rickettsial diseases of man can be divided into five main groups as shown in Table 6.3.

Most of the rickettsial diseases have a world-wide distribution, and are not confined to the tropics.

Table 6.3 Classification of rickettsial diseases

Disease	Causative Agent	Vector	Animal Reservoir
A TYPHUS GROUP			
(i) Epidemic	*Rickettsia prowazekii*	*Pediculus humanus*	None
(ii) Brill-Zinsser disease	*R. prowazekii*	*P. humanus*	None
(iii) Murine	*R. mooseri*	*Xenopsylla cheopis*	Rat
B SPOTTED FEVER GROUP			
(i) American spotted fevers	*R. rickettsii*	Various species ticks	Many species of small mammals
(ii) African tick typhus	*R. rickettsii* var. *pijperi*		
(iii) Fièvre boutonneuse	*R. conori*		
(iv) Siberian tick typhus	*R. siberica*		
(v) Queensland tick typhus	*R. australis*		
(vi) Rickettsialpox	*R. akari*	Mite	
C SCRUB TYPHUS	*R. tsutsugamushi*	Trombiculid mites	Small mammals, mice and field rats
D TRENCH FEVER	*R. quintana*	*P. humanus*	None
E Q FEVER	*Coxiella burnetii*	None (ticks)	Cattle, sheep, goats and wild animals

The most important are epidemic louse-borne typhus, murine typhus, scrub typhus and, to a lesser extent, African tick typhus and Q fever.

1 Epidemic Louse-borne Typhus

This acute disease is caused by R. *prowazekii* and is transmitted by the louse *Pediculus humanus*. The *incubation period* is about 10 days.

Medical geography
Epidemic typhus has a world-wide distribution but the incidence of the disease is generally low in tropical countries. Endemic foci exist in central Europe, Russia, China and North Africa. In the tropics it is common at high altitudes and in deserts. Recently epidemics have occurred in Burundi, Rwanda and Ethiopia.

Epidemiology
This disease is commoner in cold climates than in the tropics. Man is the main reservoir of infection although in Tunisia serological evidence has

been obtained that the rat may also be a reservoir of epidemic typhus in that country. In Ethiopia it has lost its overwhelming dominance and epidemic typhus is now the least common of the rickettsial infections. The louse becomes infected by feeding on a person with the disease from 2 days before symptoms appear until the end of fever. The rickettsiae multiply in the cells of the louse midgut, and when these rupture the organisms are discharged in the faeces. Human infection follows contamination of breaches of the skin surface by infected louse faeces. The rickettsiae can remain viable for months on dried louse faeces, and may possibly cause infection through the conjunctiva or by inhalation, as well as percutaneously. Recovery is followed by immunity, which persists for several years. In some patients the infection appears to remain latent after symptoms have subsided and to relapse some years later (Brill's disease).

Laboratory diagnosis
This is established by the Weil-Felix reaction, in which *B. proteus* OX_{19} is agglutinated and also OX_2 to a lower titre, or more specifically by the complement-fixation test using suspensions or extracts of the specific organism.

Control

Delousing of the whole population with residual insecticidal powders is the principal control measure.

(a) *The individual*
Sporadic cases are isolated and deloused, but isolation of infected persons is not practicable in epidemics. On admission to hospital, the patient should be bathed with soap and water or a 1 per cent solution of lysol. The tetracyclines are highly specific and are given in a total dosage of 25 mg per kg, daily. They must be continued for 3 days after the temperature is normal. A single oral dose of doxycycline 200 mg is also very effective in controlling the disease. Contacts should be deloused and kept under observation for 2 weeks. The patient's clothes and bedding should be sterilised and his house sprayed with residual insecticides.

(b) *The community*
Mass delousing of the entire population controls epidemic typhus. This is carried out by blowing insecticide (commonly 10 per cent insecticidal powder) with a dusting-gun under the clothes next to the skin over the whole body, the operation occupying only a few minutes. In some areas lice have become resistant to DDT, and other residual insecticides must be used, such as BHC.

(c) *Immunisation*
Vaccines containing attenuated strains of epidemic or murine rickettsiae will give some degree of protection for about 6 months and may be used

in endemic areas before seasonal transmission starts. Dosage is 1 ml subcutaneously on two occasions at weekly intervals with booster doses every 6 months.

2 Murine Typhus

The disease is caused by *R. mooseri* and transmitted by rat fleas. The *incubation period* is 10–12 days.

Epidemiology

Murine typhus has a world-wide distribution. Flea-borne (murine) typhus is widely distributed and occurs wherever the rat lives in close association with man, e.g. grain stores, irrespective of climate. In a recent serological survey carried out in the Ivory Coast, varieties of murine typhus had an overall frequency of 4.5 per cent but were more prevalent among adults (6 per cent) and also more frequent in the coastal regions (7 per cent). Converted old rat-infested farmhouses are sometimes foci of infection. Murine typhus is essentially a rodent infection which appears sporadically in man. It exists throughout the world, and the organism *Rickettsia mooseri* is conveyed to man by the faeces of infected rat-fleas of the genus *Xenopsylla* or the rat-mite *Bdellonyssus bacoti*. The Weil-Felix test gives the same reaction as in epidemic typhus.

Control

Control of murine typhus is rarely required, but if needed the anti-rat and anti-flea measures employed in plague will be effective. Individual patients should be treated with antibiotics as in epidemic typhus (see above).

3 Mite-borne Typhus

Scrub typhus (tsutsugamushi disease; Japanese river or flood fever tropical typhus; rural typhus) is an acute febrile disease characterised by fever, a cutaneous rash which appears on the 5th day, and an eschar at the site of attachment of the trombiculid mites which transmit the disease. The causative organism is *Rickettsia tsutsugamushi* (*R. orientalis*). The *incubation period* is about 12 days.

Medical geography

Mite-borne typhus occurs in Japan, Thailand, other countries in East and South-East Asia, some Pacific islands and Queensland in Australia. The distribution of scrub typhus is closely related to certain physical and ecological factors which produce 'scrub typhus country', resulting in a recurring cycle of passage of rickettsiae between rodents and mites with a spillover into man.

Epidemiology

'Scrub typhus' is enzootic in wild rodents and the two most important vectors are the larvae of *Trombicula akamushi* and *T. deliensis*. In Indonesia the rat flea is the vector. The reservoir of infection are rodents, and man becomes infected when the larval mites feed on blood. Only the larval mites feed on the vertebrate hosts' blood, and since the larva only feeds once, the rickettsiae persist through the nymph, adult and egg stages into the larval stages of the next generation, which are thus infective. Man contracts the disease by exposure, e.g. walking or resting in infected foci, particularly after slight rain or heavy dew.

The disease may be encountered in grassy fields, along river banks, in abandoned rice-fields, in forests or jungles, and in the neglected shrubby fringes between field and forest. The different epidemiological patterns of the disease are related to the influence of climatic variations on the life cycle of the trombiculid mite vectors. The seasonal occurrence of tsutsugamushi disease in Japan corresponds exactly with the time of appearance of each species of vector, *T. akamushi* in summer; *T. scutellaris* in autumn and winter; and *T. pallida* in winter and early spring. While the terrain of *T. akamushi* is limited to places along the rivers, other vectors seem to extend far beyond river banks. In Malaysia, scrub typhus occurs throughout the year. Man is only an accidental host, while field-mice, rats, possibly other small mammals, and ground-frequenting birds are the natural hosts responsible for the continuing transmission of *R. tsutsugamushi* from infected to uninfected mites. The mites function both as vector and reservoir since transovarial transmission of rickettsial infection occurs.

The presence of scrub-typhus infection in rodents or trombiculid mites in unusual habitats in West Pakistan—e.g. alpine terrain at 3200 m, semi-desert and desert 'oasis greenhouse'—has been reported.

Laboratory diagnosis

A diagnosis of scrub typhus can be made by recovering R. *tsutsugamushi* from the blood of a patient during the febrile period by culture in living-tissue culture media, or in the yolk-sac membrane of developing chick embryos. Intraperitoneal inoculation of blood or of tissue into white mice results in fatal illness, and on autopsy there is a white peritoneal exudate with numerous organisms in the peritoneal cells. The organism can also be recovered from human tissue taken at post-mortem.

The most widely used serological test for the diagnosis of scrub typhus is the Weil-Felix reaction. Agglutinins for Proteus OXK, but not for Proteus OX_{19} or OX_2 appear in the patient's serum about the 10th day of the disease reaching a maximum titre by the end of the third week, after which they rapidly decline. Serial examination reveals a four-fold or greater rise in titre. The complement-fixation test has also been used for diagnostic and sero-epidemiological surveys. Indirect immuno-fluorescence employing smears of rickettsiae as antigen can be used for the specific diagnosis of scrub typhus.

The results obtained by Weil-Felix tests from patients with various forms of typhus are summarised in Table 6.4.

Table 6.4 Weil-Felix reaction in typhus fevers

Typhus fever	Standard strains		
	OX_{19}	OX_2	OXK
Mite-borne	−	−	+ + +
Tick-borne	− to + +	− to + +	−
Louse-borne ⎱ Flea-borne ⎰	+ + + to −	+ + to −	−

In the majority of cases of louse-borne and flea-borne typhus OX_{19} is agglutinated to a high titre; while in tick-borne typhus OX_{19} and OX_2 are only agglutinated to a low titre.

Control

Control measures are based upon (i) control of the ecology, (ii) anti-mite measures and (iii) chemoprophylaxis and treatment of individual cases.

(i) *Control of the ecology*

The ecology of scrub typhus must be clarified in each area where it occurs before control measures can be successful. The ecology will differ in different geographical areas, from the abandoned rubber plantations of Malaysia to the scrub typhus oases of Pakistan.

Known endemic areas which are often localised to small geographical sites should be avoided for the construction of camps and living-quarters. These areas are frequently second-degree growths in de-forested areas. Prospective camp sites may be prepared by cutting all vegetation level with the ground and burning it. After thorough clearing, the ground dries sufficiently in 2 or 3 weeks to kill the mites. If the site is required immediately, it should be sprayed with dieldrin or gamma Benzene hexachloride (1 kg per 4000 m^2).

(ii) *Anti-mite measures*

Clothing must be rubbed or impregnated with dimethyl or dibutyl phthalate, benzyl benzoate or benzene hexachloride. These kill the mites on contact. Particular care should be given to those parts of the clothing that give access to the interior of the garment.

(iii) *Chemoprophylaxis*

Tetracyclines 3 g orally once weekly, will permit individuals to remain ambulatory even though rickettsiaemia will occur from time to time.

The drug must be continued for 4 weeks after leaving the endemic area, otherwise clinical disease will occur within a week of withdrawal of the drug. Clinical cases respond to tetracyclines 3 g (loading dose) followed by 0.5 g 6-hourly until the temperature is normal. Doxycycline is also effective in the treatment of individuals suffering from scrub typhus at a single dose of 200 mg orally, and is more convenient for obvious reasons.

4 African Tick Typhus

This is found in Africa south of the Sahara, West Africa, East Africa (Kenya), South Africa, the Sudan, Somalia and Ethiopia.

The disease is contracted by man from ticks in the bush, where the reservoirs are wild rodents. Occasionally, the infection may be brought into suburban areas by dog ticks on domestic dogs. Transovarial transmission occurs in the tick. African tick typhus is a mild disease in man and deaths are almost unknown. A primary eschar is found at the site of the tick bite. Inapparent infections do not occur, although mild abortive attacks without a rash are not uncommon.

Control

No quarantine measures are necessary. Tetracyclines are specific in treatment as for scrub typhus. If antibiotic therapy is given at the time of appearance of the primary eschar, the attack will be aborted. Breaking the tick/man contact is the most effective control measure. Known endemic areas should be avoided during the tick season when they are most active. When camping in these areas, individuals should sleep off the ground on camp beds. Where dogs act as tick carriers, then the animals, if they are household pets, should be regularly examined for ticks, which must be removed. Proper clothing should be worn, and the shirt tucked inside the trousers. Socks and high boots should be worn outside the trousers. Since ticks rarely transmit the infection until they have fed for several hours, an important precaution is to remove the clothes and search both body and clothing twice daily, removing the ticks gently with a gloved hand or with forceps.

5 Q Fever

This infection due to *Coxiella burnetii* has a world-wide distribution. The rickettsiae are distributed widely in nature in ticks, human body lice, small wild mammals, cattle, sheep, goats, birds and man. The epidemiology varies in different parts of the world, according to the local geographical and environmental factors present.

The infection is maintained in domestic animals, mainly by wild animals, ticks, domestic animal association, and man acquires the infection as an occupational hazard by direct contact with milk. Secondary cases are caused by the inhalation of infected dust or from human carriers, when the infection is transmitted from man-to-man, via the respiratory tract. Many mild and inapparent infections undoubtedly occur.

The epidemiology of Q fever is complex, but most human infections are acquired directly or indirectly from domestic animals (see p. 238).

Control

Control of the disease on a community basis rests upon control of the disease in domestic animals either by immunisation or by antibiotics. This requires a large economic effort. Milk from goats, sheep, and cows should be pasteurised. Calving and lambing processes in endemic areas should be confined to an enclosed area which can be decontaminated after the products of parturition have been disposed of. Immunisation is the most effective control measure from the individual point of view.

Vaccination will prevent infection with Q Fever amongst high-risk laboratory workers and in heavily exposed industrial groups, such as farm workers in endemic areas and workers handling farm products such as meat and milk. A standard vaccine Q-34, prepared by Cox's method from formolised *C. burnetii* and containing 10 complement fixing units per ml is given in 1 ml doses as 3-weekly subcutaneous injections. Preliminary skin testing with 0.1 ml of a 1/50 dilution of the vaccine should be performed to avoid reactions. Successful vaccination is shown by the development of a positive skin reaction after 40 days.

Typhus Fevers—Summary

	Louse-borne	Flea-borne	Mite-borne
1 *Occurrence*	Central Europe, China, North Africa	World-wide	South-East Asia, Far East
2 *Organisms*	*R. prowazekii*	*R. mooseri*	*R. orientalis*
3 *Reservoir of infection*	Man	Rodents, man	Rodents
4 *Mode of transmission*	Contamination by infected louse faeces	Contamination by infected rat faeces	Bites of mites
5 *Control*	(i) Mass delousing (ii) Personal hygiene	(i) Anti-flea measures (ii) Anti-rat measures	(i) Control of ecology (ii) Anti-mite measures (iii) Chemoprophylaxis

THE BACTERIAL DISEASES

PLAGUE

Plague is a rapidly fatal disease due to *Yersinia pestis* which can manifest itself in a variety of ways—bubonic, pneumonic and septicaemic forms. The *incubation period* is 2–4 days.

Medical geography
Although the number of cases of plague have gradually declined, foci of the disease still exist in the Indian subcontinent, China, South-East Asia, Africa, South America and the Middle East. A noteworthy feature has been the continuing importance of the disease in Vietnam. The principal endemic foci are India, China, Manchuria, Mongolia, Burma, Vietnam, East Africa, Malagasy Republic, Brazil, Bolivia, Peru and Ecuador.

Bacteriology
The organisms are small, Gram-negative, ovoid bacilli showing bipolar staining. *Yersinia pestis* is easily destroyed by disinfectants, heat and sunlight but in cold or freezing conditions it can survive for weeks or months.

Epidemiology
The reservoir of infection is rats and non-domestic rodents. The bubonic disease which is the commonest is transmitted by the bite of an infected rat flea *Xenopsylla cheopis* while pneumonic plague spreads from person to person by droplet infection.

(a) Bubonic Plague

The occurrence of plague in a human population is always preceded by an enzootic in the rat population and hence any unusual mortality among rats should be looked into promptly. Plague spreads rapidly wherever the human population is congested, living in insanitary conditions where rats are numerous and have access to food. When a flea ingests infected blood the plague bacilli multiply in its gut and may gradually block the flea's proventriculus. As a result, the flea cannot feed, becomes hungry and tries repeatedly to bite, regurgitating plague bacilli into the puncture at each attempt. These so-called 'blocked-fleas' are a very important factor in the dissemination of human disease. In temperate climates plague is common in the warmer months (i.e. summer), while in the tropics it appears in the colder months (i.e. winter). The efficiency of flea transmission declines with increasing temperatures. All ages and either sex may be infected. Plague spreads from region to region chiefly through rats in ships and strict surveillance is needed in busy seaports. Serological evidence indicates that there are a substantial number of asymptomatic plague infections.

Plague also occurs in non-domestic rodents—*wild rodent plague*—and epizootics affect many different species throughout the world. The infection is transferred to rats living in urban areas from wild rodents and thence to man. In rural areas man, e.g. hunters and trappers, can be infected in the field, bring the disease home, infect their own domestic rats and fleas and thereby their families.

(b) Pneumonic Plague

Pneumonic plague is transmitted from person to person by 'droplet infection' from patients suffering from primary pneumonic plague or from individuals with bubonic plague who develop terminal plague pneumonia—neither rats nor fleas play a part in the spread of the disease. Overcrowding favours dissemination of pneumonic plague. Some years ago in Vietnam, a mixed pneumonic bubonic plague outbreak occurred and *Y. pestis* was recovered from the throats of asymptomatic healthy carriers.

Laboratory diagnosis

Y. pestis may be detected in smears of material aspirated from buboes, from sputum, or even from the blood stained by Gram's method. Culture and animal inoculation should be performed. Smears from the spleen are positive at necropsy. Specimens of material aspirated from buboes, throat swabs and sputa can now be placed in a special holding medium which maintains the organisms in a viable condition during transport to distant laboratories. Fluorescent antibody, complement fixation, and haemagglutination techniques have also been used.

Control

Plague is a notifiable and quarantinable disease and the quarantine period laid down by the International Health Regulations is 6 days.

(a) *The individual*

Cases of **bubonic** plague should be removed to hospital and isolated. Care should be taken in the nursing of such cases in case they develop pneumonia and hence masks and gowns should be worn by attendants. Contacts should be kept under surveillance for 6 days and dusted with DDT powder. All patients should be treated with streptomycin (2–4 g daily up to a total of 20 g) or the broad-spectrum antibiotics of the tetracycline series, (2–6 g daily up to a total of 40 g) as early as possible. The overall fatality rate of untreated bubonic plague is between 20 and 75 per cent while untreated pneumonic plague is almost invariably fatal. Prompt and adequate therapy reduces the overall mortality to less than 5 per cent.

Pneumonic plague is a highly infectious disease and immediate and strict isolation is vitally important. The patient, his clothing, his house and everything he has been in contact with must be disinfected. Medical and nursing staff attending such patients must wear protective clothing, including goggles. Strict surveillance of all contacts must be carried out daily and prompt isolation and treatment of infected cases carried out. While in hospital the strict 'current disinfection' must be done throughout the course of the disease.

All personnel engaged in flea or rat control during an epizootic must wear protective clothing impregnated with DDT, while dead rats should be sprinkled with DDT, and handled and disposed of carefully.

(b) *The community*
The immediate and widespread use of DDT and BHC in dusting rat-infested areas and thus eliminating the fleas is the most important single control measure that interrupts transmission. In areas where resistance to one or both of these materials occurs dusts of carbanyl (2 %), diazinon (2 %), or malathion (5 %) should prove effective. Dusts of DDT and BHC should contain 10 % and 3 % of the active ingredient respectively. An evaluation of the efficiency of dusting programme is mandatory. The elimination of fleas is coupled with the systemic destruction of rats which should commence on lines extending radially from the centre of infection in order to delimit the enzootic area. All rats caught should be examined for evidence of plague and any new foci infection found treated with DDT. The systemic rat trapping and destruction is followed by measures such as rat-proofing of houses and buildings, protection of food and sanitary disposal of refuse. Rat-proofing of ships and general maintenance of ship hygiene should be encouraged. Port health authorities are particularly responsible for supervising this and constant vigilance is required especially in busy ports such as Singapore.

(c) *Immunisation*
Personal protection is provided by the use of a dead vaccine or attenuated live vaccine of *Y. pestis*. The latter is given in a single dose while two doses of the dead vaccine are required at weekly intervals. Protection commences a week after inoculation and lasts for about 10 months. Most authorities also recommend *chemoprophylaxis* for all contacts of both forms of plague—tetracyclines 2 g daily for 1 week or sulphadimidine 3 g daily for 1 week.

Plague—Summary

1 *Occurrence*—South-East Asia, South America, Middle East, Africa
2 *Organisms—Y. pestis*
3 *Reservoir of infection*—Rats (bubonic), man (pneumonic)
4 *Modes of transmission*—Flea bite (bubonic), droplet (pneumonic)
5 *Control*— (i) Isolation
      (ii) DDT for elimination of fleas
      (iii) Rat destruction
      (iv) Raising standards of environmental hygiene

THE RELAPSING FEVERS

Relapsing fever is due to infection of the blood by morphologically indistinguishable strains of spirochaetes which are transmitted by ticks resulting in endemic disease, and by body lice resulting usually in epidemic disease. The louse-borne spirochaete is known as *Borrelia recurrentis* while the tick-borne spirochaetes are often named according to their tick vector.

(1) Tick-borne Relapsing Fever

Non-epidemic relapsing fever is due to infection with *Borrelia duttoni* and is transmitted by a number of ticks, of which the African *Ornithodorus moubata* is one of the most important. The *incubation period* is 3–10 days, and recovery is followed by immunity lasting about a year.

Medical geography
The disease occurs in Central, East and South Africa as well as in North Africa, North, Central and South America, the Middle East and northern India.

Epidemiology
In most areas *B. duttoni* normally affects rodents and occurs only accidentally in man, while in central Africa it primarily affects man, in whom it is endemic. The vector in South America is *Ornithodorus rudis*. The other vector species are not domestic in habit, and they feed primarily on rodents and other small mammals. The disease, therefore, is highly endemic where the vector is domestic in habit and very sporadic in areas where human contact with the tick is in open country or caves. The tick lives in the soil of the floor, or the mud-plaster walls of African huts; they are also found in caves and in the soil of bush or scrub country. The female lays batches of eggs each of which hatches to produce a larval tick with three pairs of legs. The larval forms pass through about five moults at intervals of 2 weeks. Larval forms and adults feed by sucking blood. A proportion of the offspring of infected female ticks are infected transovarially, thus the infection may persist through several generations. During feeding a saline fluid, called coxal fluid, is excreted from glands near the attachment of the legs.

It is generally believed that the infected fluid exuded by the coxal glands, saliva and bowel contaminates the wound made by the bite of the tick and spirochaetes enter the bloodstream.

Humans entering caves, working in bush country, living in infected African huts, or sleeping in rest houses in the vicinity of infected villages are liable to acquire the infection. It seems that babies and little children are very susceptible to the disease and it appears that immunity is acquired with increasing age by those living in endemic areas. There are several reports in the literature of newborn infants developing relapsing fever within the first 10 days after birth, but no case of congenital infection has been recorded. It has been suggested that infection is transmitted after birth during the process of suckling, possibly from cracks in nipples, to abrasions in the child's mouth. Although *B. duttoni* will infect lice, no large-scale change in vector has been proved to occur under natural conditions.

Control

(a) *The individual*
In areas where transmission is by non-domestic vectors control consists in wearing protective clothing, such a high-legged boots, or in using repellents.

(b) *The vector*
Domestic vectors can be controlled by treating the interiors of houses with benzene hexachloride or dieldrin. Spray treatments (usually suspensions) have been used in dosages ranging from 0.2 up to 6 g *gamma* BHC per square metre; the higher dosage will give protection up to a year or more.

(c) *The community*
The most satisfactory control results from rehousing the people in buildings which provided no harbourage for ticks.

(2) Louse-borne Relapsing Fever

This disease is usually epidemic and has a similar geographical distribution as epidemic typhus. The *incubation period* is usually from 2 to 10 days. In an attack of louse-borne relapsing fever there are only one or two, and never more than four relapses, and death, as opposed to tick-borne relapsing fever, is often in the first attack. Fever, headache, skeletal and abdominal pain, and the usual symptoms of acute infection are common. Tachypnoea, upper abdominal tenderness with a palpable liver and spleen, jaundice and purpura occur. Hyperpyrexia, hypotension and cardiac failure can be fatal.

Medical geography
Louse-borne relapsing fever is more common in temperate than tropical climates, but outbreaks of epidemic louse-borne relapsing fever have occurred in parts of Africa, India and South America. The disease is endemic in Ethiopia.

Epidemiology
Like epidemic typhus fever, which it may accompany, it is associated with poor sanitation and personal hygiene, particularly overcrowding,

undernutrition and lice-infested clothing. It is conveyed from one man to another by the human body louse *Pediculus humanus*, and the spirochaete responsible is *Borrelia recurrentis*. The blood of a patient suffering from relapsing fever contains spirochaetes only during the febrile periods and lice become infected at this time. Man is the only reservoir of louse-borne relapsing fever, and an endemic focus, as is present in Ethiopia, is capable of starting a widespread epidemic. African epidemics in the past seem to have occurred every 20 years, the last being in 1943. In contrast to ticks, no transovarial transmission in lice occurs. Infection is conveyed to human beings not by the bite of the louse, but by contamination of the wounds (made by biting or scratching) with the body fluids of the louse. Little is known of where relapsing fever lurks between epidemics and how it suddenly springs up after silent intervals of several years.

Laboratory diagnosis
Blood should be taken during the pyrexial period and examined either by dark-ground illumination or after staining with a Romanovsky stain. *B. duttoni* is about 15 μm long and made up of spiral turns occupying 2–3 μm. The numbers present in blood film vary from case to case; at the height of the first pyrexial attack they are often numerous. Blood infection is less heavy in the tick-borne than in the louse-borne disease. The organisms may be recovered by culture or by intraperitoneal inoculation of blood into laboratory animals (e.g. mouse or rat). The Wasserman reaction may be positive.

Control

This essentially consists in mass delousing by residual insecticidal powders, as in epidemic typhus.

(a) *The individual*
The safest, most effective and economical method of treating louse-borne relapsing fever is one injection of 300 000 units of procaine penicillin followed the next day by an oral dose of 250 mg tetracycline. Severe reactions of the Jarisch-Herxheimer type can occur.

(b) *The community*
The only effective measure is to control infestation with lice with DDT as has been described for epidemic typhus (p. 175).

Relapsing Fever—Summary

	Louse-borne	Tick-borne
1 *Occurrence*	Ethiopia, parts of Africa, India, South America	Africa, South America, Middle East
2 *Organisms*	*Borrelia recurrentis*	*B. duttoni*

3 *Reservoir of*		
infection	Man	Rodents, man
4 *Mode of*		
transmission	Contamination by	Contamination by
	infected louse body	infected tick body
	fluids	fluids
5 *Control*	Mass delousing	(i) Individual
		protection
		(ii) Vector control
		(iii) Rehousing

BARTONELLOSIS

Bartonellosis appears in two distinct forms: (*a*) Oroya fever and (*b*) Verruca peruana.

Oroya fever is an acute, febrile illness associated with a rapidly developing anaemia and a high mortality.

Verruca peruana is a non-fatal disease exemplified by generalised cutaneous lesions. It usually occurs following recovery from the Oroya fever stage although it occasionally arises apparently spontaneously.

The infection is limited to Bolivia, Peru, Colombia and Ecuador. The causative organism is *Bartonella bacilliformis*. Although known since 1905 it was first cultured in 1928 by Noguchi from an acute case of Oroya fever and the culture produced the nodules of verruca in monkeys. Oroya fever is also known as Carrion's disease since Carrion, a medical student, inoculated himself with material from a verruca lesion and died from Oroya fever 39 days later. The disease is transmitted from man to man by the bites of various species of sandflies *Phlebotomus*, which live at altitudes of 2000–8000 feet and bite only at night. The disease is most prevalent at the end of the rainy season when these insects are most numerous. When a susceptible person is bitten infection follows, usually in 3–4 weeks.

The organisms are pleomorphic Gram-negative coccobacilli and are found in blood smears, either free in the plasma or within red cells, in Oroya fever. They are sparse in the nodules in verruca and culture of material on serum agar is the most reliable method of isolation.

The principal cause of mortality is a particular susceptibility of patients with Oroya fever to septicaemic infections with Salmonella organisms, commonly *S. typhimurium*. Recovery confers some resistance to reinfection, so that in endemic areas the disease is most prevalent in children.

Control

The disease has been successfully controlled by applying residual insecticides to the interior of houses and outbuildings. Personal prophylaxis consists in the use of repellents and sandfly bed-nets. As soon as Oroya fever is diagnosed the patient should be given chloramphenicol in standard doses as for Salmonella infections.

THE PROTOZOAL DISEASES

MALARIA

Human malaria is a disease of wide distribution caused by sporozoa of the genus *Plasmodium*. There are four species of parasites that infect man: *P. falciparum, P. vivax, P. malariae* and *P. ovale*. The differentiation of the species depends on the morphology and staining of the parasites and associated changes in the containing cells. The most common and important infections are those caused by *P. falciparum* and *P. vivax*. Mixed infections occur.

The arthropod hosts are females of certain species of *Anopheles* mosquito. The predominant malaria vectors are *A. gambiae, A. funestus, A. darlingi* and *A. punctulatus*. Clinically malaria is characterised by fever, splenomegaly, varying degrees of anaemia, and various syndromes resulting from the involvement of individual organs.

Medical geography
Malaria is found in regions lying roughly between latitudes 60° N and 40° S. It is still commonly found throughout most of Africa, South America, South-East Asia, the Arabian peninsula and the Western Pacific.

Applied biology
The complete life cycle of the human malaria parasite embraces (1) a period of development within the mosquito, and (2) a period of infection in man.

After ingestion of human infected blood a period of development lasting 10–14 days occurs in the mosquito resulting in the production of sporozoites. A bite infects the human host with these forms which remain in the circulating blood for 30 minutes or less then enter tissue cells notably in the liver, where the *pre-erythrocytic* cycle takes place. During the succeeding 7–9 days the sporozoites develop in the parenchymal cells of the liver. As in the short sporozoite phase no symptoms of malaria are experienced during the pre-erythrocytic cycle. The liberation of the merozoites from the liver cells and their entry into the bloodstream initiates the *erythrocytic cycle*. The plasmodium first appears in red cells as a small speck of chromatin surrounded by scanty cytoplasm, and soon becomes a ring-shaped trophozoite. As the parasite develops, pigment particles appear in the cytoplasm, and the chromatin is more prominent. Chromatin division then proceeds, and when complete there is formed the mature schizont containing daughter merozoites. The parasitised red blood cell now ruptures, releasing merozoites the majority of which re-enter erythrocytes to re-initiate erythrocytic schizogony. In *P. falciparum* the erythrocytic cycle takes 36–48 hours (subtertian); in *P. vivax* and *P. ovale* infections 48 hours (tertian); and *P. malariae* 72 hours (quartan). In response to some unknown stimulus a number of the merozoites released after erythrocytic schizogony develop into male and female forms known as *gametocytes*. Gametocytes are believed to be inert in man. They provide the reservoir of infection enabling mosquitoes to perpetuate the malaria cycle, and remain within the red cell for the duration of their survial, i.e. up to 120 days.

A certain proportion of the merozoites liberated from the schizonts of the pre-erythrocytic phase, do *not* enter the bloodstream but re-enter the parenchymal cells of the liver and are responsible for the persistence of the *exo-erythrocytic cycle* (EE). The reappearance of malaria after clinical cure results from the parasite's ability to persist in the tissues in this (EE) form. The eventual discharge of merozoites from these EE forms into the bloodstream, results in reinvasion of red blood cells so producing a relapse. The exo-erythrocytic cycle occurs in *P. vivax*, *P. ovale* and *P. malariae* infections; although doubt has recently been cast as to whether an (EE) cycle occurs in *P. malariae*. *P. vivax* can usually produce relapses up to 3 years after infection; while *P. malariae* has occasionally relapsed 10, 20 or even 30 years after infection. In *P. falciparum* malaria the liver phase is said not to persist, it follows therefore that when adequate treatment for the erythrocytic cycle is given relapses do not occur. It is therefore rare for *P. falciparum* infections to relapse after 1 year of freedom from exposure to infection, although a few authentic cases with long intervals prior to relapse have been described.

Malaria pigment is derived from the haemoglobin of the invaded red cell and is composed of haem plus denatured protein.

Epidemiology

The effect that malaria exerts on any population is largely governed by its epidemiological pattern. In this respect two epidemiological extremes are described—stable and unstable malaria. The salient differences are shown below.

Stable malaria	Unstable malaria
1 Transmission occurs throughout the year. Fairly uniform intensity of transmission. Pattern repeats itself annually with astonishing regularity, showing little variation over several years.	Transmission seasonal—intensity of transmission variable. Liable to flare up into dramatic epidemics.

2 Potent resistance in the community due to prevailing intense transmission.	General lack of immunity in the community due to the low level of transmission, which only occasionally becomes intense.
3 Main impact of disease in young children.	Impact of disease on all age-groups.
4 Difficult to eradicate.	Eradicated with greater ease than stable malaria.
5 Classical areas where it occurs—West Africa, Lowlands of New Guinea.	Classical areas—high plateau of Ethiopia or Highlands of New Guinea.

Immunity to malaria is well developed among populations living in 'stable' malaria areas and can be considered under four main headings: (a) Cellular, (b) Humoral, (c) Inherited factors in the blood and (d) Racial.

Cellular Immunity

The response of phagocytic cells in malaria was shown in early histological studies and for many years resistance to the disease was considered to be exclusively cellular in nature. The reticulo-endothelial system undergoes proliferation during malarial infection and the macrophages of the spleen, liver and bone marrow have been shown to phagocytose parasitised and unparasitised erythrocytes, isolated parasites and malarial pigment. In areas of stable malaria, large amounts of this pigment are continuously being engulfed by the reticulo-endothelial system over periods of years, and the part that this possible 'blockade' plays in the immunological mechanism of the host, both in the fields of infection and malignancy, has still to be elucidated. There is considerable evidence that T-cells are required to initiate mechanisms which lead to the elimination of malaria parasites.

Humoral Immunity

Past studies have demonstrated and stressed the importance of humoral immunity. Several workers have demonstrated that the concentration of gamma globulin in the serum of the newborn African infant is considerably higher than corresponding values reported from Europe. It was further shown that, in 'stable' areas, malarial infection contributes significantly to the maintenance of high γ-globulin levels in all subjects after the first year of life, and moreover that γ-globulin prepared from the sera of adults immune to malaria has a consistent therapeutic effect when administered to West African children suffering from heavy *P. falciparum* infection. Serum from the cord blood of infants born of immune mothers has a similar effect. It is now generally accepted that acquired malarial immunity is basically dependent upon the presence of circulating antibody which is associated with 7S γ-globulin fraction

(IgG) of serum. It is probable that the two mechanisms of defence in malaria, the cellular (through the reticulo-endothelial system) and the humoral (through IgG immunoglobulin) are interdependent.

Advances in continuous culture techniques have facilitated the use of *in vitro* assays for the study of mechanisms of action of immune serum in falciparum malaria. It has recently been also shown that humoral factors play a role in immunity to sporozoite stages of the infection.

Inherited Factors in the Blood

It has been postulated that the following hereditary red cell traits protect against the lethal effects of malaria: (1) haemoglobin S, (2) haemoglobin C, (3) haemoglobin E, (4) HbF, (5) glucose-6-phosphate dehydrogenase deficiency. The only convincing evidence of protection to date concerns sickle-cell haemoglobin and G-6-PD deficiency; while there is no evidence that HbC has any protective value. Further studies are required to assess the situation in relation to HbE and HbF.

Racial Immunity

It has long been known that Negroes in the USA had a vivax infection rate lower than that of whites and that it was more difficult to infect them with this species in the course of malarial therapy. The most evident consequence of resistance to *P. vivax* in Negroes occurs in West Africa, where, in many regions, it cannot be found in the indigenous population; yet the parasite is common in the inhabitants of the Eastern Congo and East Africa. It has recently been shown that the Duffy blood group acts as a receptor for *P. vivax* and in populations where *P. vivax* is rare, the incidence of Duffy negative persons is high.

Laboratory diagnosis

The certain diagnosis of malaria is parasitological and is made by examining thick blood films stained with Field or Giemsa stains. Although species diagnosis can be made on thick films it is usually made on thin films stained with Leishman or Giemsa stains. As a rule only ring forms and gametocytes are found in the peripheral blood in falciparum malaria unless the infection is severe, in which case, schizonts also appear. In cases of vivax, malariae and ovale malaria all forms of development of the asexual parasites are found. Various more sophisticated techniques such as the fluorescent antibody test (FAT), ELISA and haemagglutination tests are valuable adjuncts to diagnosis, but do not supersede the direct microscopical identification of the parasite in stained blood smears. These serological tests are more useful for epidemiological assessment than clinical diagnosis.

Control

The control of malaria is either designed to protect particular individuals from infection or to prevent transmission and thereby protect the whole community. Control measures are therefore aimed at the individual, against the vector or to provide communal protection.

(a) *The individual*
Individual protective measures are best based on the regular use of a prophylactic drug and of mosquito nets over the bed, to which may be added, when there is a general mosquito nuisance, house-screening and repellents such as dimethyl phthalate.

CHEMOPROPHYLAXIS   Several basic points must be emphasised at the very outset. *Firstly*, it must never be assumed that chemoprophylaxis, even when taken regularly, will certainly protect against malaria — *protection is relative.* Thus, every non-immune person residing temporarily or for longer periods in a malarious area must be warned that, if he feels ill, malaria must still be excluded as a possible diagnosis. This is particularly relevant because of the spread of resistance to many antimalarial drugs and the absence of accurate maps of the distribution of resistance to the antimalarials in current use. Evidence of resistance based on *clinical* experience often without concomitant and competent microscopic diagnosis of malaria has aggravated an already complex situation.

Secondly, accept with the greatest scepticism that any potentially malarious area is free from risk. Anecdotes that in West Africa, for example, cities are malaria-free are fraught with great danger and quite wrong.

Thirdly, malaria can be acquired at relatively short stops on a journey, e.g. refuelling of the aeroplane.

Fourthly, it is important to have adequate blood levels of antimalarials by the time a person is at risk. This can be achieved by taking a dose the day before departure. Despite this, it is considered wise to begin antimalarials one week before travelling in order to get used to the habit and to detect rare cases of idiosyncracy.

For practical purposes, the antimalarials available for chemoprophylaxis are the following:
(a) The antifolates — i.e. Proguanil and pyrimethamine.
(b) The 4-aminoquinolines — i.e. Chloroquine and Amodiaquine.
(c) The potentiating combinations — i.e. Fansidar and Maloprim.

The pharmacological basis of these mixtures is that the individual components — sulphadoxine + pyrimethamine   or   dapsone + pyrimethamine — act at different sites along the same metabolic pathway and impede folate metabolism in parasites that are resistant to single anti-folates.

(a) *Chloroquine-resistant falciparum malaria* The precise distribution of chloroquine-resistant malaria changes so rapidly that up to date advice should always be sought from WHO or other recognised centres throughout the world. The choice of antimalarial in these areas is between Fansidar and Maloprim.

1 Fansidar (pyrimethamine 25 mg + sulfadoxine 500 mg): one tablet weekly.
2 Maloprim (pyrimethamine 12.5 mg + diaminodiphenyl sulphone 100 mg): one tablet weekly.

Persons who are sensitive to sulphonamides should not receive Fansidar and be given Maloprim instead, initially under supervision, to ascertain that there is no cross-sensitivity. Those also sensitive to dapsone have to be put on chloroquine or proguanil with a clear warning that they run a greater malaria risk than if they had been able to take Fansidar or Maloprim.

(b) *Chloroquine-sensitive malaria areas* The choice of antimalarials for these areas lies between proguanil, pyrimethamine, chloroquine or amodiaquine.
1 Proguanil: 100–200 mg daily.
2 Pyrimethamine: 25 mg weekly.
3 Chloroquine: 300 mg (base) weekly.
4 Amodiaquine: 300 mg(base) weekly.

Proguanil even when taken for many years has a very low toxicity and the daily dosage regime is easier to remember. However, resistance to this drug occurs.

Pyrimethamine being tasteless is easily administrated to children. However, accidental poisoning for this very reason has occurred more often than with other antimalarials. Resistance to the drug occurs, and reported breakthroughs seem frequent.

Chloroquine is highly effective and the drug of choice for short-term visits. For those taking up residence in malarious areas for periods over three years proguanil is a good alternative.

The duration of continuing antimalarials after returning from an endemic area is *four weeks* and the need to continue for this time must be stressed.

Resistance to chloroquine and amodiaquine has been reported from parts of South America, South-East Asia, the Western Pacific and now seems to be spreading to Africa where *authentic* cases have been reported in Tanzania, Kenya, Uganda, Zambia, the Comores and Madagascar. In Africa the predominant resistance is RI (see below). A number of strains of *P. falciparum* that are resistant to the 4-aminoquinolines also show resistance to mepacrine, primaquine, quinine, proguanil and pyrimethamine. Resistance and sensitivity to chloroquine are not absolute, and a system of grading has been devised—RI, RII and RIII resistance.

RI = Clinical and parasitological response *but* recrudescence a few weeks after treatment.
RII = Clinical response but *no* parasitological response.

RIII = Neither clinical nor parasitological response.

There have been no reports of resistance to the 4-aminoquinolines in any species of human *Plasmodium* other than *P. falciparum*. An *in vitro* technique is now available for the assessment of chloroquine-resistance.

MALARIA VACCINE. The techniques which are now available for the cultivation of blood forms of the parasite represent an important step forward. Nonetheless, further development is required before cultivation of parasites can be fully exploited for vaccine production. Further work is also required on the characterisation and fractionisation of antigens and although remarkable progress is being done in this field with the development of new techniques, e.g. hybridoma, it is estimated that it will take about 10 years before a safe and effective vaccine may be available for widespread communal use.

(b) *The vector*

The control of the mosquito has been attempted in two ways, (1) attack on the adult mosquito, i.e. imagicidal control. The choice of method depends on the nature of the terrain and on the habitats of the vector mosquito and (2) prevention of mosquito breeding by larval control.

IMAGICIDAL CONTROL. Several important vector species consist in fact of a complex of sibling species with similar morphological patterns, but with specific genetic and behavioural characteristics. The amenability of vectors to imagicidal control therefore varies from area to area and this inherent biological difficulty has been compounded by the problem of widespread resistance to insecticides. Thus about 41 species of Anopheline mosquitoes are known to be resistant to Dieldrin, 24 to DDT, and many species have developed double resistance. It is finally becoming acknowledged that resistance is probably the biggest single obstacle in the struggle against vector-borne disease and is mainly responsible for preventing successful malaria eradication in many countries.

LARVAL CONTROL has, however, been used successfully to control malaria in Singapore and in urban areas of Malaysia. Control of breeding can be effected either by means of larvicides or more permanent measures such as subsoil drainage, depending on existing local conditions. Anopheline and other mosquito larvae may be killed by heavy oiling by antimalarial oil (with or without a little added insecticide) or by light spraying with kerosene containing high concentration of insecticide (e.g. 5 per cent DDT). The former treatment also kills weeds in irrigation ditches and seems to have a slightly residual action; the latter saves labour. Both liquids are intended to spread freely across water surface and must possess good spreading pressure to overcome natural contamination of pools. If drainage is used, it must be efficiently carried out and permanent drains must be kept unblocked and functional by regular supervision.

(c) The community

The post-1945 era of DDT and other synthetic insecticides saw a significant worldwide decrease in the prevalence of malaria, especially in countries in the temperate regions, in some tropical islands, and certain continental tropical areas. In many countries, however, malaria resisted the measures applied, due to complex operational, technical, administrative and financial reasons; the widespread emergence of resistance and the lack of adequate basic health services.

For the immediate future the concept of global malaria eradication has been dropped and the main thrust is to devise ways and means to reduce malaria morbidity and mortality. Thus trials are being carried out in various countries in which drug prophylaxis with chloroquine is compared with prompt systematic cure of all febrile cases, especially amongst children.

In Papua New Guinea the authorities are attempting to organise antimalarial operations using a novel decentralized approach, placing emphasis on the direct active participation of the community. The measures to be applied by *locally recruited* and trained workers include residual spraying, larviciding, and mass drug administration. The reduction of malaria morbidity and mortality in the community is the mainstay of control.

MALARIA IN PREGNANCY.   There is little doubt that, for a pregnant woman, malaria poses a greater hazard than any of the prophylactic drugs currently advocated.

In *semi-immune primiparae* there is epidemiological, clinical and laboratory evidence that a temporary attenuation of immunity occurs resulting in maternal and foetal morbidity and mortality. In endemic areas of malaria where the parasite is chloroquine sensitive, it is sound obstetric practice to administer a curative dose of chloroquine to pregnant women at their first attendance at the antenatal clinic and to continue with weekly prophylaxis either with pyrimethamine 25 mg or chloroquine 300 mg (base) weekly throughout the course of pregnancy and the first month of the puerperium. There is, to date, no evidence of teratogenicity *in humans* with either of these drugs in the dosage recommended, moreover in endemic areas indigenous pregnant women rarely attend antenatal clinics before the second month. In chloroquine-resistant areas curative therapy with Fansidar whenever indicated is a feasible alternative to regular weekly chemoprophylaxis with Fansidar or Maloprim (see above).

Malaria—Summary

1 *Occurrence*—World-wide $60°N$–$40°S$ of equator
2 *Organisms*—P. falciparum, P. vivax, P. malariae, P. ovale
3 *Reservoir of infection*—Man
4 *Mode of transmission*—Bite of Anopheles mosquitoes
5 *Control*— (i) Chemotherapy
             (ii) Vector control

THE TRYPANOSOMIASES

The trypanosome species pathogenic for man can be classified into two groups: (1) those transmitted through the bite of a blood-sucking fly, i.e. *Trypanosoma brucei gambiense* and *T. brucei rhodesiense*, which cause African trypanosomiasis and (2) those transmitted by faecal contamination from an arthropod vector, e.g. *T. cruzi*, which causes South African trypanosomiasis (Chagas' disease).

(1) African Trypanosomiasis

African trypanosomiasis is caused by either *Trypanosoma b. gambiense* or *T. b. rhodesiense*, and the infection is conveyed to man by the bites of flies of the genus *Glossina*. The *incubation period* is usually between 2 and 3 weeks but can be very much longer (6 years).

Medical geography
African trypanosomiasis is confined to that part of Africa lying between latitudes 10° N and 25° S. *T. b. rhodesiense* infection is limited to Kenya, Tanzania, Uganda, Malawi, Zambia, Rhodesia, Mozambique, Northern Botswana and South-East Angola, while *T. b. gambiense* is more widespread, extending from West Africa through Central Africa to Uganda, Tanzania and Malawi. Comparatively recent epidemics of *T. b. rhodesiense* have been reported from Botswana, the Southern Sudan, Ethiopia and Zaire. It is estimated that 35 million people and about 25 million cattle are exposed to the risk of infection.

Applied biology
In man, *T. b. gambiense* and *T. b. rhodesiense* are morphologically identical, varying in length from 10 μm to 30 μm with a pointed anterior end and blunt posterior. The cytoplasm stains blue with a Romanowsky stain, there is a large oval centrally placed nucleus, a small posteriorly placed kinetoplast, an undulating membrane projecting beyond the anterior end of the body. Other morphological forms in blood are also seen. *T. b. gambiense* and *T. b. rhodesiense* have a similar life cycle. When blood containing trypanosomes is ingested by a suitable species of *Glossina*, the trypanosomes reach the intestine of the fly and undergo cyclical development, eventually developing into infective metacyclic forms in the salivary glands. These are introduced when saliva is injected into the wound produced during the act of feeding. Multiplication of the trypanosomes occurs in the blood. The entire cycle of development in the fly, after feeding on blood containing trypanosomes, is about 3 weeks (extrinsic incubation period).

The main vectors of Gambian sleeping sickness are the riverine species of *Glossina: G. palpalis* and *G. tachinoides*; while the chief vectors of Rhodesian sleeping sickness are *G. morsitans, G. swynnertoni* and *G. pallipides*.

Epidemiology

The maintenance of human trypanosomiasis in Africa depends on the interrelations of three elements—the vertebrate host, the parasite and the vector responsible for transmission. Sleeping sickness is essentially a disease of rural populations and its prevalence is largely dependent on the degree of contact between man and tsetse, this is particularly so with Gambiense sleeping sickness. Thus at the height of the dry season, riverine species of fly are often restricted to isolated pools of water which are essential to the local human population for so many of their activities, e.g. collecting water and firewood, washing, fishing and cultivation. The sacred groves of some religions may also provide foci of intimate man/fly contact. Over recent years there has been an increasing incidence and dispersion of *T. b. rhodesiense* sleeping sickness on the north-east shores of Lake Victoria, associated with increased fishing activity and increasing and irregular settlement of the tsetse-fly belt of south-east Uganda.

Each species of tsetse has particular requirements in regard to climate and vegetation, which determine its distribution. All of them tend to concentrate seasonally in habitats offering permanent shade and humidity. The distribution of the fly thus varies with the season, and in addition it advances and retreats spatially at intervals of years. Population density affects the incidence of the disease, which is sporadic at densities below 50 per square kilometre, and is liable to become epidemic at densities up to 500 or so per square kilometre, above which it disappears because tsetse habitats are eliminated.

In general, in endemic conditions, the incidence of sleeping sickness is greater in males. In contrast to this usual picture it has been reported that in the Gambia the women and older girls were most affected because they were exposed while working in the rice fields. In epidemic conditions no clear sex difference in incidence occurs and the proportion of children infected rises sharply. Adverse environmental climatic conditions can effect the mean period between emergence of the young fly (pupa) and the taking of the first blood meal as well as the period of development of trypanosomes in the vector; these factors can influence the chance of transmission of the disease. *T. b. rhodesiense* has been isolated from a bush-buck, and so a reservoir in wild animals—long suspected—has been proved. This wild animal reservoir plays an important role in the epidemiology of the human disease (see Fig. 6.3). *T. b. rhodesiense* has been found in lion, hyena, hartebeest and domestic cattle. There is now increasing evidence confirming the suspicion that there is also an animal reservoir for *T. b. gambiense*. Organisms indistinguishable from *T. b. gambiense* have been found in domestic and wild animals using the new technique of biochemical characterisation of stains. It remains to be shown what part these infections in animals play in the epidemiology of the human disease.

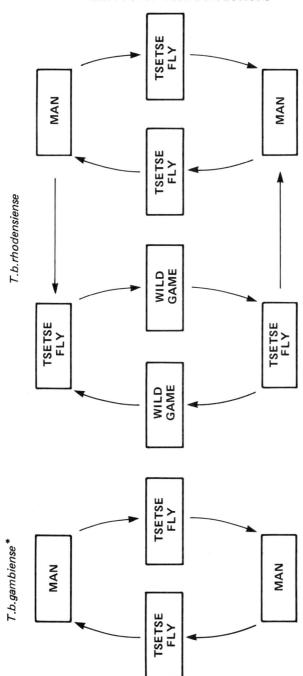

Fig. 6.3 Epidemiology of African Trypanosomiasis

*Possible animal reservoir now strongly suspected

Laboratory diagnosis

Microscopical examination of blood, lymph fluid, serous fluids, or CSF with or without concentration techniques may reveal the organism in fresh or suitably stained preparations. *In vitro* culture of trypanosomes has proved sensitive and reliable, as has the complement-fixation test. A fluorescent antibody test and a card flocculation method, for the serodiagnosis of African trypanosomiasis have been used; and numerous other sophisticated techniques have been developed for trypanosome identification. A raised serum bilirubin level, excess urobilinogen and bilirubinuria is common in early acutely febrile *Rhodesiense* patients but these indices are not raised in the late stages of the disease. The bromsulphalein excretion test is also abnormal in the acutely febrile early-stage associated with a precipitous fall in the serum albumin. In the late stages of both *gambiense* and *rhodesiense* infections the total plasma proteins are high and the γ-globulin grossly increased, except in wasted patients in whom the total serum proteins and especially albumin are low. The lymphocytes and protein content of the CSF are invariably raised and sugar low when the central nervous system is involved. The fluorescent antibody test has been applied to the CSF of patients with sleeping sickness, antibodies were found in all the samples which showed pathological changes. The test is sensitive, specific and suitable for the early detection of involvement of the nervous system.

The serum levels of IgM, IgA and IgG are raised in both *T. b. gambiense* and *T. b. rhodesiense* infections. High levels of M-antiglobulins (rheumatoid-factor-like globulins) can occur in African trypanosomiasis. EEG sometimes shows a disturbed wave pattern, and air encephalography, dilatation of the ventricles when brain involvement has occurred.

Control

This is directed against the parasite in man and against the fly.

(a) The individual

The survey of infected communities and treatment of all those found infected rapidly lowers the incidence and reduces the reservoir of infection. Medical field units have been particularly successful using this approach both in West and East Africa.

Chemoprophylaxis, using pentamidine 200 mg in one single intramuscular injection, will give protection against *T. b. gambiense* for some 6 months in individuals or in circumscribed communities, e.g. labour force. It is generally felt that chemoprophylaxis against *T. b. rhodesiense* is not effective and possibly undesirable.

The wearing of long trousers and of long-sleeved shirts gives some protection against the bites of tsetse fly. Vehicles which have to pass through heavily tsetse-infected country should be fly-proofed with mosquito gauze. Individuals who are sensitive to insect bites may find repellents (dimethylphthalate or diethyl toluamide) useful quite apart from the protection which they may give against infection, for a severe local reaction to the tsetse bite is not uncommon.

The commonly used drugs for African trypanosomiasis are pentamidine, suramin, melarsoprol and nitrofurazone. Pentamidine is often not active against *T. b. rhodesiense*. Melarsoprol is the only drug used for the routine treatment of patients with CNS involvement. Nitrofurazone can be employed in melarsoprol resistant cases. Berenil has been reported to give satisfactory results in African sleeping sickness but is at present only manufactured for veterinary use.

(b) *The fly*

Control of the fly can be effected in a variety of ways—(1) chemical, (2) land use management, (3) biological and (4) the use of traps.

CHEMICAL CONTROL   The most favoured method of tsetse control in many years is still *ground spraying* and DDT or dieldrin are usually used for this. A long-acting pyrethroid NRDC 143 has recently given most promising result. *Aerial spraying* techniques have been extensively developed in recent years applying aerosols of endosulfan or ultra low volume (ULV) formulations. The need to integrate tsetse control programmes into rural development has long been recognised. Thus organised *land settlement* has been used to control sleeping sickness in both East and West Africa. Large scale tsetse reclamation projects are motivated by the current impact of infestation and the need to accommodate a rapidly expanding human population aspiring to a higher standard of living—the development of tsetse is modified by this type of ecological control.

BIOLOGICAL METHODS   include the use of predators and parasites as well as genetic control. The genetic methods explored include hybridisation, the production of heterozygotes for chromosomal translocations, and the release of males sterilised by irradiation or chemical means.

TRAPS   Simple mechanical traps have given encouraging results in field trials and may soon be introduced as a control measure.

(c) *The community*

Pentamidine diisethionate in doses of 200–250 mg given to each labourer on engagement and thereafter at 4 to 6 months intervals is a very effective way of protecting labour forces working in trypanosomiasis-affected areas. This prophylactic measure should be applied to gangs of labourers working on road, railways or similar works in areas of high risk. Such controlled groups can be protected effectively and without difficulty.

Chemoprophylaxis for communities has been widely practised in most of the endemic areas of francophone West and Equatorial Africa, but nowhere has the hope of eradication been fulfilled and the dangers of 'cryptic infections'* are very real. The disadvantage of this control measure is that if it is used on recently infected persons who have not been diagnosed, the parasites are driven from the blood and may establish themselves in the central nervous system. It is mandatory, therefore, before using mass prophylaxis that every care must be taken to detect all infected persons.

African Trypanosomiases—Summary

1 *Occurrence*—Africa 10°N-25°S of equator
2 *Organisms*—T. b. gambiense, T. b. rhodesiense
3 *Reservoir of infection*—Man
4 *Mode of transmission*—Bite of tsetse fly
5 *Control*— (i) Treatment of tsetse fly
　　　　　　 (ii) Chemoprophylaxis
　　　　　　 (iii) Reduction of man/fly contact

(2) American Trypanosomiasis

Chagas' disease may present as congenital, acute or chronic forms. The main impact of the infection especially in children is on the heart, enteromegaly is common in chronic Chagas' disease.

Medical geography
The infection is found in Central and South America, especially in Brazil, Venezuela, Colombia and Northern Argentina.

Applied biology
The adult trypanosomes, which measure about 20 μm in length with a central nucleus and very large posterior kinetoplast, are found in the blood. When ingested by blood-sucking reduviid bugs, after a period of development in the invertebrate host's intestinal canal lasting 8–10 days, trypanosomes, known as 'metacyclic' forms reappear in the hindgut and are passed with the faeces of the insect. Infection of man takes place when faecal matter is rubbed into scratch wounds and the wound caused by the bite of the insect. Certain trypanosomes leave the bloodstream and invade various organs, especially the myocardium. Here they assume a leishmanoid appearance and rapid multiplication by binary fission takes place forming nests of Leishman-Donovan bodies. At a later stage these leishmanoid forms elongate and are eventually transformed into trypanosomes, which make their way through the tissues and into the bloodstream.

Epidemiology
The reservoir of infection is man. The most important vector bugs belong to the genera *Triatoma, Panstrongylus* and *Rhodnius*. These

---

* 'Cryptic infections' are characterised by gross abnormalities of the cerebrospinal fluid with no trypanosomes in the blood or glands.

reduviid bugs are largely disseminated throughout the rural areas of Latin America where the mud huts of the agricultural workers are their favourite habitats. The usual mode of transmission is by rubbing infected faeces into cuts of abrasions or into the intact skin or mucous membrane. Transmission occurs predominantly at night since reduviid bugs attack only in darkness. The disease is observed at any age, although children are mainly affected. Other unusual methods of infection are transplacental, by blood transfusion, and laboratory transmission from infected syringes or blood. Although an animal reservoir of infection has been established its role in the epidemiology of human disease is uncertain. Symptoms usually develop about 2 weeks after infective trypanosomes enter the skin.

Infections with another trypanosome, *T. rangeli*, have been found in various animals, and human infections with this trypanosome have occasionally also been reported. In contrast to *T. cruzi* the transmission of this disease is by the actual bite of the reduviid bug rather than through its excreta.

Laboratory diagnosis
Trypanosomes may be demonstrated in wet and stained thick blood films; in lymph gland juice, or in CSF and may be cultured on NNN medium. A complement-fixation test—employing antigen from flagellates cultivated *in vitro*—is widely used and is the most sensitive means of diagnosis. Immunofluorescence has been used in the diagnosis of Chagas' disease.

Control

Chagas' disease flourishes only where social and economic levels are low, and long-term control measures involve economic rehabilitation, in particular, better housing.

(a) The individual
Personal prophylaxis consists in avoiding sleeping in houses liable to harbour the vectors and in using bed nets. In endemic areas blood donors for transfusion should be carefully screened and rejected if infected.

(b) The community
Mud hovels with thatched roofs need to be replaced with houses of materials giving no harbourage to bugs. Residual insecticides, especially dieldrin (at $1.6\,g/m^2$) or benzene hexachloride at $(0.5\,g/m^2)$, applied to floors, walls and thatch will eliminate most of the vectors, but reinfestation occurs in a few months.

American Trypanosomiases—Summary

1 *Occurrence*—South America
2 *Organism*—*T. cruzi*

3 *Reservoir of infection*—Man
4 *Mode of transmission*—Rubbing infected reduviid bugs' faeces into
       skin
5 *Control*— (i) Better housing
       (ii) Using bed nets

THE LEISHMANIASES

It is convenient (though not strictly justifiable) to subdivide the Leishmaniases into three clinical types: the visceral, the cutaneous and the
muco-cutaneous (Table 6.5).

Medical geography
The Leishmaniases occur over wide areas of the globe from China across
Asia, India, Persia and Afghanistan, the Caucasus, the Middle and Near

Table 6.5 Classification of leishmaniases (From Peters, W. O. and Gilles, H. M. Colour Atlas of Tropical Medicine and Parasitology. 2nd edn. Wolfe Medical Publications Ltd.)

Type of Disease	Species	Main Localities	Main Vectors	Reservoirs
VISCERAL LEISHMANIASIS (KALA-AZAR) 60% betweem 10 and 20 years of age	L. donovani L. infantum complex	India China (N. of Yangtze) USSR Iraq Sudan	P. argentipes P. chinensis ⎫ P. major ⎬ P. major ⎭ P. langeroni orientalis	Man dog, ? fox ? jackal rodents, serval cat, genet
		Kenya Uganda	P. martini	rodents
INFANTILE KALA-AZAR 80–90% under 10 years old	L. infantum complex	France Mediterranean basin	P. ariasi ⎫ P. perniciosus ⎬ P. major ⎭	fox, dog.
	'L. chagasi'	Brazil Paraguay Venezuela	P. longipalpis ⎫⎬⎭	fox, dog
POST K-A DERMAL LEISHMANOID	L. donovani L. infantum complex	(as classical kala-azar)		
ORONASAL K-A	L. infantum complex	Sudan Ethiopia		may lead to man-man spread
CUTANEOUS LEISHMANIASIS (OLD WORLD)	L. tropica tropica (= minor)	India Mediterranean basin Middle East	P. sergenti ⎫⎬ P. papatasi ⎭	dog rodents,? dog, gerbils
		Iran USSR (urban)	P. ansarii P. mongolensis	dog rodents, gerbils

Table 6.5 (continued)

Type of Disease	Species	Localities	Main Vectors	Main Reservoirs
ORIENTAL SORE	L. major	Iran USSR (rural)	P. caucasicus ⎱ P. papatasi ⎰	gerbils, merions
		Saudi Arabia Libya	? ?	
	L. tropica complex	Tanzania Senegal Namibia	? P. duboscqi P. rossi	? rodents hyrax spp.
SINGLE SORE AND DIFFUSA	L. aethiopica	Ethiopia Kenya	P. longipes ?	hyrax spp. ?
CUTANEOUS AND MUCO-CUTANEOUS (NEW WORLD)	L. mexicana mexicana	Mexico Guatemala ⎱ Honduras ⎰	P. olmeca	forest rodents
SINGLE SORE AND DIFFUSA	L. m. pifanoi	Venezuela	? P. panamensis ? P. flaviscutellata	forest rodents
	L. m. amazonensis	Amazon basin ? Trinidad	P. flaviscutellata	forest rodents, opossums
	L. mexicana complex	Costa Rica ⎱ Panama ⎰ Matto Grosso ⎰	?	forest rodents
ESPUNDIA	L. braziliensis braziliensis	Brazil* Peru Ecuador Bolivia Venezuela Paraguay Colombia	P. pessoai P. intermedia P. wellcomei P. paraensis ? P. migonei ? P. whitmani ? P. anduzei	forest rodents ? forest rodents, ? paca
PIAN BOIS	L. braziliensis guyanensis	Guyanas Brazil (Nor- thern states) ? Venezuela	P. umbratilis P. whitmani	sloths and other arboreal mammals
USUALLY SINGLE SORES, SOME LYMPHATIC SPREAD	L. braziliensis panamensis	Panama ? Central America to Colombia	P. trapidoi P. ylephiletor P. gomezi P. panamensis	sloths marmoset kinkajou olingo
UTA	L. peruviana	Peru (West of Andes)	? P. noguchii P. verrucarum P. peruensis	dog

* Forested areas East of Andean chain

East, the Mediterranean basin, East and West Africa, the Sudan and South America. There is an increasing awareness of the importance of the leishmaniases as public health problems, and of the seriousness of recent outbreaks in South America, Asia and Africa. A conservative estimate of the number of new cases is 400 000 per year.

Applied biology

There are two phases in the life cycle of Leishmania: an aflagellate—*amastigote*—(leishmanial) rounded form which occurs in man and in animal reservoir hosts; and a flagellate—*promastigote*—(leptomonad) form which is found in the vector sandfly and in culture media. The former is oval (2μm × 3μm) and consists of cytoplasm, a round nucleus, and a small, more deeply staining, rod-shaped kinetoplast or rhizoplast and a vacuole. It is known as the Leishman-Donovan (L-D) body. In man leishmania multiply by binary fission. They are most commonly found in the large mononuclear cells of the reticulo-endothelial system, especially in the liver, spleen and bone marrow; leishmanial forms are also found in the leucocytes of the circulating blood.

When the appropriate sandfly feeds on an infected person, it ingests the parasites with the blood meal. These develop in its gut into the flagellate (promastigote) forms: these migrate forwards, multiply and form a mass which may block the pharynx of the sandfly. When the sandfly next feeds, some of these leptomonads become dislodged and are injected into the new host in the process of feeding; they again assume the leishmanial form. They are phagocytosed by macrophages, multiply by simple division and cause the cells to rupture. They are then carried in the circulation to the sites already referred to where they give rise to the characteristic lesions. Following specific treatment in some cases they pass from their visceral habitat—liver, spleen, etc., back to the skin, giving rise to the condition described as *post-kala-azar dermal leishmaniasis*.

The above life-history applies to *L. donovani*, which is the causative organism of visceral leishmaniasis. In cutaneous and muco-cutaneous leishmaniasis, the multiplication of the amastigote forms takes place in the skin and the appropriate sandfly vectors become infected by feeding on a cutaneous lesion.

Biochemical taxonomy, using the excreted factor (EF) serotyping, enzyme analysis and DNA buoyant density determination is being used to identify leishmanial strains from different geographical areas and to sub-divide the *L. braziliensis* complex.

Epidemiology

The epidemiology of the leishmaniases, whether visceral, cutaneous or muco-cutaneous, is in every case determined by a reservoir of infection (animal, man or both) from which local *Phlebotomine* sandflies, infect themselves by ingesting amastigote forms from blood or infected tissues. The climatic conditions of the various foci of leishmaniasis range from arid to tropical humid and the terrain and altitude are equally variable. Modes of transmission other than by sandflies, e.g. marital, blood transfusion, and intra-uterine infection, are of little epidemiological significance. With the possible exception of Indian kala-azar it is increasingly being recognised that in most endemic foci the leishmaniases are zoonoses.

VISCERAL LEISHMANIASIS

There are three distinct types of visceral leishmaniasis: (*a*) Indian kala-azar, (*b*) kala-azar associated predominantly with a canine reservoir and (*c*) African kala-azar. Kala-azar is essentially a rural disease, and *L. donovani* is now accepted as the cause of all forms of kala-azar. Post-kala-azar dermal leishmaniasis occurs as a sequel of visceral leishmaniasis. The *incubation period* of visceral leishmaniasis ranges from 2 weeks to more than 1 year.

(a) *Indian kala-azar* is unique in so far as man is the only known natural host of the infection. The vector *P. argentipes* breeds in close proximity to human habitations and feeds readily on man. All age-groups are susceptible with a peak incidence at 10–20 years. Devastating epidemics may occur. The lesions of post-kala-azar dermal leishmaniasis are of epidemiological importance since they contain numerous L-D bodies in the dermis and are readily accessible to sandflies, they are a feature of Indian kala-azar but are also seen elsewhere.

(b) *Kala-azar predominantly associated with a canine reservoir.* In the Mediterranean basin, Portugal, North Africa, the Caucasus, China, Brazil and other parts of South America, the domestic dog, fox and jackal are very important reservoirs of human infection.

Visceral leishmaniasis associated with a canine reservoir is predominantly a disease of children under 10 years. The most important vector sandflies are *Phlebotomus chinensis* in China, *P. longipalpis* in Brazil, and *P. perniciosus* in the Mediterranean.

(c) *African kala-azar.* The epidemiology of the disease in the Sudan and Kenya presents unique features differing from those described above. There is a primary stage in the skin (leishmanoma) which lasts for some time before the symptoms of kala-azar develop, and this is of prime epidemiological importance; in this area rodents may form a reservoir of infection. There is a definite relationship between the proximity of homes to termite hills and the incidence of kala-azar. The most important vectors are *P. martini* in Kenya and *P. orientalis* in the Sudan where the disease attacks all age-groups but is commoner in adults than in children. Both these vectors are out-of-doors biters. The human distribution is affected by immunity as well as by relative exposure to infection.

CUTANEOUS LEISHMANIASIS

Several varieties of cutaneous leishmaniasis have been described from the Old and New World. These include (1) oriental sore, (2) chiclero ulcer, (3) uta, (4) leishmaniasis tegumentaria diffusa, (5) Ethiopian cutaneous leishmaniasis, (6) lupoid leishmaniasis.

(1) Oriental Sore

(tropical sore; bouton d'Orient; Aleppo, Baghdad or Delhi boil; Pendah sore).

Epidemiology

This cutaneous infection is widely distributed in the Indian subcontinent, the Middle East, Ethiopia, Southern Russia, the Mediterranean countries, Nigeria, China and the Sudan. The most important vectors are *P. papatasii* and *P. sergenti*. The disease is most commonly seen in children, and in high endemic areas most of the adult population have been infected in childhood. The parasite responsible is *L. tropica* of which two varieties are recognised on clinical and epidemiological grounds, *L. tropica* var. *major*, is an infection of rodents occasionally transmitted to man which produces a disease with a short incubation period, rapid course of under 6 months, much inflammatory reaction and the 'moist' lesion it produces contains few parasites; while *L. tropica minor* is an infection of dogs, only occasionally man, characterised by a 'dry' lesion containing many parasites with a long incubation period, course of over 1 year and a mild inflammatory reaction.

Immunity to *L. tropica* follows spontaneous cure and experimental attempt at reinfection very often (but not invariably) gives negative results; moreover, 98 per cent of cases of oriental sore show a delayed hypersensitivity test (Montenegro reaction) in response to the intradermal inoculation of dead and washed leptomonads.

(2) Chiclero Ulcer

The cutaneous leishmaniases of the New World—chiclero ulcer, uta, and leishmaniasis tegumentaria diffusa—are scattered in Central and South America over an area extending from 22°N to 30°S of the equator. They are characterised epidemiologically by the fact that they are (i) zoonoses and (ii) predominatly non-urban diseases, usually confined to the forest regions or jungles.

Epidemiology

L. mexicana is the cause of 'chiclero's ulcer' in Mexico and neighbouring countries. The infection is virtually restricted to people who habitually live and work in the forests with the result that women and children are rarely infected. It is an 'occupational disease' of the chicleros who spend a considerable time in the forests bleeding the *Sapodella* trees for chewing-gum latex. The disease is almost always limited to a single dermal lesion, usually in the ear. Forest rodents are the important animal reservoirs and man is an accidental host. Transmission of *L. mexicana* is by *Phlebotomus pessoanus* in British Honduras.

With *L. mexicana* a solid and long-lasting immunity is developed from the infection and the development of this immunity occurs very early in the course of the disease.

(3) Uta

L. peruviana causes cutaneous lesions on exposed sites such as the face, arm and leg—and the disease is known as uta in Peru. The infection occurs primarily in dogs which are the reservoir from which man acquires the disease. House-dwelling sandflies, e.g. *P. peruensis*, are the vectors of infection.

(4) Leishmaniasis Tegumentaria Diffusa

L. pifanoi causes a disseminated form of cutaneous leishmaniasis in Bolivia and Venezuela. The leishmania intradermal test (Montenegro) is always negative.

(5) Ethiopian Cutaneous Leishmaniasis

This is an antimony-resistant cutaneous leishmaniasis which is endemic in Ethiopia and clinically is very similar to leprosy. The Montenegro test is negative in the 'pseudo-lepromatous' type of the disease and positive in the tuberculoid type.

(6) Lupoid Leishmaniasis

This is a relapsing form of cutaneous leishmaniasis which is common in the Middle East, and resembles lupus vulgaris. Leishmania are scarce in biopsies and the leishmania test is positive.

MUCO-CUTANEOUS LEISHMANIASIS (Espundia)

Espundia is widely distributed through South and Central America.

Epidemiology
Muco-cutaneous leishmaniasis is caused by *L. braziliensis* and the sandflies *P. whitmani, P. passoai* and *P. migonei* are proven vectors of the disease. The most important animal reservoir of infection is the spiny rat. Espundia occurs mainly among men working in virgin forest. Human infections are acquired when new settlements are started in jungle areas and small clearings are made. At first, these settlements have an intimate contact with the forest, but after a time the wild rodents are driven away and the disease dies out. The infection is often confined to the skin but metastases to mucous membrane often occur through the bloodstream. The parasite has a predilection for the nasopharynx. It appears that clinical immunity to heterologous strains of leishmania does occur, an observation in keeping with the finding that although *L. braziliensis, L. tropica* and *L. mexicana* can easily be distinguished from each other serologically they share certain common antigens. It seems, moreover, that chiclero's ulcer, oriental sore and uta produce low levels of circulating antibody in the serum despite the fact that they result in

lifelong immunity in most patients, while patients suffering from muco-cutaneous leishmaniasis possess high levels of circulating antibody.

Laboratory diagnosis of the leishmaniases

L. donovani can be demonstrated in Giemsa-stained smears from the peripheral blood (usually very scanty), spleen, liver, lymph nodes or bone marrow, and culture of material obtained from the above sources, or by inoculation into hamsters. Tests based on increase in serum gamma globulin are at best only indicative but not diagnostic of the disease (e.g. Napier, Chopra, etc.). The complement-fixation test is very useful in diagnosis of early cases. The indirect fluorescent antibody technique has been successfully used in the serodiagnosis of kala-azar, negative results were reported from *L. tropica* patients.

The diagnosis of infection with *L. tropica* is made by examining microscopically material obtained by puncture of the undivided edge of the ulcer after appropriate staining. Culture of the material in NNN-type medium should also be done. Biopsy of skin under the edge of the ulcer can provide proof of infection. Histologically the organism may be confused with *H. capsulatum* which, however, stains well with methanamine silver and thus allows differentiation. The Montenegro (leishmanin) test is positive in 95 per cent of patients with *L. tropica*; in contrast it is negative in the active stages of Indian kala-azar.

L. mexicana can be demonstrated in material obtained from the initial ulcers, from the lesions in the mucous membrane, cultured material or NNN medium. The Montenegro skin test is positive in 92 per cent of patients but negative in the disseminated form of leishmaniasis due to *L. pifanoi*.

Control of the Leishmaniases

Control of visceral leishmaniasis consists in identifying and treating infected persons, including cases of dermal leishmaniasis; and in attacking the sandfly as well as the animal reservoir of infection.

(a) *The individual*

Pentostam is the drug of choice for visceral leishmaniasis. It is easy to administer and toxic effects are low. The dose for adults is 0.6 g intravenously or intramuscularly, daily for 6 days for Indian kala-azar; and for 30 days for all other forms of visceral leishmaniasis. Resistant cases occur. The efficacy of liposome-incorporated known or potential anti-leishmanial agents is being studied in experimental laboratory animals. Sandfly bites can be partially avoided by sleeping on the upper floors of houses and using repellents.

(b) *The vector*

The breeding places of sandflies in walls can be plastered over and the rubble of broken-down hoses cleared away. The indoor biting *Phlebotomus* species are very susceptible to DDT and residual spraying of dwellings eradicates the sandfly.

(c) *The animal reservoir of infection*

Infection in dogs can be controlled and eradicated by removing all infected dogs from the community. Mass diagnosis can be carried out using the complement-fixation test. A 10 per cent infection rate in the dog community implies a substantial reservoir for human infection and suspected dogs should be individually diagnosed and destroyed if sick. In endemic areas a licensing system should be instituted whereby dogs must be examined annually and destroyed if ill. Kala-azar can be eradicated from the community in this way. Wild canine and rodent reservoirs cannot of course be controlled in this way.

(d) *The community*

Villages should be sited away from ecological environments favourable to outdoor biting sandfly vectors. Thus, in Northern Kenya, houses should be sited more than 100 yards from termite hills, which can be destroyed or treated with DDT.

Mass surveys and treatment of the human population should be undertaken. Army and police personnel working in endemic areas should consist of leishman-positive persons. When a large number of leishmaniasis-negative persons is introduced into endemic areas, epidemic of kala-azar can be expected. This is a particularly pertinent point to remember when populations are moved from one area to another as a result of the building of large dams, e.g. the Aswan dam.

Control of *cutaneous leishmaniasis* of the Old World (tropical sore) is achieved by breaking the man/sandfly contact, rodent destruction and immunisation.

Sandfly eradication by DDT spraying of houses and breeding places as above has markedly reduced the prevalence of cutaneous leishmaniasis. If this cannot be done, sleeping at night on the roof or the second floor of a house will reduce infection, since sandflies do not readily move above the ground floor. *Leishmania tropica major* mainly results from sandfly bites out of doors, and house spraying is not as effective as in *L. tropica minor*.

Since the main reservoir of infection in Asia is a communal rodent; rat destruction for a radius of 3 miles around villages should be carried out.

Since rodents cannot be eradicated from remote areas, travellers and nomads should be protected by immunisation. The immunity conferred by *L. tropica major* is virtually lifelong and protects also against *L. tropica minor*. A live culture on NNN of the gerbil leishmania is inoculated intradermally under the skin. A nodule forms which lasts 3–6 months and confers immunity to reinfection in the great majority of cases. The Montenegro test becomes positive.

Chiclero ulcer is difficult to control since both eradication of the rodent reservoir and spraying to destroy the sandflies in the forest canopy high above the ground, are both impracticable. Immunisation of gum collectors and forest workers is the only sensible remedy.

Vaccination using a live culture of *L. mexicana* protects against the chronic disfiguring lesions found on the ears.

Uta can be eradicated by residual spraying of dwellings with DDT. Since little is known of the epidemiology of the diffuse cutaneous forms of leishmaniasis, control of this infection is not yet feasible.

Muco-cutaneous leishmaniasis being a sporadic jungle forest disease with an animal reservoir is extremely difficult to control. Dwellings in new settlements in the forest should be concentrated away from the forest edge so that a barrier of clear land is maintained between the village and the forest. Temporary spraying of the forest edges with insecticides can be carried out and travellers into forests should wear protective clothing and use repellents.

Leishmaniasis—Summary

	Visceral	**Cutaneous**	**Muco-cutaneous**
1 *Occurrence*	India, Mediterranean, Middle East, Africa, South America	India, Mediterranean, Middle East, Africa, Central and South America	South and Central America
2 *Organisms*	L. donovani	L. tropica, L. mexicana, L. peruviana	L. braziliensis
3 *Reservoir of infection*	Man, dogs and rodents	Rodents, dogs	Rodents
4 *Mode of Transmission*	Bite of sandfly (*Phlebotomus* ssp.)	*Phlebotomus* ssp.)	*Phlebotomus* ssp.
5 *Control*	(i) Treatment of infected individuals (ii) Attacking animal reservoir of infection (iii) Attacking sandfly with insecticides		

THE HELMINTHIC DISEASES

THE FILARIASES

Under this generic title are grouped a variety of diseases which bear little relation to each other pathologically although they are produced by nematode worms all belonging to the superfamily Filarioidea. Man is the definitive host of several filarial nematodes. Their embryos (microfilariae) are taken up by insect vectors when feeding on man. They pass through a developmental cycle lasting about a fortnight, at the end of which infective larvae are present in the proboscis. When the insect next feeds, the larvae escape and pass through breaches of the skin surface into the tissues. The main differential characteristics of the various filarial infections are given in Table 6.6.

FILARIASIS (BANCROFTIAN AND MALAYAN)

Filariasis results from infection with the parasite nematodes *Wuchereria bancrofti* and *Brugia malayi*. It is estimated that at least 250 million people throughout the world are infected.

Applied biology

The features of the life cycles of these two filariae are practically identical. The adult worms live in the lymphatic system where the female worms, which are viviparous, produce sheathed microfilariae which are about 200–300 μm long. The microfilariae make their way to and circulate in the bloodstream where they are ingested by a mosquito. After ingestion the microfilariae escape from the sheath, penetrate the gut wall of the insect and pass to the thoracic muscles where they undergo development. After 2 or more weeks the infective larvae reach the proboscis and enter another vertebrate host when the mosquito is biting. It is not certain how they reach the lymphatics after the insect bites. Many species of mosquitoes, belonging to the genera *Culex, Aëdes, Anopheles* and *Mansonioides*, can act as intermediate hosts of *W. bancrofti* and *B. malayi*.

The microfilariae of *B. malayi* can be distinguished from those of *W. bancrofti* on morphological grounds and by their staining reaction to Giemsa.

Microfilariae of both *W. bancrofti* and *B. malayi* appear in the peripheral blood at distinct times of the day—a characteristic referred to as periodicity. The controlling mechanism for this periodicity has never been satisfactorily explained. It does not appear to depend on the parasympathetic system, nor is the microfilaria count influenced by alteration in the corticosteroid level in the blood of man, or by a general anaesthetic.

Medical geography

The geographical distribution of the parasites is determined largely by climate and the distribution of their mosquito vectors.

Epidemiology

Whereas *W. bancrofti* has so far been found only in man, *B. malayi* is a parasite of both man and animals. The most consistent sign of infection is the appearance of microfilaria in the peripheral blood and many microfilaria carriers are apparently symptom-free and remain so for many years or for life.

Table 6.6 General features of filarial worms infecting man

Species	Wuchereria bancrofti	Brugia malayi	Loa loa	Onchocerca volvulus	Tetrapetalonema perstans	Tetrapetalonema streptocerca	Mansonella ozzardi
Geographical distribution	Africa America Asia Australia Pacific Islands	Asia	West and Central Africa	Africa Central America	Africa South America	West Africa	West Indies South America
Site of adult worm	Lymphatic system	Lymphatic system	Subcutaneous tissues	Subcutaneous tissues	Body cavities, e.g. pleura, pericardium	Subcutaneous tissues	Visceral adipose tissue
Microfilaria: Periodicity	Nocturnal / Diurnally subperiodic	Nocturnal / Nocturnally subperiodic	Diurnal	Non-periodic	Non-periodic	Non-periodic	Non-periodic
Sheath	Sheathed	Sheathed	Sheathed	Unsheathed	Unsheathed	Unsheathed	Unsheathed
Site	Blood	Blood	Blood	Skin and tissues	Blood	Skin and tissues	Blood
Vectors	Culex p. fatigans Anopheles spp. / C.p.fatigans Aëdes spp.	Mansonia spp. Anopheles spp. / M. longipalpis M. annulatus	Chrysops spp.	Simulium spp.	Culicoides spp.	Culicoides spp.	Culicoides spp.
Animal reservoir	None	Doubtful / Monkeys, rodents	None	None	None	None	None
Diagnosis	Blood film (night) / Blood film (afternoon)	Blood film (night)	Blood film (afternoon)	Skin snips or scarification	Blood film (day)	Skin snips	Blood film (day)
Clinical effects	Lymphangitis, hydrocoele, elephantiasis of whole leg	Lymphangitis, elephantiasis of lower legs (mainly below knee)	Subcutaneous swellings	Dermatitis, subcutaneous nodules, blindness	Ill defined, but occur	Ill defined, but occur	Ill defined, but occur

Wucheria bancrofti

Two biologically different forms of *W. bancrofti* exist—tne nocturnal periodic form, in which the microfilariae appear in the peripheral blood between 10 p.m. and 2 a.m., and is predominantly an infection of urban communities, transmitted by the domestic night-biting mosquito *Culex pipiens fatigans*. It has an almost world-wide distribution, occurring in Central and South America, West, Central and East Africa, Egypt and South-East Asia.

The other form, which is diurnally subperiodic, i.e. microfilariae are present in appreciable numbers throughout the 24 hours but show a consistent minor peak diurnally (usually sometime in the afternoon) is restricted to Polynesia and is transmitted mainly by day-biting mosquitoes.

Brugia malayi

Human infection with *B. malayi* has only been recognised in Asia, where it is predominantly an infection of rural populations, in contrast to the usual distribution of *W. bancrofti*.

There are two forms of *B. malayi*, the periodic in which the microfilariae show markedly nocturnal periodicity in the blood (10 p.m. to 2 a.m.), and which has a tendency to occur in small endemic foci in countries extending from the west coast of India to New Guinea, the Philippines and Japan; and the subperiodic form in which the microfilariae tend to be present throughout the 24 hours with a minor nocturnl peak from 10 p.m. to 6 a.m. This nocturnally subperiodic form has been found, to date, only in Malaysia, Borneo and Palawan Island in the Philippines. The nocturnal periodic form is transmitted by the *Mansonia* mosquitoes of open swamps, lakes and reservoirs which bite mainly at night, while the nocturnal subperiodic is transmitted by the *Mansonia* of swamp forest, mosquitoes which will bite in shade at any time. The periodic form is found mainly in man, and animal infections are rare. In contrast, the subperiodic form is found in many animals (primates, carnivores, rodents, etc.) as well as man (Fig. 6.4).

Timor microfilaria

This new microfilaria was recently discovered in the Portuguese island of Timor. There is no animal reservoir and the vector is unknown. The periodicity and symptomatology are similar to that of the periodic form of *W. bancrofti*. Recently another new microfilaria has been discovered in Madagascar and named *W. bancrofti* var. *Vauceli*.

Symptoms attributable to filariasis can present many years after a relatively brief period of exposure to infection, although severe disabling symptoms for deformity are usually due to a long period of exposure and reinfection. Males are usually more frequently affected than

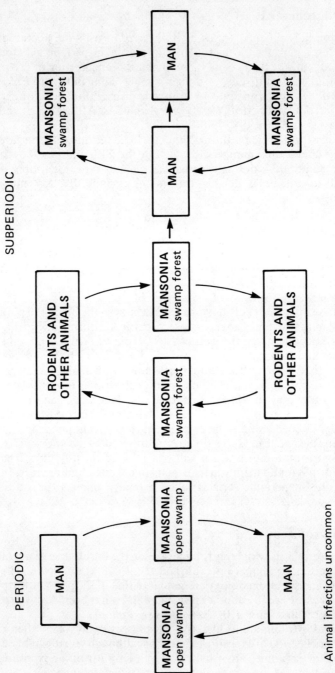

Fig. 6.4 Epidemiology of *Brugia malaya*

females. This higher incidence of microfilaraemia in males is probably due to a greater chance of infection; it is possible, however, that a hormonal influence may be responsible. Most surveys for either form of *W. bancrofti* have shown low microfilaria rates in children below the age of 5 years, probably because *W. bancrofti* takes a long time to produce a patent microfilaraemia. In contrast it has been shown that high microfilariae rates occur in children under 5 years with both the periodic and the subperiodic form of *B. malayi*; thus a low infection rate among children under 5 years usually implies low transmission for *B. malayi* in the area surveyed.

Laboratory diagnosis

The finding of microfilariae in the blood provides the certain diagnosis of filarial infection. Thick blood films should be taken at the appropriate times (e.g. at night for microfilaria *bancrofti*) and fresh cover-slip preparations examined. Simultaneously, dried, stained specimens should be made and identification of the microfilariae made according to the diagnostic criteria given in Table 6.6. Microfilariae may also be found in fluids obtained from hydrocoeles, varices, pleura, joints and in ascitic fluid. Eosinophilia is usually present. It is important to realise that microfilariae may be absent in the very early or late stages of the infection—thus in only 4 per cent of patients with elephantiasis and 30 per cent with hydrocoeles are microfilariae found in the blood. Occasionally the adult filarial worms may be found in biopsy of lymph glands, or by X-ray when calcified.

Many techniques are available for concentrating blood microfilariae.

Serodiagnostic methods for the diagnosis of filariasis have been widely used. There is a range of variation in the results obtained and these variations derive partly from differences in technique of antigen preparation. These immunodiagnostic methods are group specific (i.e. positive in any filarial infection) and on the whole still unsatisfactory with the possible exception of the filarial complement-fixation test (FCFT).

Control

The filariases may be controlled by reducing the human reservoir or by attacking the vector mosquitoes. A combination of vector control and mass treatment with diethylcarbamazine offers the best hope of eventual eradication of bancroftian filariasis.

(a) Human reservoir

The human reservoir of infection may be reduced by treatment of the infected population with diethylcarbamazine (Hetrazan), which abolishes or greatly reduces circulating microfilariae and kills some of the adult worms.

The administration of diethylcarbamazine for the purpose of control can be carried out in various ways:

(a) the mass administration of the drug to the total population at risk in a given area.
(b) the selective administration of the drug to cover a segment of the population found infected in the survey carried out prior to the campaign.
(c) the provision of medicated food, e.g. salt or beverages—soft drinks to be consumed by the population at risk.

Whatever means of drug administration is selected, an adequate total dose of at least 36 mg/kg for *Brugia* infections and 72 mg/kg for *W. bancrofti* infection should be taken by at least 80% of the *target* population in order to make a significant impact on the microfilaria rate within the population and ultimately on the control of endemicity. Sharp reactions may follow the use of diethylcarbamazine especially when microfilariae are numerous. Spaced doses over a long period, e.g. 4–6 mg/kg diethylcarbamazine citrate once weekly or once monthly for eight to twelve doses, have proved effective in South-East Asia against both forms of filariasis. These 'travelling treatment' teams have been particularly successful in Tahiti and West Malaysia. *B. malayi* seems more susceptible to diethylcarbamazine than is *W. bancrofti*. There are good reasons to believe that spaced doses of diethylcarbamazine given to a sufficient proportion of the population, and supplemented by follow-up surveys and treatment of those found infected, can bring about a long-lasting reduction in infection rates in areas of endemic filariasis due to *B. malayi*. This has been the case in many of the Pacific islands, particularly in Polynesia.

(b) *The vector*

Control measures may be taken against the aquatic stages of the mosquito by eliminating breeding places, using insecticides to kill aquatic forms, or in the case of *Mansonia* mosquitoes, destroying by herbicides or hand collection, the water vegetation on which the insect is dependent. Adult vectors may be controlled by residual insecticides using the newer ultra-low-volume spraying techniques employing either air or ground equipment. *Culex fatigans*, a common vector, is naturally tolerant of DDT and strains resistant to benzene hexachloride and dieldrin have been reported. Organophosphorus insecticides (e.g. Fenthion) can be used against the larval stages, which often breed in septic pits and drains near houses. Unfortunately, the rapid and unplanned urbanization that has occurred in most tropical cities has caused the populations of these cities to expand at rate that exceeds the ability of the authorities to provide adequate sanitation and underground waste water disposal systems—thus eliminating the breeding sites of *C. p. fatigans* by environmental control.

LOIASIS

This is an infection due to the filarial worm *Loa loa* and is characterised by transient subcutaneous swellings.

Applied biology

The adult worms live in the connective tissue of man and the females, which are about 70 mm long, produce microfilariae which pass into the bloodstream. The microfilariae are sheathed and about 300 μm in length, they appear in greatest numbers in the blood during the day. When the circulating microfilariae are taken up by suitable species of Chrysops, they pass from the stomach to the thoracic muscles and after a period of development, lasting about 12 days, present in the proboscis. When the fly next feeds on a human host the larvae penetrate the skin and migrate in the connective tissues, reaching maturity in about a year.

Medical geography

Loiasis is found in the equatorial rain-forest belt of Africa stretching from the Gulf of Guinea in the west to the Great Lakes in the east.

Epidemiology

Various species of *Chrysops* are the only known vectors of loiasis and they breed in densely shaded, slow-moving streams and swamps. The adults live in the tree tops, the females coming down to attack man at ground level or to lay their eggs on the mud and decaying vegetation of stagnant waters. The males do not feed on blood. *Chrysops* are attracted by movement, light and smoke from wood fires, they bite in daylight and seem to prefer dark to white skins. In man, all ages and both sexes are affected, although overt infection in young children is uncommon, probably due to the long incubation period of the filarial worm.

Laboratory diagnosis

Microfilariae may be found in the peripheral blood taken preferably around midday and they can be differentiated on morphological grounds from other sheathed microfilariae (see Table 6.6). Concentration techniques are useful to detect scanty infections. The adult worms may be seen wriggling under the conjunctiva. A high eosinophilia (60–80 per cent) is usually present. The filarial complement-fixation tests gives the highest incidence of positive results with loiasis, and is particularly useful in early infections before microfilariae have appeared in the blood, or in unisexual infections when microfilariae are absent. Intradermal tests are available but have the same limitations in their use as in the other filarial infections.

Control

As in the case of Bancroft's filariasis, control measures are directed against the parasite in man and against the vector fly.

Diethylcarbamazine clears microfilariae from the blood and kills the adult worm in recent infections, but it sometimes causes unpleasant reactions. The drug can be used as a chemoprophylactic at an adult dosage of 200 mg twice daily for three successive days once a month. The fly may be controlled by clearing shade vegetation at breeding sites or by applying residual insecticides to the mud in the breeding places. Personal protection against bites of *Chrysops* can be effected by screening of houses and wearing long trousers.

ONCHOCERCIASIS

This infection is caused by the nematode *Onchocerca volvulus* and is characterised by the development of skin changes, subcutaneous nodules and ocular lesions.

Applied biology

The adult worms are found in subcutaneous nodules and tissue spaces. The females, which are ovoviviparous, measure about 50 cm in length while the males are only 2–4 cm long. Worms of both sexes are found coiled together in nodules and larvae are present in large numbers near the coiled gravid female. The developed larvae (microfilariae) vary greatly in size (150–350 μm) and are unsheathed.

Microfilariae are ingested when the vector—a *Simulium* fly—feeds on an infected individual. The microfilariae develop in the thoracic muscles of the fly after escaping from its stomach, and after a series of moults become infective larvae on reaching the proboscis. When the *Simulium* next bites an undividual the larval forms of *Onchocerca* are injected under the skin. The development in the fly takes about 15 days and the common vectors are *S. damnosum* and *S. neavei* (in Africa), and *S. ochraceum, S. metallicum* and *S. callidium* (in Central America). *S. damnosum* was formerly regarded as a fairly uniform species, but chromosomal investigations have shown it to be a complex of at least 8 species. The microfilariae introduced by the fly mature in the subcutaneous tissues. In some instances a fibrous tissue reaction around the adults causes the formation of nodules. After about a year the female worm produces microfilariae. The microfilariae remain in the skin and do not enter the peripheral blood.

Medical geography

Onchocerciasis has a focal distribution in both African and tropical America. It is endemic in West Africa, in equatorial and East Africa, and in the Sudan. One of the largest endemic areas occurs in the Volta River Basin area, which incorporates parts of Benin, Ghana, Ivory Coast, Mali, Niger, Togo and all of Upper Volta. This is the area of the Onchocerciasis Control Programme (OCP – see p. 223).

In Latin America endemic onchocerciasis occurs in Mexico,

Guatemala, Colombia, Venezuela and Brazil. It is endemic in the southern part of Yemen, in and around Taiz and this focus may extend north into Saudi Arabia.

Onchocercial infection in man produces nodules, a wide variety of skin changes, lymphatic pathology and some systemic effects.

The prepatent interval of *O. volvulus* in man varies between 3–15 months.

Epidemiology

Although *O. volvulus* has been found in primates, in most endemic areas the infection is maintained by man-to-man transmission. *Simulium* can breed at high altitudes (610 m or more) and the larvae and pupae are found attached to submerged vegetation and stones in highly oxygenated waters. They are also found at sea-level along the banks of very large rivers such as the Niger. The larvae of *S. neavei* have been found adherent to the carapace of aquatic crabs. Though some species of *Simulium* have a long flight range, the infection is mainly concentrated near the breeding sites, and thus tends to be focal. Man is the only reservoir of infection.

The period of greatest transmission is in the rainy season coinciding, as might be expected, with the period of maximal *Simulium* breeding. The disease is widespread and males are infected more frequently than females, but this is probably on occupational hazard. The incidence of infection increases with age and in an endemic area 75 per cent of persons might be infected by middle age. No clear relationship is necessarily found between the number of microfilariae in the skin and the extent or degree of the lesions. Comparisons between African and Central American onchocerciasis reveal certain epidemiological and clinical differences. Thus in some parts of Africa there is tendency for the microfilariae to be most numerous in the most dependant parts of the body; while in Guatemala microfilariae are abundant in the upper parts of the body. A relationship seems to exist between the site of biting of the vector and the localisation of nodules. As would be expected, in Africa the majority of nodules are found in the lower parts of the body, whereas in Central America as many as 70 per cent are found on the head. Bony lesions of the occipital region of the skull produced by these nodules are found in 5 per cent of patients.

In Central America infection is acquired at an early age and in the Cheapas State of Mexico 50 per cent of children are infected by the age of 14 years. Both in Mexico and Guatemala 'erysipela de la costa' is found in children and young persons and 'mal morado' in the older age-groups. Both these syndromes are associated with high microfilaria densities.

OCULAR LESIONS   There is now no doubt that the lesions of the eye listed below are directly caused by infection with *O. volvulus*, and that their prevalence and severity are clearly related to the prevalence and intensity of infection and particularly to the density of microfilariae found in the head region and in the eye. The same ocular lesions are found in Africa and Latin America. The types of lesion are—(a) 'fluffy' corneal opacities, (b) sclerosing keratitis (c) anterior uveitis with or without secondary glaucoma and cataract (d) chorioido-retinal, (e) optic neuritis and postneuritic optic atrophy.

In West Africa the risk of blindness is higher among communities living in savanna than in rain-forest. The major differences in the epidemiology of the disease in the rain-forest and savannah regions of Africa and in Latin America are probably multifactional and include the following—(1) distinct geographical strains of the parasite with differences in their vector infectivity and in their pathogenicity, (2) the social and behavioural patterns of the human host, (3) the state of immunity of the individual, (4) the intensity of transmission, (5) unidentified nutritional features and (6) exposure of the eye to sunlight.

Laboratory diagnosis

Microfilariae of *O. volvulus* are identified by examination of skin or conjunctival snips (see Table 6.6). They are most easily found in samples of skin taken from the region of the nodule. Alternatively, the skin snip is teased, immersed in saline, and the deposit examined after centrifugation. Excision of nodules for histological examination will reveal the adult worms, while aspiration of fluid from nodules will occasionally show microfilariae. Microfilariae may also be seen in the anterior chamber of the eye with an ophthalmoscope or slit lamp. A moderate eosinophilia is usually present.

Various serological tests have been used with variable success in the diagnosis of onchocerciasis—these include: complement fixation; intradermal; precipitin; immunofluorescence ELISA and a haemagglutination reaction.

Simple qualitative information is of little value. It is necessary to express the results quantitatively, either as the number of m/f per skin snip or, preferably as the number of m/f per milligram or per unit surface area, or volume of skin. Several quantitative techniques are available.

Control

Control is most commony carried out by attacking the *Simulium* fly.

(a) The vector

Control of the fly by attacking its breeding sites has to be continued for some 20 years before the disease can be expected to die out in the affected communities because the life span of the adult female worm is around 15 years, and that of the microfilariae between 6–30 months. The largest control operation is being undertaken in the savannah area of the Volta River Basin in West Africa. It covers approximately 700 000 square kilometres with about 10 million inhabitants. It is estimated that of these at least 70 000 are blind, mainly from onchocerciasis, while many more have serious visual impairment. The governments of the seven West African countries concerned have recognised that onchocerciasis is the most important single deterrent to large-scale development of the potentially fertile river valleys in the area, which now lie uninhabited and unproductive. Furthermore, the serious effects of drought in the Sahel for 6 successive years have gravely disturbed the delicate socioeconomic balance in the Volta River Basin area. The Onchocerciasis Control Programme (OCP) as it is widely known is in its second quinquennial period. Because many of the breeding sites of *S. damnosum* are inaccessible by land the only feasible method of insecticide application is by aircraft. For large, open rivers light fixed-wing planes can be used, but for narrow, twisting waterways and for those overhung by forest, helicopters are needed. After years of research the insecticide finally selected for OCP is a biodegradable insecticide. Abate, which in suitable formulations combines high effectiveness against the blackfly larvae with very low toxicity for man, non-target fauna and plants.

Monitoring of the effects of insecticide application to the large target area is shared with a specially created, independent Ecological Panel, which advises the programme director and the governments concerned on appropriate measures to ensure the satisfactory protection of the environment.

The control operations are being implemented progressively in 3 stages and, when the complete area is covered, approximately 14 000 km of river will be under treatment. Helicopters and fixed-wing aircraft are being used to apply the larvicide to the rivers weekly in amounts calculated to give an effective concentration of 0.05 mg/l for 10 minutes in the rainy season, and 0.10 mg/l for 10 minutes in the dry season. The insecticide is deposited in a single mass by means of a rapid-release system specially designed for the Programme. Drop points in the large rivers are approximately 30 km apart during the rainy season, when the riverine discharge is sufficient to transport the larvicide downstream. In the dry season applications are made just upstream from each breeding site.

The epidemiological evaluation is made by 2 teams, each with its own epidemiologist, ophthalmologist, and sociologist, which operate in about 150 selected villages throughout the area. There are 2 types of investigations. The first is designed to measure changes in the incidence, prevalence and intensity of infection, as well as in visual acuity, in all the selected villages. These villages will be re-examined at 3-year intervals. The second type of investigation will involve more detailed clinical and laboratory studies of a subsample. The intensive epidemiological follow-up studies are carried out in close cooperation with the entomological teams in order to obtain data on the dynamics of transmission. The information from these combined studies will also be used to test and improve mathematical models of onchocerciasis dynamics, such as those being developed by WHO. Results are already showing that the reduction in transmission is associated with a reduced incidence of blindness.

Bacillus thurigiensis has proved successful as a biological method of control and is now being mass produced for the purpose.

(b) *The human reservoir*
Individual therapy may well be beneficial for patients who can be selected as being at serious risk of becoming blind. Removal of the subcutaneous nodules reduces the incidence of eye lesions, and mass treatment with diethylcarbamazine of all infected persons in the community kills the microfilariae and reduces transmission, but there is the danger of exacerbating occular complications. Suramin kills the majority of adult worms, but the microfilariae disappear slowly.

A possibility, which has not yet been widely tested, is to use small weekly doses of diethylcarbamazine (50–200 mg) to reduce the microfilarial concentrations in the skin and to maintain this for long periods. For the first 3 to 4 weeks of this regime reactions of declining severity occur and, thereafter, once the main load of microfilariae has been eliminated, the weekly dose can be taken by most persons without inconvenience. Transmission of infection is reduced but the administrative and economic problems of such a campaign make this measure of control rather impracticable in endemic areas.

Tetrapetalonema perstans
T. perstans has an extensive distribution throughout Africa, tropical America and the Caribbean. The adults have been reported in the liver, pleura, pericardium, mesentery, perirenal and retroperitoneal tissues. The microfilariae are non-periodic and are unsheathed (Table 6.6). The intermediate vectors are *Culicoides austini* and *C. grahami* in Africa. The detailed epidemiology has not been studied, but it is known that many individuals in some African villages may harbour the parasite.

Tetrapetalonema streptocerca
This parasite lives both as an adult and as a microfilaria within the skin. In West Africa the vector is *C. grahami*. Both the adult worms and microfilariae are susceptible to diethylcarbamazine.

Mansonella ozzardi
This filarial worm is confined to the New World and is found in South and Central America and in certain foci in the Caribbean. The adult worms are embedded in visceral adipose tissue. The vectors are *Culicoides* spp.

Dirofilariasis
Various species of *Dirofilaria* have been reported from the Mediterranean basin, the Balkans, South America, Turkey, Africa and the United States. They include *D. conjunctivae*, *D. repens*, *D. magalhaesi* and *D. louisanensis*. The life cycle of these parasites in man is not

fully known and it seems probable that mosquitoes or fleas are the natural intermediate hosts.

The adults do not develop normally in man.

Control

Control of *T. perstans, T. streptocerca* and *M. ozzardi*, which is dependent on controlling the vector species of *Culicoides*, has not been seriously attempted.

INSECTICIDES IN PUBLIC HEALTH

Most of the insecticides manufactured are used in agriculture, many of them affect insects of public health importance and may cause poisoning in man.

Insecticides in public health are used either for a quick knock-down or for a residual effect.

(1) Knock-down Insecticides

Most knock-down insecticides contain pyrethrum (sometimes with addition of DDT to improve their efficiency). They are used, usually as a fine spray, to get rid of adult insects quickly, but the effect lasts for only a short time. They can be used when rapid control is required, as in an epidemic of an insect-borne disease, or to kill insects in aircraft. This quick knock-down can be achieved with insecticidal fogs, smoke and aerial spraying.

(2) Residual Insecticides

For long-continued effect (e.g. 6 months' duration) residual insecticides are used, DDT for example, applied to wall surfaces at a dose of 2 g/m^2, will kill mosquitoes that rest indoors—providing they are still susceptible.

DDT the oldest, is probably still the best, certainly for malaria control. It is relatively non-toxic. **BHC** (HCH) is less long-lasting; **Dieldrin** is too toxic for general use without strict precautions.

Various organic phosphorus insecticides have been used in situations where DDT is not effective. These vary enormously in their toxicity, from parathion which is very dangerous indeed (it is used in agriculture but seldom in public health) to malathion which is only slightly more toxic than DDT. They are less long lasting and more expensive than DDT.

Methods of Application

The insecticides can be applied in many ways, depending on the objective to be achieved. Some of these formulations are:

(1) *Aerosols, fogs, vapours, smokes*
These are used where penetration is required but does not give a long-lasting residual effect. Recently ultra-low volume (ULV) aerosols have been popular, dispensing about 0.1 litre per minute of concentrated insecticide.

(2) *Aerial spraying*
Spraying from low levels (up to 100 m) by slow-flying (250–320 km/h) aeroplanes, or by helicopters, may be useful for treating large or inaccessible breeding grounds of some pests, such as mosquito larvae in large swamps, or tsetse flies in extensive bush. Air spraying can be done only during stable air conditions. In tropical countries ground heating during the day produces violent air convection, which restricts spraying to about an hour either just after sunrise and just before sunset. Aerial spraying is very useful in epidemic situations.

(3) *Larvicides*
These have been successfully used in the control of mosquitoes (see p. 195) especially when breeding sites are restricted or close to houses, e.g. *Aëdes aegypti* (see p. 174). They have also been successful in controlling *Simulium* (see p. 223).

The decision which insecticides and formulation should be used depends on the circumstances of the particular problem.

(4) *Water-dispersible powders (WDP)*
These are used for applying insecticides to wall surfaces. They are cheap but messy, leaving a white deposit of inert powder on the wall. Most malaria eradication campaigns use 5 per cent DDT (WDP).

(5) *Solutions, emulsions*
These have the same effect as water-dispersible powders. The solvent evaporates, leaving the insecticide on the wall. On some surfaces however, e.g. mud, soakage takes place and the insecticidal effect is markedly lessened.

Resistance

Insects of public health importance can have developed resistance to insecticides. House flies rapidly become resistant (therefore good sanitation is the control method of choice); anopheline mosquitoes are less liable to become resistant to DDT, than to dieldrin or BHC. The only measure to overcome resistance is to change the insecticide. The mechanisms of resistance are complex and beyond the scope of this book.

Toxicity

All the residual insecticides are toxic to man, but the degree varies enormously. DDT and BHC are only slightly toxic; parathion is extremely toxic.

Common-sense precautions, e.g. not eating when using insecticides, washing and changing clothes at the end of the day's work, avoiding contact with concentrated insecticides especially when in solution or emulsion, must be taken by everyone involved in spraying operations. Special precautions must be taken when anything more toxic than DDT or BHC is being applied.

Other Effects of Insecticides

There is a world-wide controversy about the relative damage caused by residual insecticides to wild-life and the benefits they give by increasing food production. It is important to appreciate in this context that indoor spraying does not contribute materially to the pollution of the environment and that pesticides widely used for agricultural purposes are a far greater hazard in this respect. The decision as to the choice of insecticides, timing of application, dosage and formulation demands a careful study of each situation. Unless this is done money may be wasted and the desired result may not be achieved.

Biological control

Because of the anxiety that has developed over the widescale use of insecticides, numerous attempts at biological control are being tried both in the laboratory and in the field. Biological control may be defined as the set of control measures designed to restrict the development of insect pests by (1) modifying their biotype (ecological control), (2) exposing them to their predators and parasites, and (3) disrupting their reproductive processes (genetic control). See tsetse control, p. 200.

FURTHER READING

1 WHO Tech. Rep. Ser. No. 549: *Expert Committee on malaria.*
2 WHO Tech. Rep. Ser. No 597: *Epidemiology of Onchocerciasis.*
3 WHO Tech. Rep. Ser. No. 585: *Resistance of Vectors and Reservoirs of Disease to Pesticides.*
4 WHO Tech. Rep. Ser. No. 542: *Expert Committee on Filariasis.*
5 WHO Tech. Rep. Ser. No. 579: *Developments in malaria immunology.*
6 Trop. Dis. Res. Ser. No. 1: *The Role of the Spleen in the Immunology of Parasitic diseases.* Schwalse & Co. AG. Basel.
7 Trop. Dis. Res. Ser. No. 2: *The Membrane Pathobiology of Tropical Diseases.* Schwalse & Co. AG. Basel.
8 Trop. Dis. Res. Ser. No. 3: *The in vitro Cultivation of the Pathogen of Tropical Disease* Schwalse & Co. AG. Basel.
9 WHO Special Programme for Research and Training in Tropical Diseases: *Hybridoma Technology with Special Reference to Parasitic Diseases*

CHAPTER 7

AIRBORNE INFECTIONS

Infections of the respiratory tract are acquired mainly by the inhalation of pathogenic organisms.

INFECTIVE AGENTS

The infective agents which cause respiratory infections include viruses, bacteria, rickettsiae and fungi (Table 7.1). The spread of infection from the respiratory tract may lead to the invasion of other organs of the body. Bacterial meningitis is often secondary to a primary focus in the respiratory tract, e.g. infections due to *Streptococcus pneumoniae*, *Haemophilus influenzae* or *Mycobacterium tuberculosis*. In the case of meningococcal infection, there are usually no local symptoms from the primary focus of infection in the nasopharynx.

These pathogens vary in their ability to survive in the environment. Some are capable of surviving for long periods in dust, especially in a

Table 7.1 Examples of pathogens which cause airborne infection

Viruses of	*Rickettsiae*	*Bacteria*	*Fungi*
Smallpox*	*Rickettsia burnetti*	*Mycobacterium tuberculosis*	*Histoplasma capsulatum*
Chickenpox*		*Streptococcus pneumoniae*	
Measles		*Neisseria meningitidis*	
Rubella		*Streptococcus pyogenes*	
Mumps		*Haemophilus pertussis*	
Psittacosis		*Corynebacterium diphtheriae*	
Atypical pneumonia		*Haemophilus influenzae*	
Influenza		*Yersinia pestis* (Pneumonic	
'Common Cold'		plague)	

* See Chapter 5.

dark, warm, moist environment, protected from the lethal effects of ultraviolet rays of sunshine. For example, *M. tuberculosis* can survive for long periods in dried sputum.

Man is the reservoir of most of these infections but some have a reservoir in lower animals, e.g. plague in rodents. Carriers play an important role in the epidemiology of some of these infections, e.g. in meningococcal infection carriers represent the major part of the reservoir.

Mode of Transmission

There are three main mechanisms for the transmission of airborne infections—droplets, droplet nuclei and dust.

Droplets
These are particles which are ejected by coughing, talking, sneezing, laughing and spitting. They may contain food debris and micro-organisms enveloped in saliva or secretions of the upper respiratory tract. Being heavy, droplets tend to settle rapidly. The transmission of infection by this route can only take place over a very short distance. Because of the relatively large size, droplets are not readily inhaled into the lower respiratory tract.

Droplet nuclei
These are produced by the evaporation of droplets before they settle. The small dried nuclei are buoyant and are rapidly dispersed. The droplet nuclei are also usually small enough to pass through the bronchioles into the alveoli of the lungs.

Dust
Dust-borne infections are important in relation to organisms which persist in dust for long periods and dust can act as the reservoir for some of them. The organisms may be derived from sputum, or from settled droplets. Streptococci or staphylococci may also be derived from skin and infected wounds.

Host

A number of non-specific factors protect the respiratory tract of man. These include mechanical factors such as the mucous membrane which traps small particles on its sticky secretions and cleans them out by the action of its ciliated epithelium. In addition, the respiratory tract is also guarded by various reflex acts such as coughing and sneezing which are provoked by foreign bodies or accumulated secretions. Mucoid secretions which contain lysozyme and some biochemical constituents of tissues have anti-microbial action.

Specific immunity may be acquired by previous spontaneous infection or by artificial immunisation. For some of the infections, a single attack confers life-long immunity (e.g. measles) but in other cases, because there are many different antigenic strains of the pathogen, repeated attacks may occur, e.g. influenza.

CONTROL OF AIRBORNE INFECTIONS

The main principles involved in the control of respiratory infections are outlined under three headings—infective agent, the mode of transmission and host factors.

A Infective Agent

1 Elimination of human and animal reservoirs.
2 Disinfection of floors and the elimination of dust.

B Mode of Transmission

1 *Air hygiene* through good ventilation and in special cases, air disinfection with ultraviolet light.
2 *Avoid overcrowding*—in bedrooms of dwelling-houses, and in public halls.
3 *Personal hygiene*—avoid coughing, sneezing, spitting or talking directily at the face of other persons. Face masks should be worn by persons with respiratory infections to limit contamination of the environment.

C Host

1 *Specific immunisation*, e.g. (a) *Active immunisation* against measles, whooping cough, influenza, etc.; (b) *Passive immunisation* in special cases, e.g. gamma globulin for the prevention of measles.
2 *Chemoprophylaxis*, e.g. Isoniazid in selected cases for the prevention of tuberculosis.

MEASLES

Measles is an acute communicable disease which presents with fever, signs of inflammation of the respiratory tract (coryza, cough), and a characteristic skin rash. The presence of punctate lesions (Koplik spots) on the buccal mucosa may assist diagnosis in the early prodromal phase. Deaths occur mainly from complications such as secondary bacterial infection, with bronchopneumonia and skin sepsis. Post-measles encephalitis occurs in a few cases.

The *incubation period* is usually about 10 days, at which stage the patient presents with the prodromal features of fever and coryza. The skin rash usually appears three to four days after the onset of symptoms.

Geographical distribution

Measles is a familiar childhood infection in most parts of the world. Until recent years there were a few isolated communities in which the infection was unknown, but the disease is endemic in virtually all parts of the world.

Virology

The aetiological agent is the virus of measles.

Epidemiology

Man is the reservoir of infection. Transmission is by droplets or by contact with sick children or with freshly contaminated articles such as toys or handkerchiefs. The outcome of measles infection is largely determined by host factors, in particular the state of nutrition of the child. Measles tends to be a severe killing disease in malnourished children; the infection not infrequently precipitates severe protein – calorie malnutrition ('kwashiorkor'). It has been shown that measles has an immunosuppressive effect; one attack confers lifelong immunity. Babies are usually immune during the first few months of life through the transplacental transmission of passive immunity from immune mothers.

The disease tends to occur in epidemic waves; in some areas, large epidemics occur on alternate years in densely populated urban areas but at longer intervals in sparsely populated rural areas. The explosive outbreaks seem to occur only when there has been a sufficient accumulation of these susceptible children.

Control

Isolation of children who have measles is of limited value in the control of the infection because the disease is highly infectious in the prodromal coryzal phase before the characteristic rash appears. Thus often by the time a diagnosis of measles is made or even suspected, a number of contacts would have been exposed to infection.

The best means of reducing the incidence of measles is by having an immune population. Children should be vaccinated at 6 months, and given one dose of live attenuated measles virus vaccine. The protection conferred appears to be durable (12 years). During shipment and storage, prior to reconstitution, measles vaccine must be kept at a temperature between 2–8 °C and must be protected from light.

Measles infection may be prevented or modified by artificial passive immunisation using immune gamma globulin. If the gamma globulin (0.25 ml/kg) is given early, within 3 days of exposure, the infection will be prevented; if a smaller dose (0.05 ml/kg) is given 4 to 6 days after exposure, the infection may be modified, the child presenting with a mild infection which confers lasting immunity. Since passive immunity by itself gives only transient protection, it is more desirable to achieve a modified attack rather than complete suppression of the infection unless the presence of some other serious condition in the child absolutely contraindicates even a mild attack.

Measles—Summary

1 *Occurrence*—World-wide
2 *Organism*—Measles virus
3 *Reservoir of infection*—Man
4 *Modes of transmission*—Droplets, airborne, contact
5 *Control*— (i) Active immunisation with live attenuated virus
          (ii) Improvement in the nutrition of the children

RUBELLA ('GERMAN MEASLES')

Rubella or German measles is an acute viral infection which presents with fever, mild upper respiratory symptoms, a morbiliform or scarlatiniform rash and lymphadenopathy usually affecting post-auricular, post-cervical and suboccipital lymph nodes. The illness is almost always mild, but infection with rubella during the first trimester of pregnancy is associated with a high risk (up to 20 per cent) of congenital abnormalities in the baby.

The *incubation period* is 2 or 3 weeks.

Geographical distribution
World-wide.

Virology
The aetiological agent is the rubella virus.

Laboratory diagnosis
Clinical differentiation from other mild exanthematous fever may be difficult or impossible. The rubella virus can be isolated from culture of the throat washings in the catarrhal phase.

Epidemiology
Man is the reservoir of infection and the infection is spread from person to person by droplets or by contact, direct or through contamination of fomites. Infection results in lifelong immunity. Infection during early pregnancy may cause such abnormalities as cataract, deaf mutism and congenital heart disease in the baby.

Control

The main interest is to prevent the infection of women who are in the early stages of pregnancy, and thus avoid the risk of rubella-induced foetal injury. One practical approach is the deliberate exposure of pre-pubertal girls to infection with rubella or vaccinating them with a single dose of vaccine. Pregnant women should avoid exposure to rubella, especially during the first 4 months of pregnancy; those who have been in contact with such infections should be protected with gamma globulin.

MUMPS

This is an acute viral infection which typically affects salivary glands, especially the parotids but may also involve submandibular or the sublingual salivary glands. Pancreatitis, orchitis, inflammation of the ovaries or meningo-encephalitis may complicate the infection; some of the complications occasionally occur in the absence of obvious clinical symptoms or signs of the salivary glands.

The *incubation period* varies from 2 to 4 weeks; usually it is about $2\frac{1}{2}$ weeks.

Geographical distribution
World-wide

Virology
The infectious agent is the mumps virus.

Epidemiology
Man is the reservoir of infection. The virus is present in the saliva of infected persons; it may be isolated as early as 1 week before clinical signs occur, and it may persist for 9 days after the onset of signs. Healthy carriers, who remain asymptomatic throughout the infection, may also transmit the infection. The source of infection therefore, includes sick patients, incubatory ('precocious') carriers and healthy carriers.

The infection is transmitted by droplets or by contact, directly or indirectly, through fomites.

One infection, whether clinical or subclinical, confers lifelong immunity. Artificial active immunisation with live or inactivated vaccine provides protection for a limited period of a few years.

Laboratory diagnosis
The typical case can be identified clinically but confirmation of diagnosis may be required in atypical cases. Serological tests; haemagglutination, neutralisation and complement-fixation tests are available; the organism may be cultured from saliva, blood or cerebrospinal fluid.

Control

The sick patient should be isolated, if possible, during the infectious phase; strict hygienic measures sholuld be observed in the cleansing of spoons, cups and other utensils handled by the patient, and also in the disposal of his soiled handkerchiefs and other linen. A live mumps virus vaccine is available.

Routine vaccination of the general public is not recommended but this measure may be of value in protecting susceptible young persons in residential institutions in which epidemics occur frequently.

Mumps—Summary

1 *Occurrence*—World-wide
2 *Organism*—Mumps virus
3 *Reservoir of infection*—Man
4 *Modes of transmission*—Droplets and contact
5 *Control*—Isolation of cases and active immunisation

PSITTACOSIS

This may present as an acute severe pneumonia which may prove fatal but mild, subclinical infections do occur.

The *incubation period* is about 4 to 14 days.

Medical geography
The distribution of the disease in man is determined by infection in parrots, budgerigars and other psittacine birds. These birds are found in Australia, Africa and South America, but may be imported as pets to other parts of the world.

Virology
The causative agent is a large virus of the psittacosis-lymphogranuloma venereum group.

Laboratory diagnosis
The organism may be isolated on culture of sputum, blood or vomitus on yolk sacs of embryonated eggs or by inoculation into mice.

Serological tests on paired sera may show rising titres in complement fixing, neutralisation or agglutination tests.

Epidemiology
Psittacosis is basically a zoonotic infection of birds. The affected birds excrete the organisms in their faeces, and through the respiratory tract. Man acquires the infection by inhalation of the infective agent from bird faeces; those who own and handle such birds are at high risk. Person-to-person spread may occur in close contacts.

Control

The importation of these birds should be strictly controlled. They can be held in quarantine to ensure that they are free from infection; infected birds can also be detected on serological tests. Broad-spectrum antibiotics, e.g. tetracycline, can be used to eliminate the carrier state. In case of human infection, the source of infection should be traced and the bird destroyed.

Psittacosis—Summary

1 *Occurrence*—World-wide
2 *Organism*—Psittacosis virus
3 *Reservoir of infection*—Birds, e.g. parrots
4 *Modes of transmission*—Airborne, contact
5 *Control*— (i) Quarantine of imported birds
(ii) Antibiotic therapy to eliminate carriers
(iii) Destruction of infected birds

INFLUENZA

This is an acute respiratory infection which is characterised by systemic manifestation—fever, rigors, headache, malaise and muscle pains, and by local manifestations of coryza, sore throat and cough. Secondary bacterial pneumonia is an important complication. The case fatality rate is low but deaths tend to occur in debilitated persons, those with underlying cardiac, respiratory or renal disease, and in the elderly.

The *incubation period* is usually 1 to 3 days.

Virology
There are three main types of the influenza virus—Influenza A, B and C; A and B types consist of several serological strains. An important feature of the epidemiology of influenza is the periodic emergence of new antigenically distinct strains which account for massive pandemics. Sporadic cases and limited outbreaks occur yearly throughout the world.

Laboratory diagnosis
The virus can be isolated on culture of throat washings. Serological tests include complement-fixation and haemagglutination tests; these can be performed on sera of acute and convalescent patients to show the rising titre of antibodies.

Epidemiology
Man is the reservoir of infection of human strains of the influenza virus. The infection is transmitted by droplets, and also by contact both direct and indirect through the handling of contaminated articles.

All age-groups are susceptible, but if the particular strain causing an epidemic is antigenically related to the cause of an earlier epidemic, the older age-group with persisting antibodies may be less liable.

Deaths occur mostly in cases with some underlying debilitating disease.

Massive epidemics of influenza periodically sweep throughout the world with attack rates as high as 50 per cent in some countries. The pandemic may first appear in a specific focus ('Asiatic 'flu', 'Hong Kong 'flu') from which it spreads from continent to continent. Rapid air travel has facilitated the global dissemination of this infection.

Control

Active immunisation with inactivated influenza virus protects against infection with that specific strain. Polyvalent vaccines are also available but they are only effective if they contain the antigens of the particular strain causing the epidemic. Sometimes, it may be possible to prepare vaccine from strains which are isolated early in the epidemic for use in other areas or countries which have not been affected. Based on serological surveys and antigenic analysis WHO recommends vaccine formulations on a year to year basis.

Influenza—Summary

1 *Occurrence*—World-wide; local endemic/epidemic picture; massive pandemics
2 *Organism*—Influenza virus
3 *Reservoir of infection*—Man
4 *Modes of transmission*—Airborne, contact
5 *Control*—Killed vaccine, identical antigenic strain

ACUTE UPPER RESPIRATORY INFECTION

Acute infection of the upper respiratory tract is a common but mainly benign disease. The most typical manifestation, 'the common cold', presents with coryza, irritation of the throat, lacrimation and mild constitutional upset. Local complications may occur with secondary bacterial infection and involvement of the para-nasal sinuses and the middle ear. Infection may spread to the larynx, trachea and bronchi.

The *incubation period* is from 1 to 3 days.

Medical geography
The distribution is world-wide.

Microbiology
These symptoms can be induced by infection with various viral agents, including the rhinoviruses, certain enteroviruses, influenza, para-influenza, adeno-viruses, reoviruses and the respiratory syncitial virus. Superinfection with various bacteria may determine the clinical picture in the later stages of the illness.

Laboratory diagnosis
Some of the viruses can be isolated from the throat washings or stool but this diagnostic test is not routinely done.

Epidemiology
Man is the reservoir of these infections. Transmission is by airborne infection, or by contact both direct and indirect (contaminated toys, handkerchiefs, etc.). All age-groups are liable but the manifestations

and complications tend to be severe in young children. Repeated attacks are very common.

Epidemics occur commonly in households, offices, schools and in other groups having close contact.

Control

No specific control measures are available. Infected persons should avoid contact with others. The exposure of young persons to infected persons should be avoided if possible.

Acute Upper Respiratory Infection—Summary

1 *Distribution*—World-wide
2 *Organisms*—Rhinoviruses, reoviruses, some enteroviruses, etc.
3 *Reservoir of infection*—Man
4 *Modes of transmission*—Airborne, contact
5 *Control*—Avoid exposure of young children to infected persons

INFECTIOUS MONONUCLEOSIS

This is an acute febrile illness which is characterised by lymphadeno-pathy ('glandular fever'), splenomegaly, sore throat and lymphocytosis. A skin rash and small mucosal lesions may be present. Occasionally jaundice and rarely meningo-encephalitis may occur.

The *incubation period* is from about 4 days to 2 weeks.

Medical geography
Isolated cases and epidemics of the disease have been reported from most parts of the world.

Virology
The causative agent is probably a virus, but it has not been definitely identified.

Laboratory diagnosis
In the acute phase, there is marked leucocytosis mainly due to an increase in monocytes and large lymphocytes. Heterophile antibodies to sheep red cells can also be demonstrated.

Epidemiology
Man is presumed to be the reservoir of infection, with the sputum being regarded as the most likely source of infection. Transmission may be airborne or by person-to-person occurring in closed institutions for young adults, there is some suggestion that kissing may be an important route. Infection occurs mostly in children and young adults.

Control

No satisfactory control measures are available.

Infectious Mononucleosis—Summary
1 *Distribution*—World-wide
2 *Organism*—Unknown virus
3 *Reservoir of infection*—Probably man
4 *Modes of transmission*—Airborne, contact
5 *Control*—No effective measures are available

Q FEVER

This is usually present as an acute febrile illness with chest symptoms but minimal clinical signs; involvement of the lungs occurs in the form of atypical pneumonia.

The *incubation period* is from about 14 to 21 days.

Medical geography
It is probably endemic in most parts of the world, but it is likely that its frequency has been underestimated in areas with poor laboratory facilities.

Microbiology
The causative agent is *Rickettsia burnetii* (*Coxiella burnetii*). The organism survives adverse physical conditions, e.g. drying; pasteurisation at 60°C for 30 minutes.

Laboratory diagnosis
The organism can be recovered on culture in eggs or animal inoculation of blood taken soon after the onset of the illness. Serological tests may show rising titre of antibodies in the complement-fixation test using yolk-sac antigen. The Weil-Felix reaction using strains of proteins is negative in Q fever.

Epidemiology
The reservoir of infection is in birds, goats, sheep and cattle. Transmission is mainly by airborne infection, but infection may occur from ingestion of milk. The soil may be contaminated from the excrement of infected sheep. The pregnant uterus and the products of conception are also important sources of infection. Most infected persons will recover spontaneously, and with antibiotic chemotherapy (tetracycline or chloramphenicol), death is rare.

Control

Susceptible persons who are at risk can be protected by immunisation with inactivated vaccine. Pasteurisation of milk at high temperature (62.9°C for 30 minutes or 71.7°C for 15 seconds) will destroy the rickettsiae. The infection should also be controlled in animals by vaccination (see p. 181).

Q Fever—Summary

1 *Distribution*—World-wide
2 *Organism*—*Rickettsia burnetii*
3 *Reservoir of infection*—Domestic animals, ticks
4 *Modes of transmission*—Airborne, milk
5 *Control*— (i) Immunisation of man and animals
             (ii) Pasteurisation of milk at high temperature

TUBERCULOSIS

Tuberculosis remains one of the major health problems in many tropical countries; in some countries the situation is being aggravated by dense overcrowding in urban slums. Tuberculosis presents a wide variety of clinical forms, but pulmonary involvement is common and is most important epidemiologically, as it is mostly responsible for the transmission of the infection. On first infection, the patient develops the primary complex which consists of a small parenchymal lesion and involvement of the regional lymph node; in the lungs, this constitutes the classical Ghon focus, with a small lung lesion and invasion of the mediastinal lymph node. In most cases the primary complex heals spontaneously, with fibrosis and calcification of the lesions, but the organisms may persist for many years within this focus. In a small proportion of cases the primary complex progresses to produce more severe manifestations locally (e.g. caseous pneumonia) or there may be haematogenous dissemination to other parts of the body. Thus within a few years of the primary infection, especially during the first 6 months, there is the danger of haematogenous spread either focal (e.g. bone and joint lesions) or disseminated in the form of miliary tuberculosis and tuberculous meningitis. Apart from the primary complex and its early complications, the 'adult' pulmonary form of tuberculosis may occur either as a result of the re-activation of an existing lesion or by re-infection. Destruction of the lung parenchyma, with fibrosis and cavitation are important features of this adult form. Clinically, it may present with cough, haemoptysis and chest pain, with general constitutional symptoms—fever, loss of weight and malaise; often it remains virtually asymptomatic especially in the early stages.

The *incubation period* is from 4 to 6 weeks.

Medical geography
Tuberculosis has a world-wide distribution. Until recently, it was absent from a few isolated communities where the local populations are now showing widespread infections with severe manifestations on first contact with tuberculosis.

Medical bacteriology
The causative agent is *Mycobacterium tuberculosis*, the tubercle bacillus.

The human type produces most of the pulmonary lesions, also some extrapulmonary lesions; the bovine strain of the organism mainly accounts for extrapulmonary lesions. Other types of *M. tuberculosis*, avian and atypical strains, rarely cause disease in man, but infection with these strains may produce immunological changes in man with non-specific tuberculin skin reaction.

Tubercle bacilli survive for long periods in dried sputum and dust.

Laboratory diagnosis

The organism may be identified on examination of sputum and other pathological specimens (cerebrospinal fluid, urine, pleural fluid or gastric washings). The tubercle bacillus is Gram-positive, but because of its waxy coat it does not stain with the standard procedure. It is usually demonstrated by the Ziehl-Neelsen method, using hot carbolfuchsin stain; the tubercle bacillus like other mycobacteria resists decolour-isation with acid ('acid fast bacilli') but unlike the others it is also not decolourised by alcohol ('acid and alcohol fast').

The organism can be isolated on culture using special media, or by inoculation into guinea-pigs.

Tuberculin test

With the first infection with *M. tuberculosis*, the host develops hypersensitivity to the organism; this hypersensitivity is the basis of various tuberculin skin tests. The material used may be a concentrated filtrate of broth in which tubercle bacilli have been grown for 6 weeks ('Old tuberculin') or a chemical fraction, the purified protein derivative (PPD). The skin reaction to tuberculin is of the delayed hypersensitivity type, and the result of tuberculin test is usually read in 48 or 72 hours. In the Mantoux test, the material is injected intradermally, a positive reaction being denoted by an induration of 10 mm diameter or larger in response to five tuberculin units. The tuberculin test can also be performed using the Heaf gun.

The tuberculin test usually becomes positive 4 to 6 weeks after primary infection with tubercle bacilli; other mycobacteria may produce cross-sensitivity. A negative reaction usually indicates that the patient has had no previous exposure to tubercle bacilli but occasionally the test is negative in patients with overwhelming infection or in certain conditions which suppress allergic response, e.g. measles, sarcoidosis.

The tuberculin test can be used in various ways:
(a) *Clinical diagnosis*—the tuberculin test is usually positive in infec-ted persons, and tends to be strongly positive in cases of active disease.
(b) *Identifying susceptible groups*—a negative reaction usually indicates that the person has had no previous exposure to tuberculous infection and therefore, no acquired immunity.
(c) *Epidemiological surveys*—to determine the pattern of infection and immunity in the community.

Epidemiology

Man is the reservoir of the human strain and patients with pulmonary infection constitute the main source of infection. The reservoir of the bovine strain is in cattle, with infected milk and meat being the main sources of infection. Transmission of infection is mainly airborne by droplets, droplet nuclei and dust; thus it is enhanced by overcrowding in poorly ventilated accommodation. Infection may also occur by ingestion, especially of contaminated milk and infected meat.

The host response is an important factor in the epidemiology of tuberculosis. A primary infection may heal with the host acquiring immunity in the process. In some cases the primary lesion progresses to produce extensive disease locally or infection may disseminate to produce metastatic or miliary lesions. Lesions that are apparently healed may subsequently break down with reactivation of disease. Certain factors such as malnutrition, measles infection, use of corticosteroids and other debilitating conditions predispose to progression and reactivation of the disease.

Control

In planning a programme for the control of tuberculosis, the entire population can be conveniently considered as falling into four groups:
1 Those who have had no previous exposure to tubercle bacilli. They would require protection from infection.
2 Those with healed primary infection. They have some immunity but must be protected from reactivation of disease and reinfection.
3 Those who are known to have active disease. They must have effective treatment and remain under supervision until they have recovered fully.
4 Those who have active disease but are as yet undiagnosed. Without treatment the disease may progress with further irreversible damage and also as potential sources of infection, they constitute a danger to the community.

The control of tuberculosis can be considered at the five levels of prevention:

(1) *General health promotion*

Improvement in housing (good ventilation, avoidance of overcrowding) will reduce the chances of airborne infections. Health education should be directed at producing better personal habits with regard to spitting and coughing. Good nutrition enhances host immunity.

(2) *Specific protection*

Three measures are available: (a) active immunisation with BCG (Bacille Calmette Guerin), (b) chemoprophylaxis, (c) control of animal tuberculosis.

(a) BCG VACCINATION This vaccine contains live attenuated tubercle bacilli of the bovine strain. It may be administered intradermally by syringe and needle or by the multiple-puncture technique. It confers significant but not absolute immunity; in particular, it protects against the disseminated miliary lesions of tuberculosis; and tuberculous meningitis. BCG vaccination may be used selectively in tuberculin-negative persons who are at high risk, e.g. close contacts, doctors, nurses and hospital ward attendants. A strain of BCG which is resistant to isoniazid has been developed; this can be used in vaccinating tuberculosis contacts who require immediate protection with isoniazid.

BCG may also be used more widely in immunising tuberculin-negative persons, especially children, in the community. In some developing countries where preliminary tuberculin testing may significantly reduce coverage, BCG may be administered in mass campaigns without tuberculin tests. The disadvantage of this method of 'direct BCG vaccination' is that those who are tuberculin-positive are likely to show more severe local reactions at the site of vaccination. BCG vaccination of the newborn is widely practised in the tropics. Overall, the evidence suggests that it confers considerable protection against tuberculosis in infants and young children. The strategy introduced recently in expanded immunization programmes, is to give BCG vaccination a few months after birth. The implications of this different timing have yet to be assessed.

Various complications have been encountered in the use of BCG. These may be:
  (i) *Local*—chronic ulceration, discharge, abscess formation and keloids.
 (ii) *Regional*—adenitis which may or not suppurate or form sinuses.
(iii) *Disseminated*—a rare complication.

One disadvantage of BCG vaccination is the loss of the tuberculin test as a diagnostic and epidemiological tool.

(b) CHEMOPROPHYLAXIS   Isoniazid has proved an effective prophylatic agent in preventing infection and preventing progression of infection to severe disease. Treatment with isoniazid for one year is recommended for the following groups:
  (i) Close contacts of patients.
 (ii) Persons who have converted from tuberculin-negative to tuberculin-positive in the previous year.
(iii) Children under 3 years who are tuberculin-positive from naturally acquired infection. The tuberculin-negative person may be protected by BCG or INH; the decision as to which method to use would depend on local factors, the acceptability of regular drug therapy and the availability of effective supervision.

There are now available several drug regimens which offer virtually certain 'cure' of tuberculosis. Shortening the total duration of chemotherapy is a potential means of combating the major problem of 'non-compliance'. In choosing such a short course chemotherapy (SCC) regimen one must aim to achieve—(1) a similar 'cure' rate, (2) no increase in drug toxicity, and (3) no appreciable increase in cost. A combination of rifampicin, isoniazid and ethambutol has recently been advocated, but the prohibitive cost of rifampicin given for 20 weeks is unlikely to make this approach widely used in most of the third world. (c) CONTROL OF BOVINE TUBERCULOSIS The ideal is to maintain herds that are free of tuberculosis. Infected animals can be identified by the tuberculin skin test and eliminated. Milk, especially from herds that are not certified tuberculosis free, should be pasteurised. After slaughter carcasses of cattle should be examined for signs of tuberculosis. Such infected meat should be condemned.

(3) *Early diagnosis and treatment*
Case-finding operations should aim at identifying active cases at an early stage of the disease. This would depend on maintaining a high index of suspicion in clinical practice and also by carrying out routine screening, especially of high-risk groups. Screening methods include tuberculin testing, sputum and chest X-ray examination. The interpretation of the tuberculin test would depend on local epidemiological factors; microscopic examination of Ziehl-Neelsen stained smears of sputum is a simple cheap screening technique which is particularly useful in rural areas of developing countries where resources are limited. Mass miniature radiography (MMR) has been widely applied and has been particularly valuable in detecting pre-symptomatic disease, but it is relatively expensive to establish and run, it requires highly trained personnel and it has little specificity, showing many lesions which are definitely non-tuberculous or of doubtful origin.

High risk and special groups that should be screened include:
(a) Contacts of tuberculous patients both household contacts and workmates
(b) Persons who have cough persisting for 3 weeks or more
(c) Workers in hospitals and sanatoria
(d) Teachers, food handlers and other persons who come into contact with the public.

Drug treatment
Drug therapy usually commences with three drugs, Streptomycin, para-amino salicylic acid PAS (or thiacetazone) and isoniazid (INH). After 3 months (when the sensitivity of the organism to these drugs may be known) the patient may be maintained on two oral drugs, PAS (or thiacetazone) and INH, if the organism is sensitive.

Treatment must be maintained for 1 year or more. Surgery may be indicated for dealing with destructive lesions of bones or the lungs.

Ambulant treatment has proved succesful; in-patient care is required for only a few special cases. It is important to have adequate supervision by home visitors of out-patient treatment.

(4) *Limitation of disability*

Apart from early diagnosis and effective drug treatment, steps should be taken to limit the physical, mental and social disability associated with the disease. The physical aspect may require active physiotherapy, e.g. breathing exercises, appropriate exercises and support for diseased bones and joints. The mental disability may be limited by suitable diversional or occupational therapy and by simple reassurance or more expert psychotherapy.

(5) *Rehabilitation*

This should, as always, commence from the beginning of the treatment of the patient. Most patients recover sufficiently well to return to their former occupation. Where chronic physical disability is unavoidable, the patient can be re-trained for alternative employment.

Careful health education of relatives and the community by breaking down prejudices will assist the rehabilitation of patients.

Surveillance of Tuberculosis

For effective control of tuberculosis, there should be a surveillance system to collect, evaluate and analyse all pertinent data, and use such knowledge to plan and evaluate the control programme. The sources of data will include:

(a) Notification of cases
(b) Investigation of contacts
(c) Post-mortem reports
(d) Special surveys—tuberculin, sputum, chest X-ray
(e) Laboratory reports on isolation of organisms including the pattern of drug sensitivity
(f) Records of BCG immunisation—routine and mass programmes
(g) Housing, especially data about overcrowding
(h) Data about tuberculosis in cattle
(i) Utilisation of anti-tuberculous drugs.

Usually these data are co-ordinated by one central tuberculosis authority which has the overall responsibility for the control of the disease.

Tuberculosis—Summary

1 *Occurrence*—World-wide
2 *Organism*—*Mycobacterium tuberculosis* (human and bovine strains)
3 *Reservoir of infection*—Man, cattle
4 *Modes of transmission*—Airborne, droplets, droplets nuclei and dust. Milk and infected meat
5 *Control*— (i) General improvement in housing, nutrition and personal hygiene
　　　　　(ii) Immunisation with BCG
　　　　　(iii) Chemoprophylaxis
　　　　　(iv) Case finding and treatment

PNEUMONIAS

A variety of organisms may cause acute infection of the lungs. The non-tuberculous pneumonias are usually classified into three groups:
(a) Pneumococcal
(b) Other bacterial
(c) Atypical

(a) PNEUMOCOCCAL PNEUMONIA

Pneumococcal infection of the lungs characteristically produces lobar consolidation but bronchopneumonia may occur. Typically the untreated case resolves by crisis, but with antibiotic treatment there is usually a rapid response. Metastatic lesions may occur in the meninges, brain, heart valves, pericardium or joints.

The *incubation period* is 1 to 3 days. The disease is usually notifiable. Pneumonia and bronchopneumonia are two of the major causes of death in the tropics, especially in children.

Geographical distribution
The aetiological agent is *Streptococcus pneumoniae*, a Gram-positive lancet-shaped diplococcal organism. It is enveloped in a polysaccharide capsule. There are 75 or more antigenic types of pneumococcus, the typing being done by the effect of the specific serum on the capsule.

Epidemiology
Man is the reservoir of infection; these include sick patients as well as carriers. Transmission is by airborne infection and droplets, by direct contact or through contaminated articles. It may persist in the dust for some time.

All ages are susceptible, but the clinical manifestations are most severe at the extremes of age. Negroes seem to be more susceptible than Caucasians.

Pneumonia may complicate viral infection of the respiratory tract. Exposure, fatigue, alcohol and pregnancy apparently lower resistance to this infection. On recovery, there is some immunity to the homologous type.

Epidemics of pneumococcal pneumonia occur in prisons, barracks and work camps.

Laboratory diagnosis
The organism may be recovered on culture of the sputum, throat swab and, less commonly, the blood. The specific type can be identified by direct serological testing of the sputum or, later, the organisms isolated on culture.

Control

The general measures for the prevention of respiratory infections apply—avoidance of overcrowding, good véntilation and improved personal hygiene with regard to coughing and spitting. Prompt treatment of cases with antibiotics would prevent complications. Chemoprophylaxis with sulphonamide is indicated in cases of outbreaks in institutions. Polyvalent polysaccharide vaccine has recently been licensed in the United States.

Pneumococcal Pneumonia—Summary

1 *Occurrence*—World-wide; epidemics occur in work camps, prisons
2 *Aetiology*—*Streptococcus pneumoniae*
3 *Reservoir of infection*—Man
4 *Modes of transmission*—Droplets, dusts, airborne contact, fomites
5 *Control*— (i) Avoid overcrowding
 (ii) Good ventilation
 (iii) Improve personal hygiene (spitting, coughing)
 (iv) Chemoprophylaxis to control institutional outbreaks

(b) OTHER BACTERIAL PNEUMONIAS

The other bacteria which can cause pneumonia include *Streptococcus pyogenes* (Group B beta paemolytieus): *Staphylococcus aureus; Klebsiella pneumoniae; Haemophilus influenzae.*

Geographical distribution
World-wide

Bacteriology and laboratory diagnosis
Although in some cases one particular organism predominates, it is not unusual to encounter mixed infections especially in persons with chronic lung disorders. The organisms can be isolated on culture of the sputum or occasionally from blood.

Epidemiology
These infections often complicate influenza, measles and other viral infections of the respiratory tract. These organisms are commonly found in man and in his environment, the occurrence of infection is largely determined by host factors, such as the presence of debilitating illness such as diabetes or chronic renal failure. Patients suffering from chronic bronchitis are also particularly liable. Transmission is by droplets, airborne infection and contact.

Control

The frequency of these bacterial pneumonias can be diminished by:

(a) Prevention of predisposing viral infection, e.g. by vaccination against measles and influenza.
(b) Prompt treatment of upper respiratory infection especially in children and in the elderly.
(c) Prevention and treatment of chronic disease of the lungs.
(d) Improvement in housing conditions.

Other Bacterial Pneumonias—Summary

1 *Occurrence*—World-wide
2 *Aetiology*—*S. pyogenes, S. aureus, K. pneumoniae, H. influenzae*
3 *Reservoir of infection*—Man
4 *Modes of transmission*—Airborne, contact
5 *Control*— (i) Prevention of predisposing viral infections
       (ii) Prompt treatment of upper respiratory infection in children and elderly people
      (iii) Prevention and treatment of chronic respiratory diseases

(c) ATYPICAL PNEUMONIA

This is an acute febrile illness usually starting with signs of an upper respiratory infection, later spreading to the bronchi and lungs. Radiological examination of the lungs shows hazy patchy infiltration.

The *incubation period* is usually about 12 days, ranging from 7 to 21 days.

Geographical distribution
World-wide

Infective agent
The infective agent is *Mycoplasma pneumoniae* (pleuro-pneumonia-like organism).

Epidemiology
Man is the reservoir of infection. It is transmitted from sick patients as well as from persons with subclinical infection. Transmission is by droplet infection and by contact. Only a small proportion of infected persons (1 to 30) show signs of illness. After recovery, the patient is immune for an indefinite period.

Laboratory diagnosis
The diagnosis can be established by showing a rising titre of antibodies to *M. pneumoniae*. The organism can also be identified by collecting throat swabs or washings at an early stage of the infection. During the convalescence, patients usually develop cold agglutinins and agglutinins for Streptococcus.

Control

General measures for the control of respiratory diseases are advocated. Treatment with tetracycline is advocated in cases of pneumonia.

Atypical Pneumonia—Summary

1 *Occurrence*—World-wide
2 *Aetiology*—*Mycoplasma pneumoniae*
3 *Reservoir of infection*—Man
4 *Modes of transmission*—Droplets, contact
5 *Control*— (i) General measures for controlling respiratory infection
   (ii) Treatment of patients with tetracycline

MENINGOCOCCAL INFECTION

A variety of clinical manifestations may be produced when human beings are infected with *Neisseria meningitidis*; the typical clinical picture is of acute pyogenic meningitis with fever, headache, nausea and vomiting, neck stiffness, loss of consciousness and a characteristic petechial rash is often present. There is a wide spectrum of clinical manifestations ranging from fulminating disease with shock and circulatory collapse to relatively mild meningococcaemia without meningitis presenting as a febrile illness with a rash. The carrier state is common.

The *incubation period* is usually 3 to 4 days, but may be 2 to 10 days.

Medical geography

There is a world-wide distribution of this infection. Sporadic cases and epidemics occur in most parts of the world, e.g. South America and the Middle East, including the developed countries of the temperate zone. Massive epidemics occur periodically in the so-called 'meningitis belt' of tropical Africa, a zone lying 5-15°N of the equator and characterised by annual rainfall between 300 and 1100 mm. In this zone, the epidemic comes in waves followed by periods of respite.

Bacteriology

N. meningitidis (Meningococcus) is a Gram-negative, bean-shaped, diplococcal organism. It is differentiated from other Neisserial organisms, including the commensal *N. catarrhalis*, by fermentation reactions. Six major antigenic strains, A, B, C, D, X and Y, have been identified on serological testing. In the 'meningitis belt' of Africa, type A is the major causative agent of most epidemics but outbreaks due to type C have also occurred.

Epidemiology

Man is the reservoir of infection. The carrier state may be 5 to 20 per cent or even higher, during epidemics. Transmission is by airborne droplets or by direct contact. It is a delicate organism; it dies rapidly on cooling or drying, and thus indirect transmission is not an important route.

Children and young adults are most susceptible, but in epidemics all age-groups may be affected. In institutions such as military barracks, new entrants and recruits usually have higher attack rates than those who have been in long residence.

In the epidemic zone of tropical Africa, the outbreaks usually begin in the dry season, reaching a peak at the end of the dry season, and end sharply at the onset of the rains.

Laboratory diagnosis
The organism can be recovered from bacteriological examination of nasopharyngeal swabs, blood and cerebrospinal fluid. The cerebrospinal fluid will, in addition, show the typical changes of pyogenic meningitis (cloudy fluid, numerous pus cells, raised protein content, low or absent glucose).

Control

There are three basic approaches to the control of meningococcal infections:
(a) The management of sick patients and their contacts
(b) Environmental control designed to reduce airborne infections
(c) Immunisation.

(a) *Sick patients and their contacts*
The most effective and simplest treatment for the individual case is a single injection of 3 g of long-acting chloramphenicol (Tifomycine).

To prevent disease among *close* contacts rifampicin can be used coupled with mass immunisation (see below), or immunisation alone if rifampicin is ruled out because of economic considerations.

Sulphonamide resistance is now so widespread that it is inadvisable to use these drugs either for treatment or prophylactically.

(b) *Environmental control*
Overcrowding should be avoided in institutions such as schools, boarding-houses and military barracks; the dormitories should be spacious and well-ventilated. In areas where people tend to live in cramped overcrowded accommodation, they should be advised to sleep out of doors so as to limit the risk of transmission of infection.

(c) *Immunisation*
Group A and C capsular polysaccharide vaccines are now available and controlled field trials have demonstrated their efficiency in many areas. Thus, after a single dose, they provide a safe means of producing immunity for a certain period against the two most important serotypes responsible for epidemics in the tropics. Immunisation provides us with the most effective means of controlling an epidemic. In malarious areas

the concomitant use of anti-malarial drugs (e.g. single oral dose of 4 tablets of chloroquine) may enhance the antibody response to the vaccines.

A number of practical problems have to be solved in dealing with outbreaks of meningitis in rural Africa. The cases tend to overwhelm the local health services and they are usually supplemented by mobile teams which can be organised and rapidly deployed to deal with the emergency. A 'cold chain' must be maintained. In the most peripheral units, the management of cases may have to rely mainly on auxiliary personnel.

For the effective control of this disease, a system of epidemiological surveillance must be established. Data derived from treatment centres, hospitals, laboratories and special surveys must be collated, evaluated, analysed and disseminated to those who have to take action in the field. National data on epidemics should be made available to neighbouring states and co-ordinated through the World Health Organisation.

Meningococcal Infection—Summary

1 *Occurrence*—World-wide; massive epidemics occur in a zone of tropical Africa—'the meningitis belt'; epidemics among recruits in military barracks
2 *Organism*—Neisseria meningitidis
3 *Reservoir of infection*—Man
4 *Modes of transmission*—Airborne, droplets, direct contact
5 *Control*— (i) Avoid overcrowding
　　　　 (ii) Mass immunisation

STREPTOCOCCAL INFECTIONS

Streptococcus pyogenes, Group A haemolytic streptococci can invade various tissues of man—skin and subcutaneous tissues, mucous membranes, blood and some deep tissues. Some strains produce an erythrogenic toxin which is responsible for the characteristic erythematous rash of scarlet fever. Rheumatic fever and acute glomerulonephritis result from allergic reactions to streptococcal infections. The common clinical manifestations of streptococcal infection include streptococcal sore throat, erysipelas, scarlet fever, and puerperal fever.

Geographical distribution
Streptococcal infections have a world-wide occurrence, but the pattern of the distribution of streptococcal diseases varies from area to area.

Bacteriology
There are at least 40 serologically distinct types of Group A streptococci; some of these specific serological types tend to be associated with particular forms of streptococcal disease, e.g. Type 12, Group A is

frequently associated with glomerulonephritis. Apart from Group A, other groups of streptococci, B, C, D and G, have been identified.

Epidemiology

Man is the reservoir of infection; this includes acutely ill and convalescent patients, as well as carriers, especially nasal carriers. The sources of infection are the infected discharges of sick patients, droplets, dust and fomites. The infection may be airborne, through droplets, droplet nuclei or dust. It may be spread by contact or through contaminated milk. Although all age-groups are liable to infection, children are particularly susceptible. Repeated attacks of tonsillitis and streptococcal sore throat are common but immunity is acquired to the erythrogenic toxin and thus it is rare to have a second attack of scarlet fever with the scalartinous rash.

Laboratory diagnosis

The organism can be isolated by culture of bacteriological swabs taken from the throat, nose or pus. The particular group and serological type can be identified from cultures grown on blood agar. Organisms can also be isolated from blood culture. A rising titre of the anti-streptolysin O antibody is also evidence of current streptococcal infection.

Control

The general measures for the control of airborne infections are applicable. In addition, such measures as the pasteurisation of milk and aseptic obstetric techniques are of value. Specific chemoprophylaxis with penicillin is indicated for persons who have had rheumatic fever and for those who are liable to recurrent streptococcal skin infections. The penicillin can be given orally in the form of daily doses of penicillin V or by monthly injections of long-acting benzathine penicillin. Sulphonamides can be used in place of penicillin, but they are less effective in preventing recurrences of rheumatic fever.

Streptococcal Infections—Summary

1 *Occurrence*—World-wide; varying pattern from area to area
2 *Organism*—*Streptococcus pyogenes*, Group A
3 *Reservoir of infection*—Man
4 *Modes of transmission*—Airborne, contact or milk-borne
5 *Control*— (i) As for other airborne infections
　　　　　　(ii) Pasteurisation of milk
　　　　　　(iii) Penicillin or sulphonamide prophylaxis

RHEUMATIC FEVER

Rheumatic fever is a complication of infection with Group A haemolytic streptococci. The initial infection may present as a sore throat or may be subclinical; the onset of rheumatic fever is usually 2 to 3 weeks after the beginning of the throat infection. Apart from fever, the patient may develop pancarditis, arthritis, chorea, subcutaneous nodules and erythema marginatum. Residual damage in the form of chronic valvular heart disease may complicate clinical or subclinical cases of rheumatic fever, the complication is more liable to occur after repeated attacks of rheumatic fever.

Geographical distribution
The disease has a world-wide occurrence. Although there is a falling incidence of the disease in the developed countries of the temperate zone, it is becoming a more prominent problem in the overcrowded urban areas of some tropical and subtropical countries, e.g. in South–East Asia and the Middle East.

Bacteriology and laboratory diagnosis
Group A haemolytic streptococci may be isolated from the bacteriological swab of the throats of some of these patients but not from the heart or the joints which are not directly invaded by the organism. A rising titre of anti-streptolysin antibody may also be demonstrated.

Epidemiology
Rheumatic fever represents an allergic response in a small proportion of persons who have streptococcal sore throat. The factors which determine this sensitivity reaction in a small proportion are not known.

Control

The control of rheumatic fever involves the control of streptococcal infections in the community generally and the prevention of recurrences by chemoprophylaxis after recovery from an attack of rheumatic fever.

Rheumatic Fever—Summary
1 *Occurrence*—World-wide, declining in developed countries but increasing prominence in some tropical developing countries
2 *Aetiology*—Complication of streptococcal infection of the throat
3 *Reservoir of infection*—Man
4 *Mode of transmission*—See 'Streptococcal infections'
5 *Control*— (i) Control of streptococcal infections
　　　　　 (ii) Long-term chemoprophylaxis to prevent recurrences

PERTUSSIS

Infection with *Bordetella pertussis* leads to inflammation of the lower respiratory tract from the trachea to the bronchioles. Clinically, the infection is characterised by paroxysmal attacks of violent cough; a rapid succession of coughs typically end with a characteristic loud, high-pitched inspiratory crowing sound—the so-called 'whoop'.

The *incubation period* is usually 7 to 10 days but may be as long as 3 weeks.

Geographical distribution
The disease has a world-wide distribution but there is falling morbidity and mortality following immunisation programmes.

Bacteriology
The pertussis organism is a Gram-negative rod which can be cultured on blood-enriched media. It can be differentiated by immunological tests from *B. parapertussis*, the aetiology of similar but milder disese.

Epidemiology
Man is the reservoir of infection. Transmission of infection may be airborne or by contact with freshly soiled articles. Children under 1 year old are highly susceptible and most deaths occur in young infants.

Laboratory diagnosis
The organism can be recovered from infected patients during the early stages of the infection, from nasopharyngeal swabs or from cough plates, followed by culture on special media.

Control

The sick children should be kept away from susceptible children during the catarrhal phase of the whooping cough; isolation need not be continued beyond 3 weeks because the patient is no longer highly infectious even though the whoop persists.

Routine active immunisation with killed vaccine is highly recommended for all infants. The pertussis vaccine is usually incorporated as a constituent of the triple antigen (Diphtheria-Pertussis-Tetanus) which is used for the immunisation of children starting from 2 to 3 months.

Pertussis—Summary

1 *Occurrence*—World-wide
2 *Organism*—Bordetella pertussis
3 *Reservoir of infection*—Man
4 *Mode of transmission*—Airborne
5 *Control*—Active immunisation with killed vaccine

DIPTHERIA

This disease is caused by infection with *Corynebacterium diphtheriae* (Klebs–Loeffler bacillus). There may be acute infection of the mucous membranes of the tonsils, pharynx, larynx or nose; skin infections may also occur and are of particular importance in tropical countries. Much faucial swelling may be produced by the local inflammatory reaction and the membranous exudate in the larynx may cause respiratory obstruction. The exotoxin which is produced by the organism may cause nerve palsies or myocarditis.

The *incubation period* is 2 to 5 days. It is usually included in the list of diseases which are notifiable nationally.

Medical geography

Although there is a world-wide occurrence of the disease and it was a common epidemic disease in childhood, it is now well controlled in most developed countries by routine immunisation of infants.

There is evidence to suggest that in some parts of the tropics a high proportion of the community acquires immunity through subclinical infections, mainly in the form of cutaneous lesions.

Bacteriology

C. diphtheriae is a Gram-positive rod, with a characteristic bipolar metachromatic staining. Virulent strains produce a soluble exotoxin which is responsible for the systemic manifestations and the sequelae of the disease. Three major types, *gravis, intermedius* and *mitis*, have been differentiated, as associated with severe, moderately severe and mild clinical manifestations respectively.

Epidemiology

Man is the reservoir of infection; this includes clinical cases and also carriers. The infective agents may be discharged from the nose and throat or from skin lesions. The transmission of the infection may be by:

(a) Airborne infection
(b) Direct contact
(c) Indirect contact through fomites
(d) Ingestion of contaminated raw milk.

All persons are liable to infection but susceptibility to infection may be modified by previous natural exposure to infection and immunisation.

The newborn baby may be protected for up to 6 months through the transplacental transmission of antibodies from an immune mother.

The most severe illness is associated with faucial or laryngeal infection in children; nasal infections tend to be more chronic and less severe; and the cutaneous lesions which are often not recognised produced immunisation of the host with low morbidity.

Susceptibility to infection may be tested by means of the *Schick test*: a test dose of 0.2 ml of diluted toxin is injected intradermally into one forearm, with a similar injection of toxin, destroyed by heat, into the other forearm to serve as a control. A positive *Schick test*, consists of an area of redness 1–2 cm diameter at the site of the test dose, reaching its maximum size in 3–4 days, later fading into a brown stain. This positive reaction is confirmed by the absence of reaction at the site of the control injection. Redness at both sites is recorded as a pseudo-reaction, and probably represents non-specific sensitivity to some of the protein substances in the injection. A negative Schick test is recorded when there is no redness at either injection site. Both the pseudo-reaction and the negative Schick test are accepted as indicating resistance to diptheria infection.

Laboratory diagnosis

Clinical diagnosis can be confirmed by bacteriological examination of swabs of the nose and throat or of skin lesions.

Control

(a) *The individual*

Active immunisation with diphtheria toxoid has proved a reliable measure for the control of this infection. It is usually administered in combination with pertussis vaccine and tetanus toxoid (DPT or triple antigen) for the immunisation of infants, starting from the 2 to 3 months old. A booster dose of diphtheria toxoid is recommended at school entry and this may be given in combination with typhoid vaccine.

In case of an outbreak of infection, anti-toxin should be given promptly on making the clinical diagnosis and without awaiting laboratory confirmation. Treatment with penicillin or other antibiotics may be given in addition to, but not instead of, serum. The patient should be isolated until throat cultures cease to yield toxigenic strains.

Non-immune young children who have been in direct contact with the patient should be protected by passive immunisation with anti-toxic serum and at the same time, active immunisation with toxoid is commenced. Susceptible (Schick-positive) adult contacts should be protected with active immunisation and a booster dose can be given to immune (Schick-negative) persons.

(b) *The community*

The search for carriers and their treatment with antibiotics may be indicated in the special circumstances of an outbreak in a closed community such as a boarding school, but the major approach to the control of this infection is routine active immunisation of the susceptible population.

Diphtheria—Summary

1 *Occurrence*—World-wide, but now largely controlled in developed countries
2 *Organism—Corynebacterium diphtheriae*
3 *Reservoir of infection*—Man

4 *Modes of transmission*—Airborne, contact—direct and indirect, contaminated milk
5 *Control*—Vaccination with toxoid

HISTOPLASMOSIS (HISTOPLASMA CAPSULATUM INFECTION)

The classical form of histoplasmosis due to *Histoplasma capsulatum* presents a variety of clinical manifestations. Infection is mostly asymptomatic, being detected only on immunological tests. On first exposure there may be an acute benign respiratory illness, which tends to be self-limiting, healing with or without calcification. Progressive disseminated lesions may occur with widespread involvement of the reticulo-endothelial system; without treatment this form may have a fatal outcome.

The *incubation period* is from 1 to $2\frac{1}{2}$ weeks.

Medical geography
The infection is endemic in certain parts of North, Central and South America, Africa and parts of the Far East.

Mycology
The causative agent is *H. capsulatum*, a dimorphic organism (both yeast phase and mycelial phase occur). In the host tissues, only the yeast phase is found. Spores can survive in the soil for long periods. They flourish particularly well in soil that is manured by bird or bat droppings, especially in caves.

Laboratory diagnosis
The organism can be isolated on culture of pathological specimens—sputum, or biopsy material—by culture on selective media, e.g. enriched Sabouraud's medium. The skin test with histoplasmin is useful epidemiologically to detect inapparent infections, including old infections. Serological tests (e.g. complement fixation) are also positive on infection, a rising titre may indicate recent exposure or current disease.

Epidemiology
The reservoir is in soil especially chicken coops, bat caves and areas polluted with pigeon droppings. The infection is acquired by inhalation of the spores. Person-to-person transmission is rare. It is not clear why in some patients the infection progresses to severe disease.

Control

The main measure is to avoid exposure to contaminated soil and caves. Infected patients with significant disease can be treated with Amphotericin B.

Histoplasmosis—Summary

1 *Distribution*—Parts of America, Africa, Asia and the Pacific
2 *Organism*—*Histoplasma capsulatum*
3 *Reservoir of infection*—Soil, especially those contaminated with bird droppings
4 *Mode of transmission*—Airborne from spores in soil
5 *Control*—Avoid exposure to infected areas

FURTHER READING

WHO Tech. Rep. Ser, No. 588: *Cerebrospinal Meningitis Control.*

CHAPTER 8

NUTRITIONAL DISORDERS

Ann P. Burgess, Formerly Senior Lecturer, and
Dr. H. J. L. Burgess, formerly, Professorial Lecturer,
Department of Nutrition, Institute of Public Health,
University of the Philippines.

Malnutrition is one of the World's major problems. It is estimated that more than 500 million people, or over 16% of the population are undernourished. Most of these live in the developing nations of Asia, Africa and Latin America where those most gravely affected are young children and pregnant or lactating women from low income families.

Undernutrition, except mild iron deficiency, rarely occurs in communities with a reasonable standard of living. However, in both rich and poor nations there is an increasing prevalence of the diseases associated with dietary affluence (e.g. obesity, cardiovascular disease, diabetes). Thus nutritional disorders are a problem to some extent in all strata of society.

The cost of malnutrition has to be measured, not only in terms of increased rates of morbidity and mortality, but also as reduced productive capacity, diminished mental potential, higher expenditure on health and unnecessary human suffering. Rarely has the planner taken into account the tremendous economic wastage caused by malnutrition and only recently has the attainment of social improvement, such as the control of malnutrition, become an acceptable goal in development planning.

THE CONTROL OF MALNUTRITION

Essentially the cause of malnutrition is an imbalance between the individual's nutrient requirements and his dietary intake.

Most types of malnutrition will only be eliminated if food supplies are adequate, the means to obtain sufficient food are available to all and each individual is healthy enough to utilise it properly. This implies national and international measures to redistribute wealth and services; to create jobs; to improve the marketing and production of food, especially by the small farmer, and to ensure that the benefits of development programmes do not by-pass the poor.

The role of the health team

At both national and local level the control of malnutrition requires the joint efforts of many disciplines (agriculture, planning, economics, education, health, etc.) as well as strong community or consumer participation. The precise role of the health team will vary with circumstance but should include:

(1) *Nutritional surveillance*

This implies monitoring the nutritional status of the community and the vulnerable individuals in it. Repeated surveys are sometimes useful but of much more practical importance is the utilisation of routinely available data such as morbidity reports, age-specific mortality rates (1 – 2 or 1–4 year old), birth weights, weights for age (or height) of preschoolers, and heights at school entry age. From such information malnourished individuals can be identified and the extent, location and characteristics of malnutrition in the community can be determined. This is used to focus the efforts of the health team, to guide the development plans of other sectors and evaluate their outcome.

(2) *Nutrition intervention*

At its simplest this means the integration of nutrition into the routine health care delivery system, especially the MCH service. All health staff should be able to:
— give practical nutritional advice particularly at crucial periods such as breastfeeding, weaning and pregnancy, based on a knowledge of local foods and customs.
— recognise malnutrition early in the individual or group.
— rehabilitate the malnourished individual or group.

The enthusiastic health worker will also encourage more ambitious programmes such as the use of mass media for nutrition education, the control of harmful advertising, the setting up of low cost nutrition rehabilitation centres, the distribution where necessary of dietary supplements, and the fortification of food with micronutrients such as iron, iodine and vitamin A.

(3) *Nutrition training*

Obviously nutrition should be included in the basic training of all staff in the health and related sectors. However, real ability is only acquired through practice and it is the duty of every doctor to make sure that each of his staff has the opportunity to improve their nutritional skills through informal in-service training. For instance this might involve rotating staff postings so that each has a chance to discuss cases, trying out teaching techniques, undertaking supervised home visits and generally gaining ideas. Nutritional principles are simple, the prime skill is in devising effective systems for delivery.

PROTEIN-ENERGY MALNUTRITION [PEM]*

PEM is the term used to describe all degrees of energy and protein deficiency, from early growth failure (or mild PEM) to severe cases of marasmus or kwashiorkor. This is one of the most serious and widespread forms of malnutrition particularly among the poor in tropical developing countries. In such populations the majority of preschool age children may exhibit growth failure; blatant clinical cases are frequent and mild PEM is quite common among school age children and pregnant or nursing women.

Significance

(1) *Morbidity and mortality*
Severe PEM is often fatal even where treatment is good. Of major importance is the strong synergistic relationship between all degrees of PEM and most infections. It is this that is responsible for the very high morbidity and mortality rates found among preschool age children in tropical countries. (A large study in the tropical Americas found malnutrition implicated in over 50 % of deaths among 0–5 year olds.) The important mechanisms involved in this synergistic interaction are:
(a) Food intake is usually reduced during an infection because the appetite is poor or the patient is offered less food, while some infections increase nutrient requirements. It is important to appreciate that an underprivileged child may spend a quarter or more of his time suffering from infections or other illness. Thus, infection is often one of the most important factors in the etiology of PEM.
(b) PEM facilitates the entry and multiplication of the infectious agent by impairing the cell-mediated immune response (also possibly the formation of antibodies) and by effecting the integrity of the epithelial tissues.

PEM in pregnancy results in offspring with low birth weights and a higher risk of perinatal mortality and neonatal morbidity.

(2) *Mental development*
Severe PEM in late foetal life and infancy has been shown to depress brain cell growth although it is not yet certain to what extent this affects function. However, it is known that PEM significantly impairs mental development *indirectly* by limiting the amount of 'stimulation' the child elicits. A malnourished child is frequently ill and, therefore, has fewer opportunities to explore, to learn and to develop motor skills and interpersonal relationships. Because he is apathetic he demands, and often receives, less attention from the family. The long term outcome may include impaired neuro-integrative skills (prerequisites for learning to read and write) resulting in poor school performances, eventual low

---

* sometimes called protein-calorie malnutrition—PCM

earning capacity and the continuation of the cycle of poverty and malnutrition into the next generation.

Cause

In most places PEM is primarily due to a deficiency of energy; protein intake is also often low and of poor quality. Typically such diets are also lacking in iron and vitamins A and B.

The young child is most vulnerable because:
— his nutrient requirements are high due to rapid growth;
— breast or cow's milk cannot provide sufficient nutrients for normal growth after the age of 4–6 months and weaning foods are often given too late and in inadequate amounts;
— if babies are bottlefed over-dilution and unhygienic preparation of the formula may lead to undernutrition and frequent infections, especially gastroenteritis;
— the food given to young children is often of low energy and nutrient density (e.g. gruels made from cereals or starchy roots) and the child is simply unable to eat enough bulk to meet his requirements. The problem is aggravated if meals are only provided infrequently;
— as the child becomes more mobile his contacts and food sources expand increasingly exposing him to new sources of infection for which he may not have yet acquired his natural active immunity. This leads to frequent illness and decreased food intake.

Alfatoxins may be implicated in the pathogenesis of kwashiorkor.

Recognition

Mild PEM

In young children this is evidenced by a slower-than-normal rate of growth. It is best detected in the individual and community by periodically weighing small children and plotting their weights on charts[1] showing the 'normal' growth curve so that deviations can be easily seen. Weighing and plotting can be done by paramedical or lay workers at clinic or community centres using inexpensive hanging scales[1] and the charts can include other pertinent data such as immunisations, medications, supplements and reasons for 'special care'.

Where only a single weight for a child is available this may be compared to a 'normal' or 'reference' weight of a child of the same age or height.[2] It is usually most useful to use the reference weight-for-height since the child who is *currently* undernourished (i.e. low weight for both age and height) can be distinguished from one who, because of *previous* chronic malnutrition, is symmetrically stunted (i.e. low weight for age

---

[1] Sample of a chart and details of a scale may be obtained from TALC, Institute of Child Health, 30 Guilford St., London.
[2] Reference weights for age and height are available for children 0–10 years from the Nutrition Unit, WHO, Geneva.

but normal weight for height)*. A child may be classified as 'under-nourished' if his weight is below 80% of 'reference' weight (for age or height) and 'severely malnourished' if below 60%.

Mild PEM in the schoolage child or adult is indicated by a low weight-for-height.

Severe PEM

Severe PEM is clinically obvious and usually presents as nutritional marasmus or marasmic kwashiorkor. Kwashiorkor is much less common but carries a higher mortality.

All severe cases exhibit *muscle wasting* which is best felt and observed over the upper arm and shoulder.

In marasmus there is also severe *fat wasting*. There is no oedema and the skin and hair are often normal. If there is no concommitant infection (which is unusual) the child may be alert and hungry.

In kwashiorkor, bilateral dependent *oedema* is always present (and unlike nephrosis there is no albumin in the urine). Additional signs often found are a 'flaky-paint' skin lesion, skin pallor and fine, sparse, pale hair. Usually the child is apathetic, miserable and anorexic.

Marasmic kwashiorkor is essentially marasmus with oedema and, sometimes, other signs of kwashiorkor.

Control

While the real control of PEM requires comprehensive and long-term national development programmes, short-term health measures can have a considerable impact especially if they are co-ordinated with the work of other sectors (particularly agriculture and education). Such measures include:

(1) SURVEILLANCE   Continuous monitoring of the nutritional status of vulnerable groups so that remedial measures can be started promptly

(2) NUTRITION EDUCATION   It is feasible to prevent and treat many cases of PEM by nutrition education alone provided there is active cooper-ation by the community and individual parents and coordination between all sources giving nutritional information. The advice given and communication or demonstration techniques used must be adapted to local conditions but the 'messages' that are usually most pertinent are:

— Breastfeed for 12 months and longer if possible;
— Start weaning of 4–5 months of age;
— Add oil (or a high-fat food) and protein-rich foods, particularly from animal sources, to the gruel or staple of young children in order to improve energy density and protein quality;
— Feed young children at least 4 times a day;
— Eat an extra 'half meal' a day during pregnancy and lactation;

---

* A child's weight-for-height level is found most easily using a 'Thinness Chart'. Details from Department of Nutrition, London School of Hygiene and Tropical Medicine, Keppel St, London.

— Add fruit and dark green leaves to the diet of the whole family;
— Give as many different kinds of food as possible;
— Prepare and store food hygienically, especially that intended for
  young children;
— Give sick children plenty of fluid and nutritious non-bulky food.

(3) CONTROL OF COMMON DEBILITATING INFECTIONS   Special attention
should be paid to the control of gastro-enteritis, respiratory infections,
measles, whooping cough and ascariasis. The use of oral home-based
rehydration fluids should be encouraged (see p. 62).

(4) OTHER MEASURES   Other measures that may be effective include
giving advice on family planning, encouragement of local food production and income generating activities, and supplementary feeding
programmes.

NUTRITIONAL ANAEMIAS

Iron-deficiency anaemia is a problem in most countries but is particularly widespread among poor families in tropical developing nations.
Women of child bearing age and preschool age children are most
frequently affected, but some degree of anaemia is often found among
school age children and adult males. Although iron deficiency is the
commonest cause of nutritional anaemia, folate deficiency can be a
contributory factor among pregnant and lactating women.

Significance

The full significance of nutritional anaemia is not yet known, but it is
established that even quite mild degrees can reduce productivity and the
capacity for physical work. Since anaemia affects large numbers of the
working population in the tropics its economic importance is obvious.

The relationship between anaemia and infection needs clarification.
While anaemia can depress the cell-mediated response and the bac-
teriocidal activity of the leucocytes, the decreased availability of free
iron may help inhibit microbe multiplication.

Severe anaemia during pregnancy increases the risk of maternal and
foetal morbidity and mortality, and milder degrees are associated with
low birth weights and reduced iron and folate stores in the newborn.

Cause of iron-deficiency anaemia

Since the homeostatic mechanisms of the body tend to maintain
haemoglobin levels by depleting body stores of iron, and increasing the
absorption of iron from the diet, iron-deficiency anaemia only occurs
after chronic deficiency or blood loss.

The amount of dietary iron absorbed is also dependent on the total
quantity of iron in the diet and the *type* of foods eaten at the same
time. The presence of meat, fish and ascorbic acid increases the

proportion of iron absorbed from *all* the accompanying foods while vegetable foods, milk, eggs and tea tend to have the reverse effect. Iron status is also affected by blood losses such as occur in menstruation, childbirth and various parasitic diseases.

Recognition

The prevalence of anaemia in a population may be estimated using the arbitrary 'cut-off' levels of haemoglobin (or haematocrit) recommended by WHO (see Table 8.1). However, it must be remembered that there is considerable variation in 'normal' haemoglobin levels amongst individuals.

Table 8.1 WHO values for haemoglobin and haematocrit below which anaemia is said to exist (sea level)

	Hb g/100 ml	Haematocrit %
Children $\frac{1}{2}$–6 years	11	33
Children 6–14 years	12	36
Adult males	13	39
Adult females, not pregnant	12	36
Adult females, pregnant	11	33

The cyanmethaemoglobin method of measuring haemoglobin, which uses a photoelectric colorimeter, is recommended although the less accurate MRC Grey Wedge photometer may be more practical under field conditions. Alternatively, the haematocrit may be measured using a microcentrifuge.

Control

Iron-deficiency anaemia is one of the most difficult of the nutritional disorders to control. Generally only a rise in living standards brings the iron status of a community up to acceptable levels although even then many women of childbearing age may still be anaemic. The health team can encourage the following measures which, where locally practical, help to improve the iron status of the more vulnerable groups:

1 The control of contributory causes of anaemia such as hookworm, severe trichuriasis, malaria and postpartum bleeding.
2 The addition, to at least one meal a day, of small quantities of foods which are rich in bioavailable iron or which enhance the absorption of iron from other foods (i.e. the flesh and liver of animals, poultry, fish and foods rich in ascorbic acid.

3 Supplementation of the most vulnerable groups with ferrous sulphate (or a similar compound). The main problems here are maintaining an effective distribution system with adequate coverage, and ensuring the necessary long-term consumption (gastric disturbances are not uncommon).

It is recommended that 100–120 mg iron + 250 mg folic acid are taken twice a day in the last semester of pregnancy. Other groups generally need less iron and no folate. The tablets should be taken between meals, unless there is gastric irritation, since this enhances absorption.

4 The fortification of widely available foods with bioavailable iron.

VITAMIN A DEFICIENCY AND XEROPHTHALMIA

Vitamin A deficiency and its ocular clinical manifestation, xerophthalmia, is found mainly among the poor of the developing countries, particularly in southeast Asia where the rice based diets are generally low in vitamin A.

All age groups may be deficient in vitamin A but xerophthalmia is most common amongst preschool age children and is almost always associated with some degree of PEM.

Significance

Vitamin A deficiency can cause partial or total blindness in young children and is the leading cause of blindness among this age group in many developing countries. Estimates for the worldwide incidence of vitamin A related blindness range from 100 000 to 250 000 cases per year.

Cause

The liver can store quantities of vitamin A sufficient for several months and therefore deficiency only becomes apparent when inadequate intake of the preformed vitamin (retinol, found in animal foods) or its precursor (beta-carotene, found in vegetable foods) has persisted for so long that the liver stores are too depleted to supply the body's requirements. A low intake of protein and fat, needed for the absorption and utilisation of vitamin A, may aggravate the problem.

Young children, because of their high requirements, are particularly at risk and therefore xerophthalmia is most prevalent in:
— chronically undernourished preschool children,
— infants with low liver stores fed unfortified skimmed milk,
— during the early stages of recovery from severe PEM if supplements are not given.
Occasionally, breastfed infants develop the condition if the mother

has chronic vitamin A deficiency. Infection may precipitate xerophth-almia by indirectly depressing the intake of vitamin A, protein and fat, and some, such as measles, can directly aggravate the ocular condition.

Recognition

Low plasma levels of vitamin A (below 10 mcg/100 ml) indicate deficiency before clinical signs are manifest but their estimation requires laboratory facilities rarely available in the field.

Qualitative dietary surveys, repeated each season, give a crude indication of the adequacy of the diet of a community but are time-consuming and expensive.

Clinical signs only occur after chronic deficiency when the condition may be difficult to reverse. The following are the signs of xerophthalmia and all indicate the need for immediate treatment in the individual. The international code is given in brackets.

Night blindness (XN)	— inability to see in dim light.
Conjunctival xerosis (X1A)	— dryness, thickening and vertical wrinkling of the bulbar conjuctiva.
Bitot's spot (X1B)	— a small foamy, superficial plaque on the temporal conjunctiva. Unless accompanied by conjunctival xerosis it is indicative, but not necessarily symptomatic, of hypovitaminosis A.
Corneal xerosis (X2)	— the cornea appears rough and lacks lustre. Later it may look bluish and 'milky'. This condition is reversible but can progress in a few hours to irreversible ulceration and keratomalacia, and therefore must be treated *immediately*.
Corneal ulceration	— the ulcer may leave a scar that can affect vision or progress to perforation and prolapse of the iris.
Keratomalacia	— softening of the cornea that leads to permanent scarring and deformation of the cornea.

Corneal ulceration/Keratomalacia less than $\frac{1}{3}$ corneal surface (X3A).

Corneal ulceration/Keratomalacia more than $\frac{1}{3}$ corneal surface (X3B).

Vitamin A deficiency may be considered a public health problem where 0.5 % of young children aged 6 months to 6 years have Bitot's spots with conjunctival xerosis (X1B) or 0.01 % exhibit corneal xerosis, corneal ulceration and keratomalacia (X2 + X3A + X3B).

Control

The control of vitamin A deficiency can only be achieved through an improvement in the population's dietary intake of retinol or beta-carotene. This may require a change in food habits, a greater production of home or mass produced carotene-rich foods, or the fortification of one or more widely consumed foodstuffs. Fortification is effective, cheap and technically feasible once a suitable vehicle has been identified (e.g. sugar).

The health team should encourage the inclusion of locally available vitamin A rich foods such as yellow/orange fruits and vegetables, dark green leaves, red palm oil, yellow maize and sweet potato, and liver into the diet of the family and young child.

A more specific short-term measure is the oral administration of a single 'high-dose' capsule[1] containing 200 000 international units of vitamin A-in-oil to 'at risk' children 4–6 monthly. Such a programme, although simple in principle, requires a closely supervised distribution system which ensures that all vulnerable individuals are reached and that, because of the risk of toxic effects, none receive multiple doses over a short period. The practical difficulties of such a system are obvious and a first step may be to provide a high-dose capsule through the regular health channels to those at highest risk who are already being reached, e.g. young children presenting with eye signs, measles or PEM. Pregnant women should not be given more than 10 000 IU per day.

ENDEMIC GOITRE

Endemic goitre is said to occur when there is a palpable enlargement of the thyroid gland in at least 30 % of the adult population in a defined geographical locality. It is found mainly, but not exclusively, among people living on a subsistance economy in mountainous and often remote areas. Goitres usually become clinically obvious around puberty. In males there is generally a regression with age whereas in females the goitre often enlarges with each pregnancy so that the biggest goitres are seen in middle-aged or old women. In a hyperendemic area 100 % of mature females may have goitre.

Significance

In endemic goitre the thyroid usually produces adequate amounts of the

---

[1] the 'high-dose' capsule is recommended for both the prophylaxis and treatment of xerophthalmia.

thyroid hormones because hyperplasia of the gland enables sufficient iodine to be 'trapped'. Thus such goitres are mainly a cosmetic problem although if they become very large there may be obstructive symptoms. Occasionally myxoedema may occur in older women.

Of greater concern are the effects of iodine deficiency during early pregnancy on the mental development of the foetus. It has long been known that endemic cretinism only occurs in populations suffering from endemic goitre. However recently it has been suggested that the offspring of iodine-deficient mothers may be at risk of a whole spectrum of diminished mental competence ranging from slight reduction to obvious mental deficiency. If this is true, the public health significance of endemic goitre will be greatly increased.

Cause

Endemic goitre is only found where there is a low intake of iodine. This occurs where the diet consists mainly of foods grown on iodine-poor soils. Goitrogens (e.g. sulphur-containing organic compounds in water or thiocyanates in cassava) appear to play a secondary role in aggravating the condition in the community.

Recognition

Goitre in the individual is diagnosed by observation and palpation and, although subjective, the following classification is recommended:

Grade	Description of thyroid gland
O	No enlargement (i.e. neither lobe bigger than terminal phalange of the subject's thumb)
1a	Enlarged. Palpable but not visible when head thrown back
1b	Palpable and visible when head thrown back
2	Visible when head in normal position
3	Easily visible from a distance
4	Monstrous goitres

Control

Endemic goitre becomes much less common as communities on a sub-sistance economy gain access to a wider range of foods produced outside the area. However, the most effective way of eliminating endemic goitre and endemic cretinism is by the iodisation of household salt and this should be strongly encouraged wherever salt is produced in bulk. It is now possible to iodise, at negligible cost, all kinds of salt including crude, sun-dried sea salt.

Where iodisation of salt is not yet logistically practical the only other control measure is the intramuscular injection of iodised oil (containing

37% iodine) every 3–4 years (0.5 ml for infants, 1.0 ml for all above 1 year). This will prevent the development or enlargement of endemic goitre and may cause the regression of some existing goitres. If given to women before conception it prevents endemic cretinism. Since it is expensive and requires much organisation to inject all the vulnerable population, priority should be given to women likely to become pregnant and those with large goitres who might develop complications.

Mild, time-limited thyrotoxicosis very occasionally occurs after control measures are introduced, usually in elderly people with large goitres, but this problem disappears when control is established.

FURTHER READING

Methodology of nutritional surveillance. WHO Tech. Rep. Ser. 593 Geneva 1976.

Food and nutrition strategies in national development. WHO Tech. Rep. 584 Geneva 1976.

The role of the Health Sector in Food and Nutrition. WHO Tech. Rep. Ser. 667 Geneva 1981.

Control of nutritional anaemia with special reference to iron deficiency. WHO Tech. Rep. Ser. 580 Geneva 1975.

Field guide to the detection and control of xerophthalmia. A. Sommers. WHO, Geneva 1982.

Control of vitamin A deficiency and xerophthalmia. WHO Tech. Rep. Ser. 672 Geneva 1982.

The control of endemic goitre. E. M. DeMaeyer et al. WHO, Geneva 1979.

Manual on feeding infants and young children 3rd edition M. Cameron and Y. Hofvander Oxford University Press 1983.

Nutrition Intervention in developing countries—an overview Harvard Institute for International Development. Oelgeschaler, Gunn & Hain, Cambridge, 1981.

CHAPTER 9

THE ORGANISATION OF HEALTH SERVICES

INTRODUCTION

It is a painful irony that in parts of some developing countries, it is not uncommon for people to fall sick and die of diseases which are easily preventable and treatable. They do not benefit from modern knowledge and technology which could have protected and restored their health. Simple remedies of proven effectiveness are not available in some communities or where the services are provided, many fail to make appropriate use of them. Individuals and communities often lack the essential knowledge on how to keep healthy, how to recognise dangerous signs in the individual and hazardous situations in the environment, and how to mobilise resources to solve health problems.

The questions raised in this chapter are often discussed under the various titles—'Organisation of health services', 'Delivery of health care', 'Planning and management of health services'—to name a few. The central issue however is how for each individual, community and country, medical knowledge and technology can be translated into practical benefit to health.

How can health services be organised to ensure that individuals, families and communities obtain the maximum benefit from current knowledge and available technology, for the promotion, maintenance and restoration of health? What can people do for themselves, what services do they require from government and other agencies, and how can they make the best use of such services? There is no simple stereotyped formula for the organisation of health services. This chapter is intended to provide guidance through the examination of general principles and the use of illustrative examples.

TASKS FOR THE HEALTH SERVICES

In order to accomplish this process of translating knowledge into effective action, the health authorities need to perform five major tasks:

1 *Measurement of needs*
This includes all the activities directed to gathering information about the health status of the community and identifying the factors which

influence it. Such determinants include environmental, hereditary and cultural factors.

2 *Assessment of resources*
There must be a realistic assessment of resources that are available or could be made available for improving the health of the community. These resources include money, manpower and materials that can be deployed for use in the health programme. In addition to the resources that are available from government, other sources both internal, from self help and community effort, and external in the form of aid must be explored.

3 *Definition of goals*
On the basis of information obtained about the health of the community it is necessary to set realistic targets in terms of measurable improvement in the health of the community. This involves a realistic assessment of needs and opportunities and careful selection of priorities. What are the major problems? How can the problems be tackled and what is the expected impact of such interventions?

4 *Planning*
Planning involves the specification of goals and the preparation of a strategy to achieve the goals. Although the health plan is first and foremost the responsibility of the health sector in the government, the important role of other sectors must not be overlooked—thus it is necessary to include these other sectors:

(a) *Agriculture*—from the point of view of nutrition as well as such issues as the use of pesticides.
(b) *Works*—with regard to housing, drainage, community water supplies, and other aspects of environmental sanitation.
(c) *Education*—with special reference to the health of school children, the school environment, and health education in schools.
(d) *Industry and Labour*—for the health of workers, and problems of environmental pollution.

Other sectors should be involved as relevant in the local situation. This multi-sectoral approach should not be regarded as being solely for the benefit of the health sector but should be perceived as a collaborative effort of mutual advantage. Thus healthier workers may be more productive, school children who are freed from disease and disability should perform better in their academic work, and the safe use of pesticides would protect the health of farmers and the community.

The value of the involvement of the community in devising the health plan cannot be over-emphasised. The people must be consulted, they must be persuaded and they must be given responsibility in decision-making under the technical and professional guidance of health workers. The plan must not be imposed but at every step the people must participate in devising the strategies which are most compatible with their needs and resources.

5 *Evaluation*

Did the intervention occur as planned and did they have the desired effect? This process of evaluation must be built into the health programme and should be an essential feature of each health unit no matter how small. Without it, things could go far wrong for a long time without coming to the notice of the health authorities. Failure to include mechanisms for evaluation is one of the commonest causes of waste in health services. Using objective indicators, baseline data must be collected, the planned interventions must be monitored and the impact of the activities must be studied.

THE MAJOR COMPONENTS OF HEALTH SERVICES

It is convenient to group the elements within each health service into five major components:

I CURATIVE—providing care for the sick.

II PREVENTIVE—for the protection of the health of the population.

III SPECIAL SERVICES—dealing with specific problems (e.g. malnutrition) or special groups (e.g. pregnant women).

IV STATISTICS—providing information for planning and evaluating health services.

V HEALTH EDUCATION—giving the people essential information to modify their behaviour in matters affecting their health.

This classification can be used as a smiple check-list for reviewing the health services in any community regardless of the details of the organisation. These components must not be regarded as existing in water-tight compartments but they should be seen as inter-related elements (Fig. 9.1).

CURATIVE SERVICES

This component deals with the care of the sick members of the population. There is a tendency to regard it as the most important element of the health services and it is usually in greatest demand by the public. In the planning of health services there is a tendency to commit an unduly high proportion of resources into it, the urgent needs of the sick favouring such a trend. On the other hand, there is less spontaneous demand for preventive services, especially those aspects which are aimed at the protection of people who feel well. The demand for the treatment

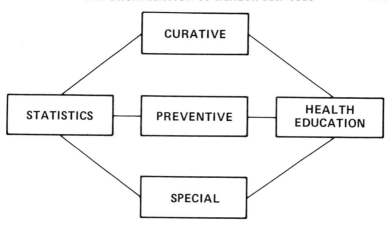

Fig. 9.1 The major components of health services

of the sick must be met but the curative services should be designed in such a way as to give maximum benefit to the population. The highest priority must be given for the most common and the most severe diseases, especially those conditions which can be significantly improved by the appropriate intervention. In selecting priorities the concept of 'Public Health Significance' can provide useful guidance. The public health significance of a disease depends on two factors:

Frequency—how many people are affected and what is the potential for spread?
Severity—how much disease, disability, and death does it cause?

The concept can be represented by this formula:

Public Health Significance = frequency × severity.

One limitation of this approach is that it does not specifically include consideration of the age of the affected persons. Obviously a disease with high morbidity and mortality in childhood and adolescence is a more serious public health problem than one that has a similar effect on elderly persons, say over the age of 80 years. An alternative approach is to compute the impact of the disease by calculating the number of useful years lost. In addition to allowing for the age of onset of the disease, this approach can also take account of partial disability.

Even without making such detailed calculations, it should be possible to identify the most commonly occurring diseases. The curative services must be equipped to cope with them. Simple, cheap, symptomatic relief must be provided for benign self-healing conditions. Early and appropriate interventions must be available to deal with serious, life threatening disease. Such conditions must be detected as early as possible preferably before irreversible damage has occurred and in the case of communicable diseases, before the infection has spread to affect others. In order to ensure early detection it is important to educate the public to make people aware of danger signals that could indicate serious illness and to encourage them to seek help whenever these occur, e.g. chronic cough, abnormal bleeding, lump in the breast. Secondly, facilities must be provided for the detection of diseases of local importance, e.g. staining of sputum to identify acid fast bacilli; simple microscopy of urine, blood and other specimens to detect parasites; serological tests for common infectious diseases. In some cases, a special survey may be indicated for the active detection of cases. The survey method may include history taking (e.g. haematuria), physical examination (e.g. hypopigmented hypoaesthetic patches and thickened nerves indicative of leprosy) or special investigations (e.g. chest X-ray, serology, cervical smear).

Finally, the staff should be trained to recognise and treat the most commonly occurring diseases in the population, and they should be equipped to do so either in the local health unit or at referral centres.

PREVENTIVE SERVICES

Preventive services are designed to maintain and protect the health of the population. They include personal protection (e.g. immunisations), environmental sanitation (e.g. provision of safe and adequate supply of water, sanitary disposal of wastes) and control of specific diseases both infectious (e.g. typhoid, tapeworm) and non-infectious (e.g. goitre).

Unlike the curative services which are provided for the sick, the preventive services are directed at the entire population. Whereas people generally appreciate the value of curative services, it is often difficult to persuade them of the value of preventive services. Furthermore whereas sick persons, especially those experiencing uncomfortable symptoms will readily seek medical care, it is not always easy to persuade healthy persons to take precautionary measures for the their own protection. It is an important duty of the health personnel to educate individuals and the community on the value of preventive services, to persuade the community to make appropriate investments in environmental sanitation or susceptible individuals to accept immunisations.

SPECIAL SERVICES

Apart from the components of the health programme that are made available to all members of the community, special services are designed to cope with the needs of specific groups and to deal with problems which deserve particular attention. Services for special groups include those for mothers and children; for workers generally or for specific groups such as migrant labourers; for the elderly or for the handicapped.

Services may be provided to deal with special problems like tuberculosis, leprosy, malnutrition, mental illness, blindness and sexually transmitted diseases. Through such special services the specific needs of sections of the population can be more adequately met and difficult problems can be more effectively tackled.

At the national level, special services may be prvided and monitored by a Division within the Ministry of Health, e.g. a malaria service. The special Division may have its own central organisation and peripheral units. In a small unit such as a rural health centre, special services can be provided by setting apart a particular time and place for dealing with the group or the specific problem. It is common to find that such small units run general clinics on most working days but schedule special clinics (nutrition, family planning, etc.) for specific days.

STATISTICS

Statistics are essential for the proper management and evaluation of the health services. The types of data, their collection and analysis have been described in more detail in Chapter 2. They serve to provide essential information about:

—the *needs* of the population as derived from demographic and epidemiological data;
—the *demand and utilisation* of services by the target populations.
—the *effectiveness and cost* of the services.

Much information is usually collected in the course of the operation of health services. Such data should be obtained and processed in such a way as to provide suitable guidance for the management of the health programmes. The information collected should be selective, concentrating on the data which can be used for making decisions. Forms for collecting information should be reviewed, pruned and simplified, limiting the items to the essential information that can be and will be used. The forms should be simple to complete and it should be easy to abstract data from them.

The data should be analysed in a relevant manner relating events to the population at risk. For example, it is common to count the number of visits by pregnant women to ante-natal services. The information is of little value when it is presented in this form. It is preferable to relate the number of pregnant women using the antenatal services to the number of pregnant women in the area. This ratio is a meaningful indicator of the coverage of the services; it provides a means of comparing the performance of the services from one area to the other and also to monitor changes over time. Simple indicators of this type should be used to monitor each component of the health services. For example, in the case of the curative services it would be of interest to determine what proportion of children who die have been treated by the health services in the course of their last illness. What proportion of newborn children are vaccinated against the common infectious diseases of childhood? What proportion of the population have access to safe potable water and how much is available per head of population? What proportion of women in the childbearing age goup accept family planning devices and what proportion continue to use them?

For each important health activity, appropriate indicators should be selected with regard to the *input*, i.e. the services offered and the *output*, i.e. the impact on the health of the population.

HEALTH EDUCATION

The aim of health education is to encourage people to value health as a worthwhile asset and to let them know what they can do as individuals and communities to promote their own health. In effect health education is designed to alter attitudes and behaviour in matters concerning health. The more people know about their own health, the better they are able to take appropriate measures in such personal matters as diet, exercise, use of alcohol, and hygiene. They are also enabled to make the most appropriate use of the health services and they can participate in making rational decisions about the operations of the health services within their community.

The variety of methods used in health education are described in more detail in Chapter 12. No single method can be wholly successful and because of the wide range of response from place to place methods must be tested and evaluated within the local setting. Above all the example set by health personnel is of great importance especially in such matters as personal hygiene, and social habits.

LEVELS OF CARE

It is convenient to classify the health services available to the community into three levels (See Fig. 9.2):

(1) PRIMARY This refers to the point at which the individual normally makes the first contact with the health services. In a rural area, it may be a health centre, a dispensary or a health post. In an urban area it could

be a general medical practitioner's clinic, a polyclinic or a health centre or even the outpatient department of a hospital.

(2) REFERRAL Most problems can be dealt with at the primary health care level but more difficult cases will be referred for more detailed evaluation and for more skilled care.

(3) SPECIALIST Specialist services, often backed by high technology, are provided for dealing with the most difficult problems, for example most pregnant women can be cared for at the primary level, high risk groups, e.g. primgravidae and grand multigravidae, go to the referral unit, and usually difficult cases including those presenting with serious complications, need specialist services.

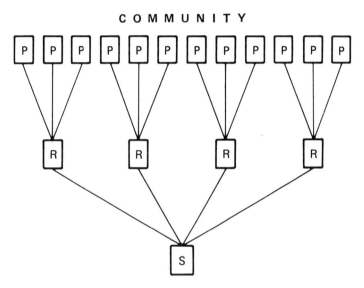

COMMUNITY

S = Specialist services
R = Referral services
P = Primary health care unit

Fig. 9.2 Primary health care and other services

In recent years, there has been increasing recognition of the pivotal role of the primary health care. The definition of this role culminated in the Alma-Ata declaration in 1978 which is reproduced in full as it represents a global consensus among governments on this important issue:

DECLARATION OF ALMA-ATA

The International Conference on Primary Health Care, meeting in Alma-Ata this twelfth day of September in the year Nineteen hundred and seventy-eight, expressing the need for urgent action by all governments, all health and development workers, and the world community to protect and promote the health of all the people of the world, hereby makes the following Declaration:

I

The Conference strongly reaffirms that health, which is a state of complete physical, mental and social wellbeing, and not merely the absence of disease or infirmity, is a fundamental human right and that the attainment of the highest possible level of health is a most important world-wide social goal whose realization requires the action of many other social and economic sectors in addition to the health sector.

II

The existing gross inequality in the health status of the people particularly between developed and developing countries as well as within countries is politically, socially and economically unacceptable and is, therefore, of common concern to all countries.

III

Economic and social development, based on a New International Economic Order, is of basic importance to the fullest attainment of health for all and to the reduction of the gap between the health status of the developing and developed countries. The promotion and protection of the health of the people is essential to sustained economic and social development and countributes to a better quality of life and to world peace.

IV

The people have the right and duty to participate individually and collectively in the planning and implementation of their health care.

V

Governments have a responsibility for the health of their people which can be fulfilled only by the provision of adequate health and social measures. A main social target of governments, international organizations and the whole world community in the coming decades should be the attainment by all peoples of the world by the year 2000 of a level of health that will permit them to lead a socially and economically productive life. Primary health care is the key to attaining this target as part of development in the spririt of social justice.

VI

Primary health care is essential health care based on practical, scientifically sound and socially acceptable methods and technology made universally accessible to individuals and families in the community through their full participation and at a cost that the community and country can afford to maintain at every stage of their development in the spirit of self-reliance and self-determination. It forms an integral part both of the country's health system, of which it is the central function and main focus, and of the overall social and economic development of the community. It is the first level of contact of individuals, the family and community with the national health system bringing health care as close as possible to where people live and work, and constitutes the first element of a continuing health care process.

VII

Primary health care:
1 reflects and evolves from the economic conditions and sociocultural and political characteristics of the country and its communities and is based on the application of the relevant results of social, biomedical and health services research and public health experience;

2 addresses the main health problems in the community, providing promotive, preventive, curative and rehabilitative services accordingly;

3 includes at least: education concerning prevailing health problems and the methods of preventing and controlling them; promotion of food supply and proper nutrition; an adequate supply of safe water and basic sanitation; maternal and child health care, including family planning; immunization against the major infectious diseases; prevention and control of locally endemic diseases; appropriate treatment of common diseases and injuries; and provision of essential drugs;

4 involves, in addition to the health sector, all related sectors and aspects of national and community development, in particular agriculture, animal husbandry, food, industry, education, housing, public works, communications and other sectors; and demands the coordinated efforts of all those sectors;

5 requires and promotes maximum community and individual self-reliance and participation in the planning, organization, operation and control of primary health care, making fullest use of local, national and other available resources; and to this end develops through appropriate education the ability of communities to participate;

6 should be sustained by integrated, functional and mutually-supportive referral systems, leading to the progressive improvement of comprehensive health care for all, and giving priority to those most in need;

7 relies, at local and referral levels, on health workers, including physicians, nurses, midwives, auxiliaries and community workers as applicable, as well as traditional practitioners as needed, suitably trained socially and technically to work as a health team and to respond to the expressed health needs of the community.

VIII

All governments should formulate national policies, strategies and plans of action to launch and sustain primary health care as part of a comprehensive national health system and in coordination with other sectors. To this end, it will be necessary to exercise political will, to mobilize the country's resources and to use available external resources rationally.

IX

All countries should cooperate in a spirit of partnership and service to ensure primary health care for all people since the attainment of health by people in any one country directly concerns and benefits every other country. In this context the joint WHO/UNICEF report on primary health care constitutes a solid basis for the further development and operation of primary health care throughout the world.

X

An acceptable level of health for all the people of the world by the year 2000 can be attained through a fuller and better use of the world's resources, a considerable part of which is now spent on armaments and military conflicts. A genuine policy of independence, peace, détente and disarmament could and should release additional resources that could well be devoted to peaceful aims and in particular to the acceleration of social and economic development of which primary health care, as an essential part, should be allotted its proper share.

* * *

The International Conference on Primary Health Care calls for urgent and effective national and international action to develop and implement primary health care throughout the world and particularly in developing countries in a spirit of technical cooperation and in keeping with a New International Economic Order. It urges governments, WHO and UNICEF, and other international organizations, as well as multilateral and bilateral agencies, non-governmental organizations, funding agencies, all health workers and the whole world community to support national and international commitment to primary health care and to channel increased technical and financial support to it, particularly in developing countries. The Conference calls on all the aforementioned to collaborate in introducing, developing and maintaining primary health care in accordance with the spirit and content of this Declaration.

The primary health care concept is not intended to represent second best medicine acceptable only to the rural poor or the dwellers of urban slums. Rather, it is 'essential care for all based on practical, scientifically sound and socially acceptable methods and technology . . .'. It is not a stopgap solution to be replaced by something better at a later stage. Rather, the primary health care approach is intended to be a permanent feature of all health services; the quality of care should steadily improve, and at all times it should be appropriate to the resources and the needs of the community. Thirdly, primary health care is not intended to function in isolation but in collaboration with the referral and specialist services. These various services should be mutually supportive. Without good primary health care, the referral services cannot function efficiently as they would be overwhelmed by problems which could have been dealt with efficiently at the primary level. Another effect of poor primary health care services is that the referral services are often confronted with cases of advanced diseases or with complications which could have been prevented by early detection of the problem and prompt care at the primary unit. On the other hand primary health care requires the support of the referral services to cope with problems which are beyond the scope of the peripheral units.

RESOURCES FOR THE HEALTH SERVICES

The resources required by the health services include money, manpower, materials and management.

Money

The financing of the health services takes many different forms. In some countries, health care is provided as a welfare service which is paid for almost exclusively from government revenue or compulsory insurance schemes. At the other extreme, some general public health services are provided by government, but individuals and communities must pay for other items of health care. In most communities there is a mixture with some services being subsidized by the government and other services are paid for by individuals either directly or through voluntary insurance schemes.

In developing countries, the funds available for the health sector are very limited and inadequate to provide all the services that are desired by the community. Difficult and painful choices have to be made in allocating these scarce resources. Ideally such judgements should be made objectively, giving highest priority to the most cost effective way of achieving the desired goals and distributing the resources with a sense of social justice, ensuring that the most needy are well served. The community should be encouraged to participate in making these difficult decisions and when appropriate they should be encouraged to make additional contributions from their resources.

Manpower

Several questions need to be answered with regard to the provision of health personnel. How many are required and can be employed? What is the role of each category of staff and what tasks are they expected to perform? What training do they require to enable them to fulfil their respective roles?

Materials

It is necessary to determine what buildings and capital equipment are required for the efficient delivery of health care, and drugs, vaccines, and other consumables must be provided. A difficult issue to resolve is the correct balance between expenditure for buildings and capital equipment on the one hand and the running costs of the services on the other hand. In many developing countries, there is a tendency to invest too heavily in lofty buildings and expensive equipment which are poorly maintained, whilst relatively few funds are left for the purchase of drugs, vaccines and other essentials. Careful planning is also required in the purchase, storage and distribution of drugs and vaccines. Each health authority should produce a basic list of essential drugs which would meet the most important needs of the service, concentrating initially on simple, safe remedies of proven value at reasonable cost.

Management

The resources available to the health authorities should be skillfully managed at all levels from the most peripheral unit to the central office at the headquarters of the Ministry of Health. Training in management is essential for health workers, especially those who are placed in position of authority and supervision. In small units, the health workers would need to devote some of their time to dealing with administrative and other managerial issues. In large units, particularly, trained administrators can make a useful contribution to the management of the services.

HEALTH PERSONNEL

The terminology used in classifying health personnel is wide and varied, reflecting differences in local practices and in organisation. Often different titles are given to personnel who perform essentially the same function and in other cases the same title is used for workers who perform different functions. Terms such as medical personnel, health personnel, professional, para-medical personnel, sub-professional and auxiliaries have been subject to varied interpretations. However, there are important general principles which can be widely applied.

In looking at the question of health personnel three issues must be carefully examined:

1 What *tasks* need to be performed?
2 What *types* or categories of personnel should perform the tasks?

3 What *training* must they be given to ensure that they can perform the tasks efficiently?

Tasks

The tasks to be performed include
1 *leadership* in health matters;
2 *health promotion* within the community;
3 *education* of the public;
4 *specific interventions* especially those requiring technical knowledge and skill, e.g. prophylaxis, diagnosis, treatment including surgery and rehabilitation.

There is a tendency to overlook the first three tasks and to think of the function of the health personnel solely in terms of the performance of technical interventions.

Types of Health Personnel

Each component of the health services requires a team of personnel with different skills who are working together in pursuance of common goals. Some members of the team are usually described as professionals, whilst others are variously described as sub-professional or auxiliary personnel. It is not possible to provide rigid criteria for separating these categories. At one end of the spectrum, the auxiliary health worker is trained to perform a number of specific tasks, of limited scope under supervision. He could be a monovalent worker in a special programme, e.g. a vaccinator, a yaws scout, etc., or he could be a multi-purpose health auxiliary who can perform a list of stereotyped tasks in accordance with clearly defined guidelines. At the other extreme, the professional worker is expected to have acquired sufficient basic knowledge and skills to be able to identify and analyse problems and arrive at independent judgements of situations, e.g. doctors, dentists, nurses, midwives, and so on. Regardless of the nomenclature and classification, the important issue is to recognise the need for team effort with allocation of tasks on the basis of skill and experience.

Supervision

One important aspect of the management of health services is the appropriate supervision of staff. This is an essential function to be performed by the leader of each group or sub-group. For effective supervision, the leader must know what tasks need to be performed and what skills are possessed by the workers under his supervision. Experience has shown that best results are obtained if supervision is positive, not only blaming when things go wrong but also praising and rewarding good performance. The supervisor's role also includes teaching his colleagues as well as learning from them. Spot checks of performance should be carried out regularly to prevent slackness in procedures.

COMMUNITY PARTICIPATIOÑ

The role of the community in the planning, organisation, operation and control of health services has been repeatedly emphasised and is highlighted in the Alma Ata Declaration:

'Primary health care is essential health care . . . made universally accessible to individuals and families in the community through their full participation and at a cost that the community and country can afford to maintain at every stage of their development in the spirit of self-reliance and self-determination.'

The role of the community in making choices and decisions with regard to priorities and strategies should be adequately supported by health education. With regard to the implementation of health services, one direct contribution that individuals can make is to function as voluntary health workers and perform a variety of simple but essential tasks. More generally, however, for the success of each activity, the community should provide optimal support and collaboration. The degree of collaboration required to ensure success depends on the particular method of implementation. At one end of the spectrum, the sole responsibility lies with individuals and families; the role of the health personnel is to provide guidance, e.g. personal hygiene, nutrition, social habits. In these cases, the individual must learn and then do the things himself. At the other end of the spectrum the tasks are such that the members of the community cannot participate directly. It is possible in such cases that specific intervention can be undertaken even if the community is indifferent or hostile, e.g. aerial spraying of insecticides. Even though a specific intervention can be carried out in spite of opposition from the community, this is most undesirable; it could destroy the rapport which should exist between this community and health workers. Rarely, if ever, should compulsion be used to override opposition.

The range of community attitudes to a specific health measure can be classified into five levels:
1 Self-reliance
2 Active collaboration
3 Indifference
4 Passive resistance
5 Extreme hostility with violent reject

This concept is schematically illustrated in Fig. 9.3. Health education is shown as the means of changing attitudes in a positive direction. For some health programmes the ultimate aim is complete self-reliance at the level of the individual and the family—as, for example, nutrition, including the feeding of infants, smoking, the use of alcohol, sexual behaviour, exercise, personal hygiene and sanitation in the home. The health workers should give advice, teach, demonstrate the best methods and encourage the people in various ways, but in the final analysis the individual and the family must do these things on their own. For such activities, the minimal level to ensure success is total self-reliance within the family.

Indoor spraying of houses with long-acting insecticides has been extensively used in the control of malaria control programmes. It is technically too difficult for each individual and each family to learn how to do it efficiently and safely. In this case, self-reliance is an unrealistic goal at the family level but the active collaboration of the families is essential for success. It is just possible to spray the houses if the community treats the matter with indifference, not helping and not impeding the sprayers. It would fail if a high proportion of families show passive resistance by locking up their houses during the visit of the spraying teams. For indoor spraying of houses, the desired level of community participation is active collaboration and the programme can be frustrated by passive resistance.

Fluoridation of municipal water supplies cannot be safely undertaken on a do-it-yourself basis and it does not call for a specific response from the individual or family. It could succeed in controlling dental caries even if a proportion of the community is indifferent on this issue. Passive resistance may however take the form of utilising other sources of water and those who are hostile to the idea may actively campaign against the continuation of the service.

Aerial spraying of insecticides for the control of arthropod vectors during an epidemic could theoretically be carried out even if there is strong opposition by the local community. It cannot be done on the

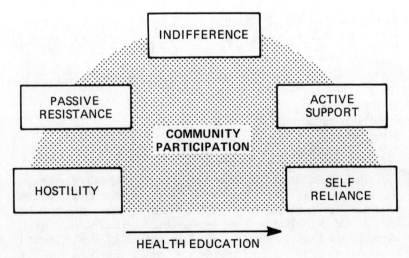

Fig. 9.3 Community attitudes to health measures

basis of self-help nor does it call for active co-operation of the community.

In all cases it is important to ensure that the community is well informed about action that is proposed, that their agreement is sought and obtained, and their involvement in the implementation is at the optimal level.

The examples given illustrate the varying degrees of community participation required for success.

Conclusion

The contents of this chapter are meant to provide general guidance about the nature and organisation of health services. In conclusion three points need emphasis:

1 *The need for planning*—This involves a careful assessment of needs and resources, a definition of goals and a strategy for achieving them.
2 *The coverage of the population*—Coverage should be measured in terms of the actual services delivered to the people rather than in terms of buildings, staff and other resources provided.
3 *Evaluation*—The performance of the health services should be kept under review, and appropriate adjustments should be made to render them more efficient and more effective in achieving the desired goals.

FURTHER READING

WHO proc. 13th CIOMS Round Table Conference. (1980). *Economics and Health Policy.* ed. A. Griffiths and Z. Bankowolli.

On being in charge. A guide for middle-management in primary health care. McMahon, Rosemary, *et al.* (1980) WHO, Geneva

Wld. Hlth. Stats. Quart. Vol. 33, No. 2. (1980). *World Trends in Health Manpower Development. A Review.* A. Mejia

DAVEY and LIGHTBODY'S *Control of Disease in the Tropics*, 4th edn. (1971). ed. T. H. Davey and T. Wilson. H. K. Lewis and Co. Ltd., London.

Control of Communicable Diseases in Man. ed. A. S. Benenson. 12th edn. (1975). American Public Health Association, Washington, D.C., 20036

Epidemiologic Methods. (1972). B. McMahon, T. F. Pugh and J. Ipsen. Little, Brown & Co., Boston.

CHAPTER 10

FAMILY HEALTH

The family health services include three components:
Maternal Health
Child Health
Family planning
The care of pregnant women, mothers and their children deserve the highest priority in every community. The reasons for giving such emphasis to these services can be briefly summarised:

(1) *High risk group*
Pregnant women and children represent a high risk group within the population. The situation is particularly serious in developing countries where the statistics show very high mortality and morbidity in these groups as compared with the rest of the population and with similar groups in developed countries and in privileged sections of their own country. In some rural communities in developing countries, the infant mortality rate may be 10 times, the child death rate (1–4 years) may be 40 times and the maternal mortality rate may be 80 times as high as in developed countries.

(2) *Need for prophylaxis and early diagnosis*
Many of the serious ailments occurring in pregnancy are best approached by prophylaxis and or by early diagnosis and treatment. For example, eclampsia is best controlled by detecting pre-eclamptic toxaemia at an early stage and taking appropriate action. Puerperal and neonatal tetanus are controlled by immunisation with tetanus toxoid and ensuring hygienic conditions during delivery and the puerperium. Children can also be protected against a number of common childhood infections by vaccination, e.g., measles, whooping cough, poliomyelitis.

(3) *Interrelated problems*
Because of the close relationship between the mother and her child, their health problems are interrelated. Illness in the pregnant woman can have adverse effect on the foetus. The care of the pregnant woman is therefore in effect, early care of her child. In early infancy the mother is usually most directly responsible for the care of the child, both feeding and general care.

(4) *The health of the next generation*
The care of children deserves high priority so as to ensure that they grow

up into fit and healthy adults. Close attention to maternal and child care is therefore an important investment in the next generation.

(5) *Operational convenience and continuity of care*
It is usually convenient for mothers and their children to be attended at the same clinic and where possible, the same team of health workers. The care of the child can be managed as a continuous process starting from early pregnancy, through delivery of the mother, to early infancy and through childhood.

Objectives of family Health Care

The objectives of the maternal services are to ensure that as far as possible women remain healthy throughout pregnancy, that they have healthy babies and recover fully from the effects of pregnancy and delivery. The child health services aim at ensuring that children remain fit and healthy and that they achieve optimal growth and development both physical and mental. The objective of family planning services is to enable couples to have children that they want when they want them and also to avoid unwanted pregnancies; and to encourage them to space the pregnancies and limit their number in the interest of the health of the family.

Maternity Services

The maternal health services include three components:
Ante-natal care
Delivery services
Post-natal care

ANTE-NATAL CARE

The provision of ante-natal services is the most valuable measure for protecting the health of pregnant women and ensuring a successful outcome of pregnancy. Ante-natal care should include the following elements:

1 Assessment of the risk status of the pregnancy

The ante-natal services should provide care for all pregnant women with special attention to the most vulnerable groups, who are most likely to develop complications. Such persons are said to be 'at risk' and the characteristics or circumstances of such groups or persons are known as 'risk factors'. Although these risk factors vary from place to place, in most parts of the world some of them are regularly associated with a poor outcome of pregnancy: first pregnancy; high parity (> 5), frequent pregnancies; age, with high-risk at both extremes, the very young and the older woman; previous child loss; malnutrition.

The risk factors can be identified by careful epidemiological studies, relating variables in the woman and her environment to the outcome of pregnancy. Statistical analysis of such data can provide estimates of the importance of various risk factors. A simple scoring system, devised by the World Health Organisation, can be modified for local use (see Table 10.1).

Table 10.1 Simple scoring system

	Characteristics	*Points*
Age	Under 19, over 40	4
	Between 30 and 39	2
	Between 20 and 29	0
Number of children	10 or more	4
	0 to 1	2
	2 to 9	0
Interval between deliveries	Less than 24 months since last delivery	1
	24 months or more since last delivery	0
Medical history	Previous obstetrical complications, perinatal deaths, etc.	3
	Diabetes heart disease, renal disease, psychoses, etc.	5
Maternal education	Illiterate	1
	Can read and write	0

The points are added up to give a total score and decisions taken as follows:

1 Highest risk, referral obligatory	5 points or more
2 High risk, referral recommended	3 to 4 points
3 Usual risk, usual local care	0 to 2 points

The risk status of the woman must be kept under review throughout pregnancy. The occurrence of a complication, e.g. abnormal presentation, may alter the risk category.

2 Education

The visits to the ante-natal clinic provide a valuable opportunity for the education of the pregnant woman on how to look after herself during pregnancy, what to expect during delivery, and also how to prepare for the care of her new baby. Generally, pregnant women are very receptive to health education because of their anxiety to have healthy babies. Advantage should be taken of this interest to teach them about nutrition, personal hygiene, and environmental sanitation. They should learn how to obtain a balanced diet using locally available foodstuffs. They should become aware of the dangers associated with dirt, and should appreciate the value of personal hygiene and good environmental sanitation. Apart from lectures and demonstrations at the clinics, where feasible, the pregnant woman should be visited at home by the community nurse or other health personnel. In this way, she can be guided to use the resources available to her in improving the sanitary condition of her home and in making other preparations for the arrival of the baby.

The pregnant woman should also learn about the normal changes which occur during pregnancy and she should be alerted about the danger signals such as the swelling of her feet and vaginal bleeding. She would then be able to seek help early should any complication occur or threaten.

3 Preventive Measures

Pregnant women are particularly susceptible to certain infections and other diseases. Depending on the local problems, specific prophylactic measures may be indicated. For example, in an endemic area of malaria, chemoprophylaxis may be of vital importance. Active immunisation of the pregnant woman with tetanus toxoid is highly effective in preventing neonatal tetanus, a disease which still occurs in communities where the health services are poorly developed. To reduce the incidence of anaemia of pregnancy, supplementary iron and folic acid are usually prescribed. Other prophylactic measures may be indicated by the local situation. The important principle is to do everything possible to improve the general health of the pregnant woman and to anticipate as far as possible any factor which may cause a deterioration in her condition.

4 Monitoring

Ante-natal care provides the opportunity of monitoring the progress of the pregnancy so that any deviations from normal can be detected at an early stage before serious complications occur. The woman is encouraged to note and describe any symptoms or signs that she has observed since her last visit to the clinic and she can be reassured when these do not signify any serious abnormality. Simple indicators have been devised for monitoring pregnancy including measurement of body weight, haemoglobin, and blood pressure, examination of urine for protein and sugar, and physical examination including specific obstetric observations.

Where resources exist, more sophisticated investigations can be used to follow the development of the foetus and to detect abnormalities. For example, because of the higher risk of Down's syndrome in women over the age of 35 years, obstetricians in developed countries recommend that amniocentesis be done in such cases to offer the possibility of therapeutic abortion if this is acceptable.

DELIVERY SERVICES

Most pregnant women can be safely delivered using relatively simple facilities but in some cases skilled intervention is required to ensure a favourable outcome. It is important to have a range of facilities, from the simplest to the most highly sophisticated, to match the full spectrum of risks associated with different pregnancies. The risk status of the woman with regard to delivery is determined from her past history and progress during pregnancy. The situation could alter dramatically in the course of delivery; emergency services providing skilled intervention should always be available regardless of the initial estimate of the risk.

In many developing countries, traditional birth attendants play an important role in the delivery of pregnant women. These are people, usually women, who have acquired their skill in delivering women by working with other traditional birth attendants and from their own experience. In some countries, formal programmes have been devised for further training of these traditional birth attendants and incorporating them within the health services. In favour of such schemes is that these attendants usually belong to the local community in which they practise, where they have gained the confidence of the families and where they are content to live and serve. Their training programme is designed to improve their technique with particular reference to cleanliness, to recognise abnormalities which indicate the need for referral for more skilled evaluation and management, and to recognise their own limitations, thereby refraining from attempting to deal with problems beyond their skill. They are also supplied with simple kits which include hygienic dressings and simple equipment.

POST-NATAL CARE

During the puerperium the woman recovers from the effects and injuries, if any, associated with delivery. The physiological changes which took place during pregnancy are now being reversed and her body is restored to its pre-pregnant state. The post-natal care services are designed to supervise this process, to detect any abnormalities and to deal with them. In particular, she should be protected against the hazards such as puerperal infection, to which she is liable at this stage.

This may be a convenient service through which to introduce family planning so as to reduce the risk of the early occurrence of another pregnancy.

With regard to the child, it is important to ensure that breast feeding is satisfactorily established at this period.

CHILD CARE

In developing countries, many of the diseases which cause severe illness and death in children can be prevented or treated by simple measures. In some areas, one quarter to one half of the children die before they reach the age of 5 years. Some of the survivors of this high death rate are left with serious sequelae and other permanent effects on their health. Yet the situation can be dramatically improved by the provision of child health services. In order to be most effective, the services must reach all the children, with particular attention to the most vulnerable groups. There are three major objectives of the child health services:

1 Promotion of the health of children to ensure that they achieve optimal growth and development both physical and mental.
2 Protection of the children from major hazards through specific measures (immunisations, chemoprophylaxis, dietary supplements) and through improvement in the level of care provided by the mothers and the family.
3 Treatment of diseases and disorders with particular emphasis on early diagnosis. The aim is to provide effective remedy at an early stage before dangerous complications occur.

The role of the family cannot be over-emphasised with regard to child health. The health personnel should therefore pay particular attention to the education of mothers on the care of their children. They should use all available means to bring about changes within the family in the interest of the child. Contacts with fathers and other influential people within the household could be of value.

Promotion of Health

The growth and development of each child should be carefully monitored. It is important that the child be seen at the clinic regularly during the first five years of life. The mother would be guided on matters concerning the child's diet, hygiene and other factors affecting the child's health and safety. Simple charts showing graphs of the normal growth curve can be used effectively in monitoring the child's physical development. Experience has shown that it is better for each mother to retain her child's growth card; it increases her involvement in monitoring the child's development.

Protection

Each child should be immunised against the common communicable diseases for which vaccines are abailable (Table 10.2). Immunisation is routinely offered against tuberculosis (BCG), tetanus, whooping cough, diphtheria, poliomyelitis and measles. The choice of vaccines and the immunisation schedule should be selected on the basis of local epidemiological situations, and on the most practicable routine. The

Table 10.2 A guide to immunisation in childhood in the tropics (Modified after R. G. Hendrickse)

Vaccine	Recommended age of administration	Method of administration	Special problems associated with use	Other comments
BCG	(i) Neonatal period as a routine. (ii) Tuberculin-negative subjects of any age exposed to myco-bacterial infections.	Intradermal injection may also be given by multiple-puncture technique using modified 'Heaf Gun'.	Vaccine light and heat sensitive—risk of inactivation in unskilled hands.	(i) INH Resistant BCG may be used in special circumstances. (ii) Multiple-puncture technique recommended for use by semi-skilled personnel.
Triple antigen (combined tetanus and diphtheria toxoids and pertussis vaccine)	Start at 2 months. Give 3 shots at monthly intervals. Booster at 12–18 months.	Subcutaneous or IM injection.	None of note. Rarely encephalitis due to pertussis component of vaccine.	Where high risk of pertussis can start at age of 1 month.
Poliomyelitis vaccine (a) killed (Salk) type	Start at 2 months and monthly × 3.	Subcutaneous or IMI.	None.	May be simultaneously administered with Triple antigen in separate syringe unless combined vaccine used. Best for small local clinics.

(b) live (Sabin) type (Trivalent)	Start at 2 months and monthly × 3.	Oral.	Cool storage required. May get poor antibody response when used on small groups in tropics.	Most effective when mass vaccination campaigns undertaken.
Measles. Further attenuated vaccine	8 months.	Subcutaneous injection. Jet injection for mass immunisation campaigns.	Refrigerated storage and maintenance of 'cold chain' before use.	Expensive. Indications that reduced dosage (to $\frac{1}{5}$ recommended dose) may be effective.

Notes: (1) *Cholera* epidemics—Cholera vaccine is given subcutaneously or intramuscularly ideally in two doses of 0.5 ml and 1.0 ml 7 to 28 days apart—one injection of 1.0 ml is usually used in *mass* immunisation campaigns.

(2) *Yellow fever* epidemics—Mass immunisation is done by using a dose of 0.5 ml given subcutaneously—infants under 1 year of age should not be vaccinated.

(3) *Tetanus*—In areas of the tropics where tetanus is prevalent, tetanus toxoid should be given to as many adults as possible who have not been immunised in childhood and to all pregnant women in order to protect the infant from neonatal tetanus.

(4) Differing epidemiological conditions in various countries may require relevant alterations to the above guidelines.

vaccines should be handled with care to ensure that they preserve their potency. This is particularly important in the case of live vaccines which are sensitive to heat and must therefore be kept under refrigeration until administered. By the use of refrigerators at the main health centres and insulated cold boxes when the vaccine is being carried for use in the field, the continuous cold chain can be preserved.

In endemic areas of malaria, chemoprophylaxis is usually recommended for the highly susceptible groups including pre-school children, pregnant women and visitors. Other specific prophylactic measures may be indicated as for example, the use of dietary supplements to prevent common nutritional deficiencies.

Early diagnosis and treatment

Simple remedies should be made available for the treatment of the common diseases of childhood. Mothers should be encouraged to seek treatment early and where appropriate to institute simple therapy at home. They should for example learn how to clean simple cuts and abrasions, covering them with clean dressings so as to prevent infection. Especially in areas where they cannot gain rapid access to the clinic, mothers should learn how to prepare and administer the oral rehydration fluid in cases of diarrhoea.

Special Services

Ideally health services should reach every child within the community. It is particularly important to identify the most vulnerable or the high risk group. The factors which most accurately identify the high risk groups are best determined locally by epidemiological studies but in general high risk is associated with factors in the mother (illiteracy, poverty, past history of a child who had died) and in the child (e.g. low birth weight, haemoglobinopathy). Special attention should be given to such children with support to the family by home visits and other measures designed to improve the level of care at home.

It may be useful to provide special services for children who have specific health problems. For example, a nutrition rehabilitation service would help to supervise the recovery of malnourished children and educate the mothers on the nutrition of their children. Services may also be provided for handicapped children, for those who are maladjusted or have emotional problems.

FAMILY PLANNING

The objective of this service is to encourage couples to take responsible decisions about pregnancy and enable them to achieve their wishes with regard to:

(a) Preventing unwanted pregnancies
(b) Securing desired pregnancies
(c) Spacing of pregnancies
(d) Limiting the size of the family.

The concept of responsible parenthood should be promoted; that in the interest of the health of the family, couples should have children by choice and not by chance.

The family planning programme should be based on an analysis of the needs of the community. Available data on the reproductive behaviours of the community should be carefully examined noting especially birth rates in various groups, age of first pregnancy, average interval between pregnancies, family size, the use of contraceptive methods both traditional and modern; knowledge of these methods and attitudes to them, the frequency of induced abortions and other indications of unwanted pregnancies.

In the context of family health, this service should make available simple effective and safe contraceptive methods which are compatible with their religion and culture, and also in keeping with their needs and resources. For religious reasons, some couples cannot accept artificial methods and devices; the natural method based on the safe period should be taught to them. A variety of contraceptive devices should be available so that each couple can select the one that is most aesthetically acceptable and practicable in their circumstances.

ORGANISATION OF FAMILY HEALTH SERVICES

For reasons stated in the early part of the chapter, it is generally preferable to provide an integrated service comprising material, child health and family planning services. The details of the organisation would vary from place to place, but the important issue is to make sure that the services are provided in such a way that the community can make the best use of them. Rather than having a rigid format, the health personnel should seek innovative ways of promoting the coverage and the quality of care. For example, adjustments in the timing of clinics could make the service more easily accessible to the mothers. It may be particularly convenient for them if the services were provided in association with markets and other community activities. It may be necessary to make special arrangements for women who would not be able to utilise the normal services. For example in Moslem communities, women in Purdah may not be able to go out to the clinics in the day time but could do so at night. Evening clinics at convenient sites could solve this particular problem.

For the family health services, more than for any other component of the health services, the intimate involvement of the community is essential in making the best decisions. The resources of the community should be fully utilised, e.g. training and using voluntary health workers, and health education through women's associations.

Continuous evaluation should be built into the service using simple indicators to monitor progress. Both the inputs (services provided, activities of the health personnel) and the outputs (changes in the health status of women and children) should be monitored. With regard to inputs, one should measure coverage of each major component of the services offered. For example, what proportion of pregnant women within the community are seen at least once during pregnancy? What proportion of them deliver under supervision of the health personnel? What proportion of children receive at least one dose of vaccine, and what proportion complete the full course? With regard to outputs, the standard rates used in health statistics should be calculated—perinatal mortality, infant mortality, neonatal mortality, etc. Major complications of pregnancy, and delivery should be recorded and the rates monitored in different groups so as to identify high risk or problem groups. The incidence of measles, paralytic poliomyelitis, severe diarrhoea, and other important diseases of children would also provide useful indicators of the health of the child population. It is not feasible to monitor each and every condition and the inclusion of too many elements may reduce the efficiency of the system. It is much better to select a few indicators, concentrating for example on the top ten killing diseases in childhood. Regardless of the indicators which are selected, it is important to relate the cases or events to the population at risk. It is difficult to interpret such data (e.g. number of children immunised, number of deliveries at maternity centres, cases of measles) unless they are related to the appropriate denominators.

THE CHILD AT SCHOOL

It is universally recognised that the health of schoolchildren deserves special attention. In order to derive the maximum benefit from the educational programme, the child must be healthy physically, mentally and emotionally. It is also well known that children at school are exposed to a variety of hazards—physical injury, infection and emotional problems. School age is a period during which the child is undergoing rapid physical and mental development; a healthy environment is required to provide the child with the best opportunity of making the appropriate adjustments that are required during this critical period. The school provides a unique opportunity for health education; a means of establishing a firm foundation for the healthy habits of the future adult population. By safeguarding the health of the schoolchildren of today, one is ensuring the health of the adults of tomorrow. In many developing countries the need for good school health programmes is particularly critical. Apart from the universal reasons for having a special programme for schoolchildren, there is the additional factor that in many developing countries, the schoolchildren are the survivors of a high childhood mortality. Many of them still bear the sequelae of the diseases which were responsible for the deaths of the other children and most of them are still subject to the environmental conditions which predisposed to the high morbidity and mortality of pre-school age.

The overall objective of the school health programme is to ensure that every child is as healthy as possible so that he can obtain the full benefit from his education.

The Elements of a School Health Programme

Although the detailed organisation of a school health programme varies from place to place, the following elements are usually represented:

1 Medical Inspection of the Children

Routine, periodic medical examination is designed to detect defects which require medical attention. The medical examination also provides the opportunity of discussing with parents and teachers the health problems and needs of the children. It includes screening for defects of hearing and sight. The school examination will ascertain whether the child is fit to take part in school activities, including sports.

2 Assessment of Handicapped Children

The school health programme must include some mechanism for finding children who are physically or mentally handicapped, assessing them, supervising them and placing them in the most appropriate institution if special care is indicated. The main categories of handicapped children are:
(a) Blind and partially sighted
(b) Those with defective hearing and/or speech
(c) Epileptic
(d) Educationally sub-normal
(e) Maladjusted and psychotic
(f) Physically handicapped or delicate.

3 Health Education

The objective of the health education programme at school is to make the children value health as a desirable asset, and to know what the individual and the community can do to maintain and promote health. The course of instruction would include basic information about the normal structure and function of the human body, the agents of disease, and the role of the environment in maintaining good health. At the appropriate age-group, various aspects of sex education can be incorporated into the syllabus. All fit children should participate in a well-designed programme of physical education.

4 Environmental Sanitation

It is necessary to ensure that the school environment is maintained at a high standard in order to safeguard the health of the children and to provide them with a practical example of healthy living. The school environment must reinforce the theoretical lessons learnt in the classes on health education. The school should be sited in a safe place, in an area free from excessive noise and other nuisances such as smoke or soot. The building should be well constructed so as to minimise accidents. The classrooms should be of adequate size, well lighted and ventilated. Sanitary facilities for the disposal of wastes should be provided, and there should be an adequate supply of safe water for drinking and washing. There should be adequate facilities for recreation.

5 Control of Infection

Going to school represents for many children the first opportunity to mix with children other than close relatives and immediate neighbours. Hence, schooling often represents their first contacts with infections to which they are susceptible. The control of infection includes the exclusion of sick children from school and the protection of susceptible children against such infections as polio, diphtheria and typhoid by immunisation. Parents should be urged not to send sick children to school and teachers should, in the course of daily inspection of the children, note any sign of illness. The health of the schoolteachers and other school personnel should be kept under careful observation to ensure that they do not transmit infection to the children. For example, schoolteachers should be routinely screened for tuberculosis and food handlers for enteric infections.

6 Nutrition

The school health programme should include some mechanism for the promotion of adequate diet for schoolchildren. The programme should be designed to ensure that each child is adequately nourished and, where specific defects are noted, to provide some means of supplementation. The programme would include some health education of parents through group activities such as the Parent-Teacher Associations, or individually in cases of special problems. It may be useful to have a school meal programme; this can provide a valuable demonstration of good balanced diets, but the school meal can also be specifically designed to supplement the child's diet at home in such a way as to make up any major specific nutritional deficiencies. Practical instruction in nutrition can include the growing of food crops in the school garden and mother-craft and cookery classes especially for the girls.

7 Special Surveys

Special epidemiological surverys can be conducted to investigate specific health problems. It can also be used as part of the assessment of health needs and evaluation of the school health programme.

Operation of the School Health Programme

The detailed organisation of the school health programme varies from one country to the other. In the more developed countries, the school health services employ numerous doctors, dentists, nurses, psychologists, speech therapists and other skilled personnel. In most developing countries, such elaborate schemes are not in operation. The objective in each country should be to exploit the available resources and co-ordinate them into a national school health programme.

The following services are usually provided in school health programmes:

(a) *Medical inspection*
(b) *Screening tests for defects*
(c) *Clinics*—(i) Minor ailments, (ii) Consultation; (iii) Special clinics, e.g. orthopaedic, ophthalmological, ear, nose and throat and child guidance
(d) *Dental services*—Preventive and therapeutic.

Co-ordination of the School Health Programme

The health care of the child at school requires the co-ordinated efforts of parents, teachers, school health personnel, family physicians and local health authorities. Each has an important role to perform; skilled dovetailing of these various units will provide the most effective school health programme. Since there are overlapping functions in several areas, it is important to avoid unnecessary duplication of effort especially where resources are scarce. Even where resources are lavish, it is essential to prevent avoidable conflict and friction.

The provision of a safe healthy environment is the responsibility of the school authorities. They are also responsible for health education and physical education at school. The personnel of the school health programme are responsible for the medical inspection of the children; in some places they also undertake treatment but in other countries any defect or illness is treated by the family physician. The school health personnel are also responsible for the control of communicable diseases, although again they or the family physician may be responsible for immunisation of the children. In developing countries, many of these functions are performed by medical auxiliaries who are working under the supervision of doctors.

Assessment and Evaluation

Evaluation of the school health programme depends in the first instance on a careful definition of the objectives of the programme.

First, there should be an assessment of the work load of the various units: the number of medical inspections, the number of cases treated at the clinics, the number of children immunised, the number of school meals served, etc. The health status of the children can be assessed from an analysis of the data gathered at the medical inspections, from sickness records and from special surveys. The data generated in the operation of the school health service should be compiled and analysed. Such information as the distribution of the heights and weights of the children, the haemoglobin level, and the frequency of dental caries can provide valuable assessment of the health of the children and the effectiveness of the school health programme.

FURTHER READING

WHO Tech. Rep. Ser. No. 569: *Evaluation of Family Planning Services.*
WHO Tech. Rep. Ser. No. 623: *Induced Abortion.*

CHAPTER 11

ENVIRONMENTAL HEALTH

The objective of environmental sanitation is to create and maintain conditions in the environment that will promote health and prevent diseases. Man's external environment contains elements which are essential for life and for the maintenance of good health. In addition, the environment contains potential hazards. Man has a wide range of tolerance of environmental conditions because of his ability to adapt. Such biological adaptation has its limits, and the breakdown of adaptation represents the onset of disease. For example, the human being can tolerate wide fluctuations in environmental temperature; he has various mechanisms (sweating, shivering) for coping with these changes. If however the heat stress is excessive, then adaptive mechanisms break down and disease results may be in the form of heat stroke. Health can therefore be viewed as successful adaptation to the environment, whereas disease represents a breakdown of adaptation.

The breakdown of adaptation can be prevented by:
(a) increasing the host's ability to withstand stresses in the environment, e.g. by good nutrition
(b) reducing the hazardous and hostile elements in the environment.

Environmental Sanitation

This is the process of taming the environment so that it no longer constitutes a hazard to man. In particular, environmental sanitation deals with:
1 Provision of a safe and adequate supply of water
2 Disposal of wastes
3 Safeguarding of food
4 Provision of good housing
5 Control of insect vectors and other pests
6 Control of animal reservoirs of infection
7 Air hygiene and prevention of atmospheric pollution
8 Elimination of other hazards—noise, radiation, etc.

Many of these problems in environmental sanitation are dealt with by public health engineers, technicians and other non-medical personnel rather than by the physician. The doctor is therefore not usually required to know in detail how the various appliances are constructed and maintained. Nevertheless, he should be familiar with the basic principles involved. This would enable him to give informed support to his environmental health team and for simple projects, guidance to the health auxiliaries.

The 1980's have been designated as the International Water Supply and Sanitation decade, during which a concerted effort will be made by seven United Nations agencies to improve the environmental health of the world's poorer population (see Fig. 11.1). A better understanding of behavioural factors influencing water use and defaecation practices is a vital and hitherto much neglected component of such a programme, since not only are changes in behaviour required to ensure that facilities are correctly utilised but the interventions must be so designed that they are acceptable to the recipient community, whether it be *rural* or living in *urban fringe* areas.

Water Supplies

Each community needs a safe and adequate supply of water. Water supply technologies need to be technically and environmentally sound, economically efficient, financially affordable, and acceptable to the users from the social, cultural, and political standpoints. They need to be simple in design and easy to install, operate and maintain.

Uses of Water

(a) *Domestic*—(i) drinking and cooking, (ii) personal hygiene—for washing the body and clothes, (iii) environmental sanitation—for washing utensils, floors and for the disposal of wastes, (iv) temperature control—for heating and cooling, (v) gardening.

(b) *Industrial and agricultural.*

Sources of Water

These include: (*a*) rain water, (*b*) surface water—streams, rivers, ponds, lakes and sea, (*c*) underground water—wells, bore holes (see Fig. 11.2) and springs.

(a) *Rain water*
Rain water is pure but it may pick up impurities from the atmosphere, roofs, roof gutterings and storage tank.

(b) *Surface water*
The source is easily polluted by direct contamination by human beings and animals, or indirectly when rain washes faeces and other pollutants from the banks into the streams and rivers. Surface water must, therefore, be purified before use.

(c) *Underground water*
(1) WELLS These may be:

International Drinking Water Supply and Sanitation Decade 1981-1990

"Clean water and adequate sanitation for all by the year 1990"

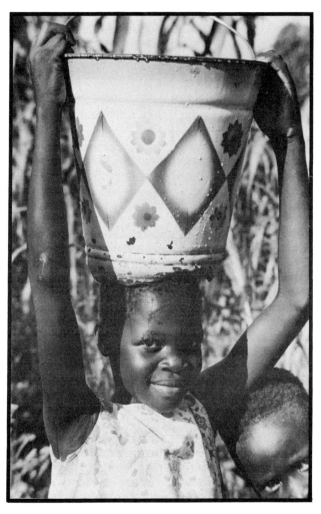

Fig. 11.1 Part of the United Nations special leaflet to promote International Drinking Water and Sanitation Decade 1981–1990

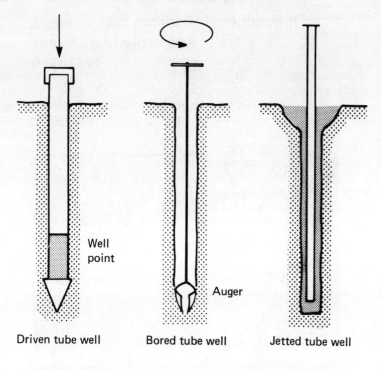

Well point

Auger

Driven tube well   Bored tube well   Jetted tube well

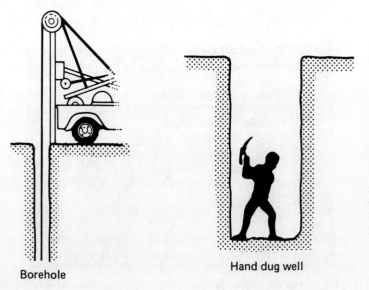

Borehole   Hand dug well

Fig. 11.2 Some commonly used methods of groundwater extraction

(a) Shallow wells—the water is collected above the first impervious layer. Shallow wells are liable to pollution by seepage from surface water.

(b) Deep wells—water is drawn below the first impervious layer.

Protection of wells. (i) The wells should be situated at least 100 feet (preferably uphill) from any potential source of pollution, e.g. pit latrine. (ii) There should be a watertight lining for at least 10 feet from the surface. (iii) There should be a parapet about 2 feet high surrounded by a concrete apron to drain the waste water away. (iv) There must be a watertight cover. (v) Water should be drawn preferably by a pump, or at least through a permanent bucket which is anchored to the well.

(2) SPRINGS   The water from a natural spring may be quite pure. It can be protected by building a concrete dam so that the water accumulates in a reservoir and is drawn through pipes.

Whatever its source, the supply of water should be:

(a) *Adequate*—A minimum of 5 to 10 gallons per person per day is required. The requirement is much higher in modern industrial urban areas (40 to 100 gallons per person per day, or more).

(b) *Safe*—It should be free from chemical and biological hazards.

(c) *Acceptable*—It should be acceptable in terms of its taste, colour and softness.

Diseases associated with Water

The water-related diseases can be broadly classified into five epidemiological groups:

Group I   Water-borne infections, e.g. cholera, typhoid, infective hepatitis.

Group II   Water-shortage diseases, e.g. skin infections, trachoma.

Group III   Water-impounding diseases, e.g. schistosomiasis, guinea-worm.

Group IV   Water-arthropod diseases, e.g. malaria, onchocerciasis.

Group V   Chemical constituents either excess or shortage, e.g. fluoride.

Purification of Water

The purification of water can be achieved by a combination of some of the following measures:

(a) *Protection of the source*

In particular, the source water should be protected from pollution from human faeces, a major source of pathogenic organisms and other human contact which could lead to contamination, e.g. with guinea-worm. Human beings and animals should be excluded from surface sources of water.

(b) *Storage*

Some of the human pathogens have a relatively short life in water, they may be absent from water that has been stored for a few days or longer. Cysts, e.g. *E. histolytica*, tend to survive for much longer periods.

(c) *Coagulation and sedimentation*

Addition of alum to water causes flocculation of the finely suspended matter; these larger particles settle more rapidly, leaving a clear supernatant.

(d) *Filtration*

Various devices are used for filtration: a thick linen cloth may remove large particles, including cyclops (intermediate host of guinea-worm), from the water; a sand filter consisting of sand and stones of graded size, with fine sand at the top and large stones at the botton; a simple domestic filter in which the water is filtered through a 'candle' filter which is made of fine clay. At best, filtration will remove bacteria, protozoal cysts and larger particles but viruses ('filterable viruses') will pass through the filter.

All filters require proper care and regular cleaning to remain effective. Some 'appropriate technology' designs for household use may well become sources of pollution themselves and require considerable health education and supervision to be effective. The same applies to porcelain and diatomaceous earth filters.

(e) *Disinfection*

Chlorination is the most widely used method of chemical disinfection of water. It may be used in the form of chlorine gas for large municipal schemes or as bleaching powder (chloride of lime), liquid bleach, or hypochlorite. *Super-chlorination* consists in the application of a dose of chlorine which considerably exceeds that required to disinfect the water. This method is often used in an emergency, e.g. during epidemics and after a suitable contact time the water is dechlorinated.

PROPERTIES AND USE OF CHLORINE   Chlorine is a germicidal and can be used to control algae and slime. It also oxidises iron, manganese and hydrogen sulphide. It cannot be used where there is heavy organic contamination or high levels of iron or manganese, but organic contamination can be reduced by pre-settlement and filtration if necessary and possible. The need for chlorination in any location must first be established and the precise requirements decided.

CHEMICAL ACTION OF CHLORINE   As chlorine is added to water the following process occurs:

1 Destruction of chlorine by reducing compounds
2 Formation of combined residual chlorine (chloramines).
3 Partial destruction of chloramines.
4 Increase in free residual chlorine.

The amount of chlorine in the water may be checked by a simple apparatus such as a colour comparator. Free residual chlorine is the main disinfecting agent and sufficient chlorine should be added to give a final residual level of 0.2 mg/1 (0.2 ppm)–0.5 mg/1. *Note* that (1) a minimum contact time of 15 minutes is required for the chlorine to be effective, and (2) chlorine in normal doses (as above) will not kill some cysts and ova or organisms embedded in solid matter.

CHOICE OF CHLORINE DISINFECTANT:

1 Liquid chlorine is generally used in main piped supplies.
2 Chloride of Lime (bleaching powder) is bulky and unstable but simple to use. It contains 20–35 % by weight of available chlorine. It must be stored in a cool, dark place in corrosion resistant containers. Since it contains insoluble solids prepared solutions should be decanted before use in drip feeds.
3 HTH (High Strength Hypochlorite) is more stable than bleaching powder. It contains 60–70 % by weight of available chlorine and is useful where large quantities are required, e.g. in emergencies.

PREPARATION OF WELLS BEFORE CHLORINATION It is important that all receptacles being used to hold chlorinated water are disinfected first. The following procedure should be used:

1 Wash and scrub lining of well with solution of chloride of lime (100 ppm available chlorine).
2 Measure the volume of water in the well. Add a solution of chloride of lime to give a chlorine dose of 50–100 ppm (100 ppm = 50 g of chloride of lime in 100 litres of water).
3 Leave for 12 hours and then pump out. The well is then ready for use.

(f) *Boiling*

This is a reliable way of eliminating pathogens for individual households but it is impracticable on a large scale. It can be used in special circumstances, e.g. when there is sudden breakdown in the treatment process of a municipal water supply. It is also advisable to boil all water to be used for feeding young infants.

Quality of Water

The quality of water is assessed by (a) physical, (b) microscopical, (c) chemical, and (d) bacteriological examination.

Chemical Properties of the Water

There should be no chemical constituent in quantities that could be a health hazard. Safety limits have been prescribed for some of the elements (Table 11.1).

With regard to fluoride, a high level (1.0 to 1.5 mg per litre) predisposes to dental and skeletal fluorosis; a low content (0.5 mg/litre) is associated with dental caries. Therefore, fluoride may be added to bring the concentration to about 1.0 mg/litre.

Table 11.1 Safety levels of common elements in domestic water

	Maximum allowable concentrations in parts per million (i.e. mg/litre)
Lead (as Pb)	0.1
Arsenic (as As)	0.2
Selenium (as Se)	0.05
Chromium (as Cr hexavalent)	0.05
Cyanide (as CN)	0.01

Biological Tests

Although pathogens such as *S. typhi* and *V. cholerae* can be isolated from water, the routine bacteriological examination of water concentrates on detecting evidence of faecal pollution of water. Coliform organisms are used as indicators of recent faecal pollution because these organisms are present in faeces in large numbers and they survive in water for relatively short periods. Faecal coli (*E. coli*) can be differentiated from other coliform organisms which occur in nature. A high coliform count ('presumptive coliform count') of 10 coliforms/100 ml or more is regarded as being suspicious or bad; and there should be no faecal coli.

DISPOSAL OF WASTES

The accumulation of waste products and their indiscriminate disposal represent a grave hazard to health. Systems of waste disposal are designed to eliminate these hazards. Village-level sanitation systems need to be culturally and politically acceptable to the users, financially affordable and technically simple to construct, operate, and maintain. It is much easier to build an excreta disposal system than to ensure its proper use. The broad objectives of a waste disposal system can thus be briefly summarised:

(a) *Eliminate hazards to man*
   (i) physical, e.g. broken bottles, empty cans
   (ii) chemical, e.g. poisonous chemicals in industrial wastes
   (iii) biological, e.g. the agents and vectors of disease harboured in wastes.

(b) *Prevent pollution of the natural environment*
The dumping of wastes on land, and the indiscriminate disposal into rivers and other surface waters, or into the air can cause destruction of the natural life.

(c) *Salvage of materials of economic value*
The following problems will be considered:
(a) Disposal of sewage
(b) Disposal of refuse
(c) Disposal of industrial wastes.

DISPOSAL OF SEWAGE

Human excreta are an important source of pathogenic organisms, especially the causative agents of diarrhoeal diseases. In addition, faeces are attractive to flies and support the development of the larval stages ('maggots') of filth flies. Apart from these hazards, the indiscriminate disposal of faeces can constitute a grave nuisance from the offensive sight and smell.

The sanitary disposal of human excreta can be achieved only where there are adequate provisions in the community for the disposal of faeces and where the people have learnt to appreciate and use them. Ideally, there should be at least one latrine for each family, and the device should be kept clean and maintained in good working order. Public latrines are also required in markets and other places where people gather in large numbers.

Qualities of the Ideal Latrine

A good latrine must possess the following qualities:
(a) There should be no handling of fresh faeces
(b) There should be no contamination of surface soil
(c) There should be no contamination of surface water or underground water that may enter springs or wells
(d) The excreta should not be accessible to flies or animals
(e) There should be no unpleasant odours or unsightly conditions
(f) The method should be simple and inexpensive in construction and operation and in relation to the resources of the community
(g) The method should be acceptable in terms of the cultural beliefs of the community.
The common methods of sewage disposal are:
(a) Bucket latrine
(b) Trench latrine
(c) Pit-hole latrine (Fig. 11.3)
(d) Bore-hole latrine
(e) Water-seal latrine of Cheugmai type
(f) Aqua privy (Fig. 11.4)
(g) Chemical closet
(h) Water-carried disposal methods—to sewage pits, septic tanks (Fig. 11.5), sewage farms or oxidation ponds.
The use of bucket latrine should be discouraged as widely as possible.

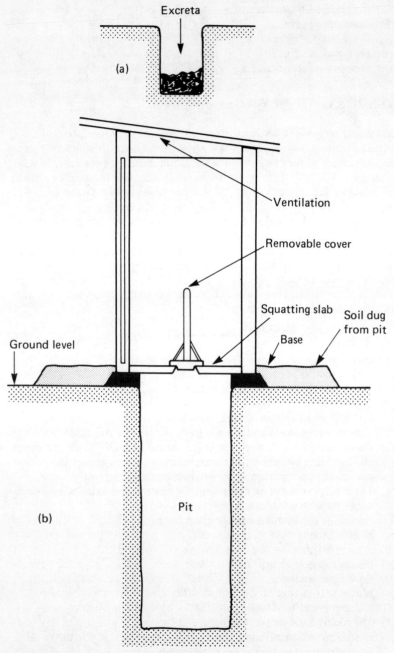

Fig. 11.3 (a) Principle of the pit-hole latrine (b) Properly constructed pit latrine

(a)

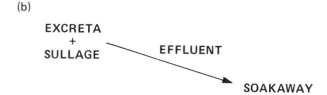

EXCRETA
+
LITTLE WATER

(b)

EXCRETA
+
SULLAGE   EFFLUENT

SOAKAWAY

Fig. 11.4 Aqua privy (a) Simplest form (b) Self-topping form

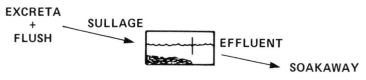

EXCRETA
+   SULLAGE
FLUSH   EFFLUENT

SOAKAWAY

Fig. 11.5 Principle of the septic tank

It often involves the handling of fresh faeces, flies and animals are attracted to and can often reach the faeces, and it tends to cause offensive odours. Where bucket latrines are in use, the single-bucket system should be replaced by the two-bucket system.

In the single-bucket system, the conservancy worker empties the bucket into a large pail or tank and returns the empty but dirty bucket to the latrine. In the two-bucket system, a fresh clean bucket is brought in to replace the dirty bucket; meanwhile the dirty bucket is removed to the depot, where it is emptied, washed and disinfected.

Various methods, such as pit latrines, septic tanks, oxidation ponds and such other methods, rely on the natural process of decomposition of faeces. Excreta, wherever deposited, decompose and ultimately become converted to an inodorous, inoffensive and stable product. In the process, many human pathogens are destroyed. Thus faeces are self-digesting and self-purifying.

The main actions of decomposition are to break down the complex organic compounds such as protein and urea into simpler and more stable forms; reduce the volume and mass (80 per cent of the decomposing material) by the production of such gases as methane, carbon dioxide, ammonia and nitrogen which are dissipated in the atmosphere, and by the production of soluble materials which leach away into the underlying soil. Pathogenic organisms are unable to survive the processes of decomposition or are attacked by the rich biological life of the decomposing mass. Bacteria play the major role in decomposition. The process may be entirely anaerobic, as it is in aqua privies, septic tanks, bottom of deep pits or entirely aerobic as in composting (see p. 315).

The long-term prevention of the diarrhoeal diseases rests largely upon the provision and use of adequate facilities for safe water and excreta disposal. The attainment of this objective requires, among other things, a large capital investment in the construction of water and sanitation facilities, and a better understanding of behavioural factors influencing water use and defaecation practices.

DISPOSAL OF REFUSE

This refers to the storage, collection and disposal of solid wastes in a community. Refuse includes various organic materials such as leaves and food remnants, and inorganic objects such as bottles, tins, and a variety of discarded objects.

Poor refuse disposal attracts flies (which then breed) and other insects, and affords food and shelter for rodents. It creates fire hazard and is a source of accidents through cuts and puncture wounds from sharp objects.

(a) *Storage of Refuse*

This involves provision of a sufficient number of containers to hold the volume of refuse produced between collections; the selection of an approved type of container; the placement of containers where they will provide maximum convenience for the user and easy access to the collection crew; and the maintenance of the containers and their surroundings in a sanitary condition. The dustbin or garbage-can should be watertight and provided with a tight-fitting lid. It should be rust resistant; structurally sound; easily filled, emptied and cleaned, and finished with side handles. The bins should rest on a concrete slab, the sweepings from which should be put in the bin and not cleared off on to the adjacent ground.

(b) *Collection of Refuse*

Where a community has no collection service, conditions are generally favourable for high fly and rat populations. Even where service is available, a careless collection employee may spill refuse on the premises or street. Rough handling may damage the container rim so that the lid may not fit properly, thereby making the refuse accessible to flies and rats.

Collection of refuse should be frequent, systematic and reliable, and bin points maintained by Government or Municipal Cleansing Services. Great improvements in collection by specially constructed vehicles have been developed in recent years.

Where combined refuse collection is practised, this service should be provided daily or at least twice a week. This practice will favour sanitary storage and will contribute to an environment adverse to flies, mosquitoes and rats. Collection crews must be properly trained.

(c) Disposal of Refuse

In any system the final disposal of refuse must be considered first, since it has an important influence on both storage and collection. Regardless of how diligently the householder attempts to control flies in his premises, he stands little chance when a nearby dump is a prolific breeding ground.

The methods of refuse disposal commonly used are:

1 *Dumping in the sea or river* This method is used in coastal cities and riverine towns, it results in littering of shore-lines with refuse and becomes a health as well as an accident hazard. It is also a deterrent to the tourist trade.

2 *Open dumping* This is cheap, it requires little planning and is therefore unfortunately too frequently found in tropical communities. It provides ideal breeding places for rats, flies and mosquitoes. Every effort should be made to eliminate this health menace and to replace it with sanitary and practical methods of disposal.

3 *Burning* Low-temperature burning of combustible refuse is frequently used. Generally speaking, burning using oil drums and cages or open burning are unsatisfactory and surroundings are frequently littered with cans and broken bottles that constitute an accident hazard to children playing in the area. The smoke and odours contribute to air pollution and it is a fire risk. Moreover, half-burnt refuse can afford breeding places for flies and provide food for rats.

4 *Composting* This is a process in which under suitable environmental conditions aerobic micro-organisms, principally thermophilic, break down organic matter to a fairly stable humus. Composting requires frequent turning, and two main methods are used: (*a*) Refuse without nightsoil, e.g. Trengganu method and (*b*) Refuse with nightsoil, e.g. Calcutta and Indore methods. The details of these various methods are available in standard textbooks of hygiene and sanitation.

5 *Controlled tipping* This is an effective and proven method for the hygienic disposal of refuse and can be used wherever sufficient and suitable land is available. Basically it consists of 4 steps: (i) depositing refuse in a planned controlled manner, (ii) spreading and compacting it in

layers to reduce its volume, (iii) covering the material with a layer of earth, and (iv) compacting the earth cover. The initial investment is low and health hazards, fire and nuisance are eliminated.

6 *Incineration* The newer incineration plants have reduced atmospheric pollution and by this method the volume of material for ultimate disposal is greatly reduced.

The final choice of method to be used for the sanitary disposal of refuse will naturally vary from rural to city areas; it will depend on the population density, the availability of land and other facilities at one's disposal.

(d) *Salvaging*

Some of the materials in refuse can be sorted and used. Thus, paper, rags, metal containers, bottles and similar objects can be salvaged.

INDUSTRIAL WASTES

Modern industrial processes produce chemical wastes which are potential hazards to man and other living things. Although each special problem cannot be examined in detail, some general principles can provide useful guide-lines.

Ideally the design of the plant should include a satisfactory means of disposal of the waste products. This may involve some processing of the effluent before it is ultimately discharged into a stream; it may require storage and final disposal by burying of solid wastes; or it may include a subsidiary process which can salvage and consume some of the waste products of the primary process.

In particular, the disposal of crude effluent into a stream should be strongly discouraged. Similarly solid wastes, such as slag heaps from mines, should not be indiscriminately dumped on land; nor should noxious fumes be blown from chimneys to cause atmospheric pollution.

HOUSING

The provision of good housing is an important aspect of environmental health. It represents:
(a) A significant part of man's environment
(b) Shelter from the elements
(c) Workshop: the kitchen for the housewife, the playroom for the children; the toolshed for the adult males.
(d) Home: the residence of the family, where this social institution carries out some of its major functions.

Good housing should minimise physical and biological hazards in the environment and should promote the health of the inhabitants. Good housing should eliminate or minimise the following hazards:

(a) Biological

The risk of the transmission of communicable diseases should be minimised. Poor ventilation and overcrowding, for example, predispose to the spread of respiratory infections. Good water supply, adequate facilities for washing utensils and other sanitary devices, good storage for food and well-designed kitchens, will help to minimise the spread of gastro-intestinal infections.

(b) Physical

Injury from falls, burns, electric shock, poisoning and similar physical hazards can be controlled by good design of homes to include appropriate safety devices. The maintenance of an equable temperature in the house, by heating in winter and cooling in the hot summer is also conducive to good health. The physical hazards include atmospheric pollution from smoky wood fires, excessive noise and poor lighting.

(c) Social

The home should be designed so that the family can function effectively in terms of its cultural background. This implies the required level of privacy for adults and a suitable setting for bringing up children.

The World Health Organisation has defined in some detail the requirements of a healthy residential environment.

The basic aspects of housing relate to the proper siting and construction of a residence which provides fundamental physiological, psychological and sanitary requirements. Types of housing in the tropics depend on the climatic environment and hence are quite different in arid zones, in savannahs, in upland jungle, in cold dry or humid high plateaux, in marshlands, in high mountain steppes and in tropical rain forest.

In many parts of the rural tropics, traditional huts are often small, ill-ventilated and lighted only through the door opening, with a smoky fireplace inside and without real furniture. Men, fowls, small and large animals may cohabit and lack of sanitation and safe water supply are all too obvious. Many model rural villages have, however, been started all over the tropical world with appropriate government help.

Housing for plantation, mining and industrial workers has been provided in many areas by employees and standards have been variable. Often government authorities have had to regulate the minimum standards including size, floor and air space, ventilation, cooking, storage, sanitary facilities and water supplies. Inspired by good management rather than by humanity or justice, industrial and agricultural companies in the tropics have learned much about the physical, biological, psychological, technical and economic problems involved in housing their employees.

For the rapid urbanising populations of the tropics provision of adequate low-cost housing is a primary responsibility of government and municipal authorities. Standards should be such that they can be made enforceable in a low income community and relate to local climate and cultural conditions.

FOOD HYGIENE

The chief aim of food hygiene is to prevent the contamination of foodstuffs at all stages of their production, i.e. collection, preparation, manufacture, transportation, storage and sale. Sometimes, despite all precautions, organisms may contaminate food, in these instances adequate refrigeration may prevent multiplication of the organisms to a level sufficient to cause clinical symptoms.

The measures to be taken to maintain high standards of catering whether in the home or in the community at large will include:
  (i) the control of primary sources of food, e.g. avoidance of use of human manure as a fertiliser.
 (ii) inspection of relevant premises, e.g. abattoirs
(iii) supervision of foodhandlers, e.g. carriers
 (iv) health education
  (v) laboratory examination of foodstuffs, e.g. precooked meats
 (vi) legislation.

DISINFECTION

The aim of disinfection is to kill noxious organisms and there are several ways of achieving this, namely by: (i) heat, (ii) desiccation, (iii) sunlight, (iv) chemical agents, (v) filtration, (vi) aerosols, and (vii) irradiation.

The destruction of the bacteria in the discharges and excreta of a patient suffering from an infectious disease, e.g. typhoid fever, and on articles in contact with him is known as 'current disinfection'. The cleansing of a room which has been occupied by a patient suffering from an infectious disease, e.g. cholera, is known as 'terminal disinfection'.

1 Heat

Heat kills bacteria and spores by coagulating their protein; moist heat is more efficient than dry heat. Thus boiling water will kill bacteria in a few minutes (5–10) and most spores in about half an hour. Pasteurisation destroys bacteria in milk without spoiling it. Steam is also an efficient method of disinfection. Burning ideally gets rid of infected fomites which are of no further use and hot air may also be used to kill bacteria although its penetrative powers are poor.

2 Desiccation

Only delicate organisms, e.g. the meningococci are killed when allowed to dry and this form of disinfection is therefore of limited value.

3 Sunlight

Sunlight, especially ultraviolet rays, are lethal to many bacteria and ultraviolet light is sometimes used for the sterilisation of air.

4 Chemical Agents

Chemical disinfectants, e.g. iodine, chlorine, hydrogen peroxide, alcohol, phenol and cresols (lysol), actively kill bacteria and are widely used for disinfection in a large variety of circumstances. 'Detergent' types of antiseptics are increasingly being utilised.

5 Filtration

See page 308.

6 Aerosols

In these days of automation aerosols are becoming extremely popular especially for the sterilisation of air, the disinfectant, e.g. sodium hypochlorite or propylene glycol being spread in a very fine spray.

7 Irradiation

Gamma irradiation (cobalt-60 as source) has been used to sterilise food and thus eliminate *Salmonellae* and other bacteria. Similarly several medical appliances, e.g. catheters, disposable syringes, etc., are being radiation-sterilised.

FURTHER READING

Ross Institute Bulletin No. 10: *Small Water Supplies.*
Ross Institute Bulletin No. 8: *Small Excreta Disposal Systems.*
Ross Institute Bulletin No. 5: *The Housefly and its Control.*
WHO Tech. Rep. Ser. No. 484: *Solid Wastes Disposal and Control.*
WHO Tech. Rep. Series. No. 225;
Wld. Hlth. Stats. Rep. Vol. 29, No. 10: *Community Water Supply and Excreta Disposal in Developing Countries—Review of Progress.*

CHAPTER 12

HEALTH EDUCATION

The objective of health education is to make people value health as a worthwhile asset and to know what they can do as individuals, families and communities to improve their own health. The more people value health, the more they might be willing to make the appropriate allocation of resources to promote and safeguard their own health. At the personal level, they would be prepared to make the effort on such matters as exercise, cleanliness in the home, diet and discipline with regard to the use of tobacco and alcohol. The community will also be more prepared to allocate resources for improvement of environmental sanitation, and for other priorities within the health services.

People need to know what they can do to remain healthy or to restore their health if they fall sick. Modern medicine has tended to interpret health in terms of medical interventions, and some people tend to over-emphasize this aspect of medical technology. It is important to promote the concept of health as the result of the interaction of human beings and their total environment (see Chapter 1). Clinical medicine seeks to restore health through the use of drugs and surgical treatment. Preventive medicine includes similar interventions with the use of immunisations and chemoprophylaxis but, more importantly, the emphasis is on alteration of the environment and of human behaviour. Individuals, families and communities should be made to understand this concept of health which can be briefly summarised as:

HEALTH, HABIT AND HABITAT

Health education relates to all aspects of health behaviour including the use of health services. It is designed to help people determine the best behaviour to adopt with regard to their personal habits and how to make the best use of the community health services.

Health education should feature as an integral part of the health services and all health personnel should accept responsibility for contributing to the programme. Specialists in health education are required to make more accurate assessments of the needs of the population, to develop suitable materials for health education and to train other workers including voluntary health workers. They would also help to evaluate local health education programmes.

Assessment of needs

The content of the health education programme should be determined by the needs of the target groups. In order to ensure that the material is relevant, information is required about the current knowledge, attitudes and behaviour of the population. An educational programme can then be designed to bring about the desired changes. For example, a health education programme should be designed after a study of the current practices and beliefs of the population. How many of the mothers breast feed their babies and for how long? When do they introduce mixed feeding, what items do they use and how is the food prepared? What foods are avoided or considered unacceptable? What substitutes are available to provide missing nutrients and are these acceptable to the mothers? Which mothers are in greatest need of education on this subject as judged by nutritional status of their infants?

Such studies aimed at identifying the needs for health education and defining the target groups. They are sometimes described as 'knowledge, attitude, practice' or 'KAP' studies.

Methods

A variety of methods, both formal and informal, are used in health education. Some are *personal*, i.e. involving a health worker in direct contact with an individual or a group. Others are *impersonal*, in which the communication does not involve such contact, e.g. the use of posters, leaflets, and the mass media (newspapers, radio, television). Each method has its advantages.

The personal methods, either in an interview on a one-to-one basis or in a group discussion, have the advantage that the content can be specifically tailored to match the needs of the individuals present. There is also the opportunity for discussion where obscure points can be clarified, objections raised and doubts expressed. The health worker can also use the opportunity to learn more local beliefs and habits. There is the opportunity for reviewing alternative approaches to the solution of specific problems, and thereby the community and the individuals can determine how best to put the new lessons that they have learnt into practice in their own circumstances. However, with the personal approach, relatively few persons can be reached by each health worker.

The impersonal methods, especially the use of the mass media, have the advantage of reaching large numbers of people who may not have direct contact with health workers. The messages can be repeated over and over again, serving as reminder and reinforcement. In some communities, material read in the newspapers or heard on the radio carries more authority than information that is obtained from local sources. Without the opportunity for questions and discussions, however, such messages may be misunderstood; constant repetition may dull their impact; and individuals may have difficulty in relating the messages to their own circumstances.

It is sometimes possible to combine the advantages of both methods. For example, wall charts, radio and television programmes and similar impersonal methods could be used as the focus for small group discussions. Alternatively, after a subject has been discussed, gifted members of the community could be encouraged to produce wall charts and other teaching materials for others in the community.

Health education materials should be pre-tested on a small scale before they are widely distributed. In this way, the material could be modified to make the message clearer.

Resistance to change

Health workers are sometimes upset and can feel frustrated when they find that people do not immediately accept their advice. They seem surprised that people do not immediately change their behaviour once new information is given to them. Especially in matters affecting personal behaviour and on emotional issues like pregnancy and child care, people are reluctant to have their ideas changed or even challenged. Although it is not always easy to change people's ideas some valuable suggestions for approaching such problems have been made:

(a) *Present the material in a new form* which is more acceptable to the people, e.g. if for religious reasons, the community does not eat meat, the health workers should devise a nutritionally balanced diet based on vegetables and, if acceptable, milk.

(b) *Associate the new idea with desired goals.* This is the approach favoured by commercial advertisers who link the use of their products with outcomes which are highly valued by the community. The general format of such advertisements is 'Use A (our product) to get B (what you want)'. The same approach can be effectively used in health education provided false claims are not made.

(c) *Draw attention to successful examples.* Individuals, families and communities may provide useful examples for others in adopting a new idea. A useful strategy for introducing a new idea is to offer it first to groups who are most likely to accept it and put it into practice. They can then serve as useful examples for others.

(d) *Work through opinion leaders.* In each community there are leaders whose views have a great influence within their society. Some of them are formal leaders holding recognised posts as political or religious leaders. Others hold important positions in local organisations such as women's clubs. There are however other influential persons, the informal leaders, who do not hold such positions but who nevertheless have considerable influence on the community. Both groups should be identified and persuaded to adopt the new ideas and also to influence others to do so.

(e) *Identify and persuade innovators.* Whereas some members of the community tend to be rigid in their views, there are others who tend to be more receptive to new ideas. It is worthwhile identifying such innovators, encouraging them and using them as instruments of change within their communities. On the whole children tend to be more receptive than adults especially the elderly. Priority should be given to the health education of children, especially school children who in the process of their general education would be prepared to accept and test new ideas. At home they can influence their parents.

(f) *Be patient and avoid confrontation.* Head-on collision and confrontation could damage relationships between the health workers and the community. Even though the health workers are very anxious that the new ideas be accepted in the interest of the health of the population, they must be patient, retaining cordial relationships with the individuals and families in the hope of winning them over eventually.

Education by example

Health personnel should reinforce the formal teaching in health education by their own example. The members of the community observe the behaviour of the health workers and compare it with what they have learnt from lectures, interviews, posters and other forms of health education. They note the standard of personal hygiene of the health workers and of environmental sanitation at health centres, clinics and other health institutions; they observe our social habits with regard to smoking and the use of alcohol; they compare the lessons that they have learnt about balanced diets with the food provided for patients in hospitals; and in many other ways they seek to reassure themselves about the value of the health education that is offered to them. If they consistently observe gross discrepancies between what is taught to them and what their teachers do, they are liable to become cynical and reject health education as a farce. It is therefore important that every contact with the health personnel and the health institutions should be a continuous exercise in health education.

FURTHER READING

EURO Reports and Studies. No. 11: *Principles and methods of health education.*

CHAPTER 13

OTHER ASPECTS OF PUBLIC HEALTH

In this chapter the following subjects will be briefly dealt with: (1) The International Health Regulations (2) Social Welfare, (3) International Health, (4) Public Health Laws, (5) Genetics and Health, (6) Mental Health, and (7) Occupation and Health.

1 INTERNATIONAL HEALTH REGULATIONS

Writing about the International Health Regulations (IHR), WHO have stressed to all national health administrations in countries bound by these regulations that (a) smallpox has been removed from the list of diseases subject to IHR and therefore an international certificate of vaccination should no longer be required from any traveller; (b) the only certificate that is now required, from a limited number of international travellers, is that for yellow fever vaccination; and (c) the requirement of cholera vaccination certificates, or indeed any other vaccination certificates, is in excess of the terms of the IHR.

It is important to note that requirements issued by embassies and consulates are not always the same as those laid down by national health authorities though it is hoped that common policies will be attained in the near future.

Most countries have a Quarantine and Epidemiology Branch at the Ministry of Health which deals with
  (i) Port health
 (ii) Airport health
(iii) Quarantine stations or hospitals and
 (iv) Vaccination.
The aim of such a division is to guard against the import and export of diseases, thus keeping the indigenous population reservoir as small as possible and *honestly* notifying WHO of the latest situation in the country irrespective of the local consequences. Unfortunately experience with cholera has shown that certain countries react most unfavourably to this concept. Although all points of entry into a country must be controlled, e.g. sea, air, road or rail, sea and airports present special problems.

Seaports

When a ship is infected, e.g. with a case of smallpox, the following action has to be taken:

(i) isolation of case

(ii) re-vaccination of passengers and crew

(iii) isolation of close contacts (14 days)

(iv) surveillance of other contacts (14 days)

(v) disinfection of patient's cabin, etc. (not whole ship)

(vi) international notification.

All passengers should have their vaccination certificates checked and those without valid certificates require vaccination and surveillance. Yellow fever and pneumonic plague suspects must be isolated. At quarantine stations and hospitals compulsory re-vaccination takes place as well as group isolation and medical surveillance.

Sanitary examination of ships, especially water, toilets, kitchen and food storage compartments should be carried out and the deratisation certificate examined. When a ship flies the 'Q' flag, no one is permitted to board or leave the ship before the Port Health Officer.

Airports

Airport health services are rapidly being developed all over the world:

(i) to perform vaccination and inoculation of passengers and crews when necessary

(ii) to examine suspected passengers

(iii) to place passengers under surveillance when necessary

(iv) to inspect aircraft coming from yellow fever infected areas for the presence of *Aëdes* and to carry out disinsectisation if necessary

(v) to vaccinate and inoculate all personnel in the airport who come in contact with aircraft coming from infected ports

(vi) to inspect and see that the airport precincts are kept in a satisfactory state including the airport restaurant and flight kitchen

(vii) to supervise the control of *Aëdes* and other mosquitoes within the control zone of the airport perimeter

(viii) to maintain and run the casualty clearing station in case of air disaster

(ix) to provide out-patient treatment facilities for cases of minor illnesses (for passengers and airport staff)

(x) to take samples of toilet wastes from planes and to send the specimens for bacteriological examination to ascertain whether adequate disinfection is being carried out

(xi) to take periodic samples of food and potable water that are supplied to the aircraft to ascertain whether these are fit for human consumption and that they have not been contaminated by bacteria or chemical substances.

Conclusion

The attitude towards the International Sanitary Regulations should be one where the security afforded to countries takes priority over the facilitation of travel. The infection status of neighbouring countries should be especially well known. Certain global trends in the spread of the quarantine diseases are very disturbing. The most notable has been the spread of El Tor cholera since 1961 across Asia, to southern Europe and the Middle East and now to Africa south of the Sahara, for the first time in history. A number of outbreaks have taken place in many countries free of epidemic diseases as a result of the rapid development of international air travel, and the frequency with which travellers move about and change planes. A reappraisal of the existing International Sanitary Regulations and their function is long overdue.

2 SOCIAL WELFARE

Departments of social welfare in the tropics provide a variable range of welfare services for the community. In some countries, e.g. Singapore, a very wide range is available while in some other countries, e.g. those of tropical Africa, social welfare services barely exist. The aim is basically to provide welfare and protection to needy children and young persons; to women and young girls with particular reference to brothels and to provide probation and aftercare services for young offenders, endeavouring to place them in employment whenever possible.

Public assistance schemes provide financial assistance to the aged, the chronic sick, the physically and mentally handicapped, the widows and orphans and the unemployed. Institutional care is provided for special cases.

Voluntary organisations have played and continue to play an important role in welfare work in the state. In some tropical countries the only welfare work available, e.g. care of handicapped children, is that provided by major voluntary organisations.

3 INTERNATIONAL HEALTH

A variety of mechanisms exist for international cooperation in the area. Some of these involve agreements between two nations; such bilateral arrangements could include financial and technical support, exchange of scientific information and various forms of assistance. The cooperation could be multilateral involving many nations in a regional or global organisation. Within the United Nations (UN) System, the World Health Organisation has the constitutional responsibility for health and it plays a leading role in this area in collaboration with other U.N. agencies as well as non-governmental organisations.

I World Health Organisation (WHO)

The Organisation was founded in 1947, and it now has 154 member states. It's headquarters is located in Geneva, Switzerland and it has six regional offices:

(a) African Regional Office (AFRO)—Brazzaville, Congo
(b) Regional Office for the Americas (AMRO)—Washington, D.C., U.S.A.
(c) Eastern Mediterranean Regional Office (EMRO)—Alexandria, Egypt
(d) European Regional Office (EURO)—Copenhagen, Denmark
(e) South East Asia Regional Office (SEARO)—New Delhi, India
(f) West Pacific Regional Office (WPRO)—Manila, Philippines

Initially WHO gave technical aid especially to developing countries, but now the new policy emphasises technical cooperation with member states with each country contributing to and deriving benefits from the Organisation. WHO has accorded the highest priority to its goal of 'Health for all by year 2000', using the primary health care approach.

WHO's activities include the following:

1 *Strengthening of health services*
WHO is cooperating with member states in the strengthening and re-orientation of their health services, with particular reference to the primary health care services. The new policy about health care was adopted in 1978 at a conference at Alma Ata, USSR.

2 *Technical services*
The Organisation provides technical services on major communicable and non-communicable diseases. These include the Malaria Action Programme, and the Parasitic Diseases Programme. There are also programmes in other communicable diseases, environmental health, mental health and health manpower development. These programmes provide support for national health authorities in specific areas.

3 *Special Programmes*
A number of special programmes have been organised to promote action in some priority areas:
Human reproduction
Tropical diseases
Control of diarrhoeal diseases
Expanded programme of immunisation

The eradication of smallpox was successfully accomplished by a special programme which is now being dissolved.

4 *Technical information*
The Organisation publishes a number of technical documents including:
(a) Technical Report Series—summarising views of expert committees and other scientific groups on specific subjects.

(b) World Health Bulletin—publishing scientific papers, either original articles or scientific reviews.
(c) World Health Forum—a new journal for reviewing and discussing public health issues and matters concerning the running of health services.
(d) World Health—a popular journal aimed at the lay public
(e) Weekly Epidemiological Records—this contains epidemiological information about the occurrence of communicable diseases.

II Other United Nation Agencies

Apart from WHO, other UN agencies play a significant role in health. WHO collaborates with these other agencies:
(a) *United Nations Childrens Fund* (UNICEF) is concerned about matters affecting the welfare of children. It co-sponsored the Alma-Ata conference.
(b) *Food and Agricultural Organisation* (FAO) collaborates in the area of nutrition and also African trypanosomiasis, an infection which affects both humans and animals.
(c) *International Labour Organisation* (ILO) deals with matters affecting the health of workers.
(d) *United Nations Environmental Programme* (UNEP) is concerned with matters affecting the environment.
(e) *United Nations Development Programme* (UNDP) coordinates UN activities in the area of development.

III Non-governmental organisations in special relationship with WHO

A variety of international organisations cooperate with WHO on a number of subjects—leprosy, epidemiology, pharmacology, to name but a few.

IV Other international organisations

Some international organisations play an important role in health:
(a) *The International Council of the Red Cross and the League of Red Cross* (Crescent) play an important part in providing relief in cases of natural disasters.
(b) *Private Foundations*—Most of these work mainly with national boundaries but some of them have substantial international activities, e.g. Rockefeller Foundation, Wellcome Trust.
(c) *The World Bank* is involved in lending funds for development. Activities such as the creation of man-made lakes and large scale irrigation schemes carry major implications for health. The World Bank is therefore involved in the assessment of the health aspects of development projects which they sponsor. A new policy indicates that the World Bank will play an increasingly active role in health.

4 PUBLIC HEALTH LAWS

Public health laws are enacted in order to protect and promote individual and community health. The enaction of these laws is very variable and is dependent on the legal system of individual countries. The application and enforcement of these laws is a function of health officers, public health inspectors and the medical officers of health, who are given certain special powers for the purpose. The number of public health laws varies from country to country and they aim at covering such topics as:

  (i) registration of births and deaths
 (ii) quarantine and prevention of disease
(iii) sales of food and drugs
 (iv) destruction of disease-bearing insects
  (v) registration of medical personnel
 (vi) registration of schools
(vii) environmental health.

Under the above laws the health officers are given power to entry into premises and to take such action as they might deem necessary to prevent the propagation of disease.

5 GENETICS AND HEALTH

In recent years interest in genetics has been greatly stimulated in the tropics and subtropics by the discovery that high gene frequencies for some genetic traits are maintained by providing a protection to the carrier against falciparum malaria. The haemoglobin genetic markers vary in importance from one area to the other, thus while haemoglobin S is the most important abnormal haemoglobin in Africa, it is superseded by haemoglobin E and thalassaemia in South-East Asia. Many other examples of the interplay between genetic factors and health are available.

Glucose-6-phosphate dehydrogenase (G-6-PD) deficiency, so common in many areas of the tropics, renders its bearer vulnerable to haemolytic anaemia on exposure to primaquine, the fava beans and other agents.

Some individuals inactivate isonicotinic acid hydrazide (isoniazid) rapidly. In these, antituberculous therapy with isoniazid is less satisfactory than in those patients in whom the drug is inactivated more slowly. On the other hand, the 'slow inactivator' is probably more likely to display toxic reactions, such as neuropathy.

It is known that a relatively high proportion of Africans lack demonstrable haptoglobins and it is reasonable to postulate that such persons are favoured by selection, but the search for such an advantage has yet to begin.

There is overwhelming evidence that patients with carcinoma of the stomach have a higher incidence of group A, and patients with peptic ulcer a high incidence of group O, than control populations from the same area.

The spread of insects resistant to DDT and other chemicals, of bacteria resistant to drugs, and of malaria parasites resistant to chloroquine are dramatic examples of changes in the genetic composition of natural populations of organisms in response to powerful selective forces.

When subjects heterozygous for two genes, e.g. (AS) are favoured by selection over both homozygotes (AA and SS), the situation is referred to as 'polymorphism'. One of the best examples of this is in fact provided by the sickle-cell gene which has remained common in parts of the world (especially in Africa), despite the fact homozygotes develop a severe anaemia from which most die in childhood. The hypothesis that the heterozygote enjoys a selective advantage against the lethal effects of *P. falciparum* malaria is now accepted and various facts confirm its veracity:

(i) The sickle-cell gene is found in its highest incidence in areas where *P. falciparum* malaria is, or was until recently, endemic

(ii) In areas of stable malaria, high *P. falciparum* densities are significantly less commonly found in children with the sickle-cell trait (AS) than in normal children (AA)

(iii) Post-mortem studies have revealed that death from cerebral malaria does not occur in the S heterozygote (AS)

(iv) There is evidence that the prevalence of the sickle-cell trait in a population increases with advancing years, which is suggestive of differential survival with a greater loss of normal genes

(v) It has been found that mothers with the sickle-cell trait had a slightly higher fertility and lower stillbirth rate, and that the birth weights of their children tended to be slightly higher than those of non-sickling mothers. This could be attributed to partial protection against *P. falciparum* malaria, as in pregnancy there is evidence that there is some lowering of immunity to this infection.

The mechanism whereby the sickle-cell haemoglobin partially protects the bearer from the severe effects of *P. falciparum* malaria is obscure. The red cell assumes the sickle shape when the oxygen tension is lowered, so it would appear reasonable to postulate that the utilisation of oxygen by the malarial parasite might enhance this effect, with consequent disposal of the young parasite and cell by the reticuloendothelial system. Maturation of the parasite would thereby be prevented. However, on estimating the incidence of gametocytes of *P. falciparum* in sicklers and non-sicklers no significant differences have been found, which implies that maturation can occur. It has also been suggested that the parasite might not be able to metabolise S as well as normal adult haemoglobin. It has been shown also that sickling children in Nigeria have significantly higher γ-globulin levels than non-sickling children which may imply that the trait enhances the antibody response against the malarial parasite. Recently, by the use of *in vitro* cultures, the increased rate of sickling of parasitised cells was confirmed, and attributed not only to oxygen uptake, but also to lowering of the intracellular pH by *P. falciparum*, resulting from loss of potassium ion.

Haemoglobin C and Malaria

The C gene occurs in its highest incidence in an area of Africa where malaria is stable. Unfortunately it also occurs in an area where the S gene is found in high incidence. The incidence of the S gene would appear to vary inversely with the incidence of C, in Northern Ghana being 12 to 18, Southern Ghana 18 to 12 and in Western Nigeria 24 to 6 per cent, the total incidence of S and C remaining very roughly constant at 30 per cent in these areas.

Pure haemoglogin-C disease (CC) causes little disability, but double heterozygosity of S and C frequently occurs and death from SC disease is not uncommon, especially in pregnancy. The C gene is therefore at a disadvantage, although the selection is much smaller than in the case of the S gene, where procreation by homozygotes (SS) is rare.

It has been suggested that, just as in the case of S haemoglobin, C may protect the bearer from the severe effects of *P. falciparum* malaria, thus offsetting the loss of C genes in SC disease. In this connection it has also been suggested that if this were so, C might have evolved from S mutation, a less harmful gene being substituted for a more lethal. It is, however, considered that, as the abnormality in both S and C haemoglobins is in the sixth position of the β chain, where the amino-acid residue glutamic acid is substituted by valine and lysine residues respectively, it is most likely that haemoglobins C and S arose as independent mutations from haemoglobin A, the mutation A to C being comparatively recent. All evidence to date points to the fact that the presence of C haemoglobin confers no partial protection against malaria.

Haemoglobin F and Malaria

It has been suggested that the presence of the 'F gene' might partially protect the bearer against the effects of *P. falciparum* malaria. An analysis of the results of various observers who have examined infants living in malarious districts of Africa reveals a comparatively low level of malaria infection in infants under 3 months of age. An apparent relationship was found in Gambian infants between the disappearance of foetal haemoglobin and the onset of malaria infection, but no definite evidence exists from population studies that haemoglobin F protects against the lethal effects of *P. falciparum*. Recent *in vitro* studies however have shown that parasite growth—as opposed to invasion—is impaired in HbF containing red cells, regardless of their source.

Haemoglobin E and Malaria

The few series of children so far investigated have failed to show any protection of haemoglobin-E heterozygotes against malaria. It has also been posited that increased iron absorption in the E-trait carrier might confer an advantage, but there is no evidence that the trait carrier does absorb more iron.

Thalassaemia and Malaria

Since the β thalassaemia gene is often lethal when homozygous, the heterozygote frequencies of 20 per cent found in some places must be explained by heterozygous advantages, and once again it has been suggested that malaria was involved. The evidence to date is inconclusive. Preliminary *in vitro* data have appeared to the effect that thalassaemia cells can be infected, but parasite development is impaired by oxidative stress, as imposed by high oxygen tension, menadione or riboflavin.

G-6-PD and Malaria

Confirmation of the malaria-protection hypothesis has been sought in various ways: gene-frequency-distribution studies in populations living in areas of different malarial endemicity; malaria-parasite-density surveys in G-6-PD normal and deficient children; induced-falciparum malaria in human volunteers; and G-6-PD deficiency among patients with severe clinical falciparum malaria. The results of recent studies have provided evidence that G-6-PD deficient heterozygotes (Gd^+/Gd^-) have a selective advantage against potentially lethal malaria infection.

Rh-negative Gene and Malaria

A most interesting hypothesis has been put forward about the possible selection against the Rh-negative gene by malaria. The incidence of the Rh gene is generally low in areas in which malaria is or was endemic. It was suggested that a population subject to a heavily malarious environment might be superior antibody producers owing to selection by elimination of poor antibody producers. If this were so, erythroblastosis foetalis should be more intense in malarious areas, and Rh-negative genes should be selectively eliminated if the frequency of the gene is or was below 0.50. Hence Rh-negative mothers in a malarious area should show a higher incidence of sensitisation to an Rh-positive foetus than their counterparts in northern areas. In Ibadan, Nigeria, over 400 Rh-negative pregnant multiparae were studied and, apart from some who had had previous transfusions of Rh-positive blood, the evidence of those sensitised by pregnancy was only 2.5 per cent—a lower incidence than the figures recorded from Europe and elsewhere. This evidence does not, therefore, substantiate the above hypothesis.

Human genetics is one of the elements that can be used in the planning of co-ordinated attacks on disease, since it can sometimes differentiate individuals who are susceptible from those who are not.

Genetic factors often determine *group susceptibility* or resistance to disease, e.g. the racial immunity to vivax malaria of West African Negroes now shown to be related to the Duffy antigen; alternatively *individual susceptibility* can be a reflection of genetic factors, e.g. twins are sometimes more liable to certain morbid conditions. In addition, immune deficiencies whether cellular or humoral, e.g. agammaglobulinaemia, are consequent on genetic factors, while genetic failure may be responsible for altered patterns of disease, e.g. defective cellular immunity in lepromatous leprosy. The clinical importance of the HLA genes in relation to transplantation and to a possible abnormal immune response to some common chronic diseases has been recently emphasized, as has the remarkable association between HLS-B27 and ankylosing spondylitis and the possible association of *S. mansoni* hepatosplenomegaly and HLA-A_1 and B_5.

Population genetic studies are a recent important expansion of the field of genetics and the knowledge thus acquired can be of practical value in preventive medicine, in the form commonly referred to as *genetic counselling*. This is particularly important in the situation as it is at present in Africa, where sickle-cell anaemia has an incidence of nearly 2 per cent in some countries and may be responsible for a childhood mortality of approximately 5 per 1000.

Genetic risks are naturally assessed in terms of probabilities. They range from the big risk of 1 in 2 with a dominant gene, or 1 in 4 with a recessive gene, through a spectrum of decreasing risks which ultimately reach very low values.

An increasing number of inherited conditions can be effectively treated if dealt with promptly, and in others treatment can at least reduce the degree of suffering. Where routine neonatal screening is possible, e.g. SS disease, there is a special obligation to make sure that early detection occurs. In some conditions, it is even possible to obtain a prenatal diagnosis of the foetus, e.g. spina bifida and β-thalssaemia.

6 MENTAL HEALTH

Throughout the world there is an increasing awareness of mental disorder as a significant cause of morbidity. This awareness has increased with the steady decline of morbidity due to nutritional disorders, communicable diseases and other forms of physical illness. There is also a better understanding of certain behavioural and social problems which had previously not been properly recognised as manifestations of mental disorder. The role of the community both in the prevention of mental disorder and the care of the mentally handicapped has now been widely recognised and it is regarded as the only appropriate basis for the development of mental health programmes.

Various forms of mental disorder are encountered:

(a) *Impaired intelligence*

Arrested or incomplete development of the mind.

(b) *Psychoses*

These include the manic-depressive psychoses and schizophrenia, and a variety of organic psychoses which are related to demonstrable lesions of the brain.

(c) *Psychoneuroses and psychosomatic disorders*

(d) *Behavioural disorders*

These include maladjustment in childhood, juvenile delinquency, absenteeism, etc.

(e) *Psychopathic disorders*

These present as irresponsible, often aggressive antisocial acts, repeated in spite of appeals, warnings and sanctions.

Objectives of Mental Health Programme

The main objective of a mental health programme is to ensure for each individual optimal development of his mental abilities and a satisfactory emotional adjustment to his community and environment. Thus, the programme will include the promotion of mental health, the prevention of mental disorder and the care of the mentally handicapped.

Promotion of Mental Health

The positive aspect of the mental health programme involves the design and creation of social and environmental situations in which mental health will grow and flourish. The factors which promote mental health are both physical and socio-cultural. The physical aspect includes the promotion of the general physical fitness of the individual and the control of environmental stresses such as excessive noise. The socio-cultural factors include the consolidation of family life, the control of economic stresses, and the resolution of conflicts within the society.

The Prevention of Mental Disorder

The prevention of mental disorder is to some extent limited because the aetiology of some of these disorders is not known. A number of underlying causes, predisposing or precipitating factors have been identified. The main aetiological groups are:

(a) Genetic factors

(b) Organic brain damage

(c) Socio-cultural factors
(d) Idiopathic group.

(a) *Genetic factors*

There has been a tendency to exaggerate the role of genetic factors in the aetiology of mental disorder. The familial occurrence of certain forms of mental disorder may be determined by social and environmental factors rather than by genetic factors. Thus, mental disorder in the child of alcoholic parents may have resulted from the stresses of an unsuitable home background rather than from genetic inheritance. There are, however, some clear examples of mental handicap resulting from genetic factors, e.g. Down's syndrome, which is determined by a demonstrable chromosomal abnormality. More subtle genetic factors which are manifested in the form of personality types, response to stresses and other behavioural patterns are recognised but are difficult to quantify. The role of genetic factors in the aetiology of the major psychoses (manic-depressive psychoses and schizophrenics) has not been clearly defined.

(b) *Organic brain damage and degenerative lesions*

Organic brain damages may result from:
  (i) *Trauma*—including birth trauma
 (ii) *Infections*—e.g. meningitis, syphilis, trypanosomiasis, kuru, and other forms of encephalitis, acute febrile illness, hyperpyrexia.
(iii) *Malnutrition*—e.g. vitamin deficiency—pellagra, beri-beri, Korsakov's psychosis; protein-malnutrition—clinical and experimental studies suggest that severe protein malnutrition in childhood may result in permanent mental retardation.
 (iv) *Toxins*—alcohol, opiates and other habit forming drugs, amphetamines, cannabis, lysergic acid.
  (v) *Degenerative lesions*—senility, specific degenerative diseases, e.g. Sydenham's chorea, changes secondary to arteriosclerosis.
    The increasing human life span has brought the problems of old age into greater prominence.

(c) *Socio-cultural factors*

The social environment of the individual plays a prominent role in determining the state of his mental health. Social stresses can often be identified as initiating and precipitating factors of acute mental disorder. This association is most prominent in relation to behavioural problems in childhood which often reflect emotional problems within the family.

Although patterns of non-organic psychoses are similar in many communities, the manifestations are conditioned by cultural factors. Thus, the recognition of mental disorder depends on a careful evaluation of the norms, beliefs and customs within the particular culture. Thus, for example, a man who would not touch a particular object because he believes that it is inhabited by evil spirits may in one culture, be manifesting signs of acute mental disorder, but in another culture, may be showing no more than reasonable caution.

(d) *Idiopathic group*
Within this group are various psychotic and psycho-neurotic illnesses, psychopathic personality problems, and behavioural disorders. It seems likely that in most cases, each condition is not the result of a single aetiological agent, rather the occurrence of disease is determined by a chain or a web of interrelated factors—a genetic predisposition, facilitating and inhibitory social, cultural and environmental factors, and the existence of various precipitating factors.

The Elements of a Community Mental Health Programme

The basic ingredient of a community health programme is community concern for the patients and their families, and community acceptance of its responsibility for the prevention and care of mental handicap. It has been rightly said that 'Community care is possible only in a community which cares'. Community health education is therefore vital to the successes of these programmes and it should be directed to the following objectives.

(i) *Eradication of superstitious fears and prejudices*
Traditional attitudes to mental disorder include superstitious fears that the ill patients are possessed by devils and evil spirits. Even in modern societies there are many social attitudes to mental disorder which are unfounded and illogical. These attitudes result in painful social stigma against the mentally handicapped and permanent prejudices against those who have fully recovered. Successful treatment and social rehabilitation of patients will be much enhanced by a tolerant and understanding attitude within the community.

(ii) *Dissemination of knowledge of the manifestations of mental disorder*
It is particularly important that the early signs of mental disorder be recognised so that remedial action can be taken promptly. The early signs may be misinterpreted by relatives, friends and society as merely anti-social behaviour calling for punishment rather than treatment. The community should be taught that 'a person who is troublesome, may be a person in trouble'.

(iii) *Participation of the community in the care and rehabilitation of the mentally handicapped*
The attitude in many communities is to seek custodial care for the mentally handicapped where the patients can be isolated for indefinite periods. The modern concept is to treat the patients as far as possible within the community, thereby minimising the effects of the disorder on the patient and his family, and also facilitating his social rehabilitation.

Patterns of Care

The prevention and curative services take many forms. Facilities are required for out-patient and in-patient care, follow-up services and general mental health promotion in the community.

Out-patient care within the community would include psychiatric out-patient clinics, a variety of special clinics (child guidance, counselling) and day hospitals. The advantages of the day hospital are that it:

(a) conserves limited in-patient hospital resources for patients who require them

(b) exploits the social dynamic forces of the community in the care of the mentally handicapped

(c) avoids the disturbing effects of the unfamiliar and artificial environment of the hospital

(d) assists in the rehabilitation of the patient in his home, family and job.

The mental health problems of the community are stratified in terms of age and other social features. The mental health programme would include measures to prevent mental disorder which are appropriate at each age-group:

(a) *Pre-natal*—to provide good ante-natal care and delivery services to ensure normal foetal development

to prevent congenital infections (e.g. syphilis)

to avoid intrapartum trauma.

(b) *Infancy*—to provide emotional security within the family circle

to care for abandoned children and children without families to prevent malnutrition, communicable and other diseases.

(c) *School age*—to provide a balanced programme of work and play

to avoid excessive fatigue—physical and mental

to encourage positive use of leisure hours

to establish satisfactory social adjustment inside and outside the family.

(d) *Adolescence*—to prevent, identify and deal with emotional problems at puberty by health education including sex-education.

(e) *Young adult*—to assist adjustment of working life, especially where rural/urban, agrarian/industrial transfers are involved.

(f) *Adults*—to provide counselling service for family life and consultant service for resolving conflicts in relation to self, family and community.

(g) *Old-age*—to provide substitute systems of care where traditional extended family systems are breaking down

to re-phrase the leadership roles of the elderly where they have been deprived of their traditional position of authority, e.g. provide ritual functions in the community.

It is clear from these examples that a successful mental care programme cannot be operated solely by professional psychiatrists and other specialist personnel, but it must include all medical and health workers, voluntary agencies and other community resources.

7 OCCUPATION AND HEALTH

The health problems of workers in developing countries are more complex than those of industrialised nations because of the high prevalence of epidemic and endemic diseases in most areas of the tropics. Modern concepts of occupational health embrace all types of employment including mercantile and commercial enterprises, service trades, utilities, forestry and agriculture. The distinction between environmental, occupational and industrial health is academic in the context of many tropical families where the husband may work in a factory while the wife and children cultivate a plot for food.

Agriculture and Health

Although industrialisation is the common path for the achievement of the fullest use of each nation's natural resources, the economy of many tropical countries is still basically agricultural and agricultural workers constitute a high proportion of the working population.

All forms of activities connected with growing, harvesting and primary processing of crops; with breeding, raising and caring of animals; and with tending of gardens and nurseries is agriculture.

Accidents take a large toll of life or result in permanent and disabling injuries. They may be associated with farm machinery or inadequate housekeeping around farms.

Infections and parasitic diseases can be contracted directly or indirecty during the course of an agricultural occupation (Table 13.1). The use of pesticides, insecticides and other chemicals has greatly increased in developing countries resulting in acute or chronic poisoning from compounds ranging from the toxic organo-phosphorus compounds, nitrate and chlorinated phenols to DDT. Besides communicable disease and exposure to chemicals, the extremes of *climatic conditions* such as temperature, humidity and solar radiation impose additional stresses upon the tropical worker.

Thus the health problems of agricultural workers are numerous and complex and methods for their prevention must be developed taking into consideration the differing conditions of every country.

Industry and Health

Most tropical countries are committed to industrialisation: it is the pace at which this is occurring which differs. Mass labour migration from rural to industrial areas immediately introduces enormous problems in housing and one is only too familiar with the growth of insanitary slums

Table 13.1 Some occupational diseases of agriculture (After who 1962)*

	A. Pricipally contracted through an agricultural occupation	B. Occasionally contracted through an agricultural occupation	C. Questionably contracted through an agricultural occupation
VIRAL	Tick-borne encephalitis Tick-borne haemorrhagic fever	Psittacosis Rabies Mosquito-borne encephalitis Mosquito-borne haemorrhagic fever	Mosquito-borne fever Tick-borne fever Cowpox Foot and mouth disease African tick-borne fever
RICKETTSIAL	Q fever	Scrub typhus	
BACTERIAL	Anthrax—Brucellosis Leptospirosis Tetanus Bovine tuberculosis Tularaemia	Plague Human tuberculosis	
PARASITIC	Ancylostomiasis Schistosomiasis	Hydatid disease Malaria	Filariasis Leishmaniasis Onchocerciasis
FUNGAL			Actinomycosis Blastomycosis— South American Histoplasmosis

* Joint ilo/who Committee on Occupational Health (who 1962).

around industrial complexes, which adversely affects the physical, mental and social well-being of the worker and his family.

Many small factories and workshops have been built where *dangerous chemicals* are being handled in a very indiscriminate and careless fashion. Lead acid battery makers and repairers are a particularly vulnerable group. In these little, often neglected workshops, a variety of occupations are going on—making; grinding, welding; cutting; moulding and painting various things.

In addition to chemicals, *heat* and *poor ventilation* are serious hazards in hot weather leading to heat cramps, heat exhaustion and fatigue resulting not only in low and faulty production but also in an increasing risk of accident. Noise induced hearing impairment is on the increase.

Compressed-air illness in divers and caisson workers on the many dams, oil rigs and bridges that are constantly being built in the tropics must be borne in mind.

With the expansion in mining and the utilisation of mineral wealth all types of *pneumoconiosis, silicosis* and *asbestosis* are on the increase in the tropics, as are the vegetable-dust diseases. *Byssinosis*, due to cottom dust, has been reported in cotton mills as well as in ginneries in Egypt, the Sudan and other tropical countries where this product is grown and exported, while respiratory diseases due to exposure to mouldy sugar cane (bagassosis), mouldy hay (farmer's lung), wool, gum acacia, ricinus, etc., are on the increase.

Accidents in factories are a major hazard, especially among the agrarian population coming into contact with industrial machinery for the first time. The danger of *cancer* in the chemical, asbestos, rubber and other industries must be borne in mind.

Thus a number of very important industrial hazards already exist in the tropics and they are likely to increase in magnitude and complexity.

Labour Legislation

Legislation covering health, safety and welfare of workers is now operative in many tropical countries and will become universal before long. Without such labour laws progress in occupational health is virtually impossible. They should cover occupational diseases, worker's compensation, medical examination, protection of women workers, protection of young persons, radiation protection and labour inspection. These labour laws must be adequately enforced and are essential prerequisites to any effective occupational health programme.

Occupational Health Programmes

The type of occupational health programme needed will vary from country to country and a constant reappraisal of the situation is required as the degree of industrialisation increases and trained personnel become available. Many countries in Africa, for example, are developing occupational health units within the Ministry of Labour, and these usually have a staff consisting of a medical specialist with a diploma in industrial health, a qualified occupational hygienist and a registered nurse trained in industrial and occupational medicine. One of the fundamental aims of achieving the objectives of occupational health programmes is the detection of environmental conditions and biological changes that are forerunners of the early stages of health impairment.

Private occupational health services are sometimes provided by big industrial enterprises in the tropics undertaking total medical care for employees and dependants.

In other areas, group occupational health services are being organised by industry itself, providing membership to companies and firms of all sizes, employing as many as 3000 employees to small enterprises employing as few as 10 workers.

Where public and private services are deficient, such a group occupational health service is welcomed by industry and fulfils a dire need.

Certain basic concepts are essential for the organisation of occupational health programmes. Management has to be convinced that the benefits of the programme justify the costs involved. The co-operation of management is also essential to ensure a high attendance rate for preventive programmes.

The collaboration of trade unions, shop-stewards, worksite committees and the individual workers sometimes is the determining factor as to whether a programme will succeed or fail. Such co-operation can only be forthcoming if the medical staff succeed in convincing labour that they are neither the tools or spies of management.

In worksites where most of the workers are non-residential, it is essential to obtain whenever possible the co-operation of general practitioners who may be able to help to complete immunization courses and give information about employees suffering from communicable diseases. Vaccination programmes should be carried out at the worksite and planned to avoid clashing with particularly busy periods. An occupational health doctor must be familiar with the disease patterns in the community outside the worksite and the whole socio-economic setting of the worker must be appreciated.

In developing and industrialising countries, health patterns are changing so rapidly that one cannot be content to sit back after devising a preventive programme, however well planned and ably executed. New priorities may have to be established in the face of some of these changes.

Summary

The essential priciples of prevention of the occupational diseases can be listed as follows:
1 Sanitation and hygiene of factories:
   (a) Cleanliness of factories
   (b) Avoidance of overcrowding
   (c) Adequate heating, ventilation and lighting
   (d) Adequate sanitary facilities
   (e) Protection against inhalation of dust fumes, e.g. by use of respirators
   (f) Protection of eyes when applicable, e.g. by suitable goggles or effective screens
   (g) Food hygiene in canteens.
2 Monitoring of the environment (e.g. radiation) and of the individual (e.g. lead workers)

3 Substitution of noxious substances or processes whenever possible
4 Limiting exposure to hazardous processes to the minimum of persons
5 Pre-employment examination
6 Notification of specified occupational diseases
7 Health education and training
8 Accident prevention, e.g. by adequate protection of machinery
9 Rehabilitation.

FURTHER READING

WHO Tech. Rep. Series. No. 571: *Early detection of health impairment in occupational exposure to health hazards.*

Symposium on Occupational Medicine. Ann. Acad. Med. Singapore. Vol. 7, No. 3. (1978)

INDEX

Accidents, domestic, 4, 317
  hazard, 315
  industrial, 338, 340
  prevention, 314, 342
Acute upper respiratory infections, 236–237
Aedes, spp, 166, 174, 213, 214
  A. aegypti, 166, 167, 170, 172
  A. africanus, 167
  A. simpsoni, 167
Airport health services, 325
Aleppo boil, 208
Amoebiasis, 69–72
Anaemia,
  diphyllobothriasis, 90
  and infection, 263
  folate deficiency, 263
  G-6-PD deficiency, 329
  hookworm, 139, 140
  iron deficiency, 263
  malaria, 189
  nutritional, 263
  Oroye fever, 188
  sickle cell, 330
Ankylostoma brazilienze, 137
  A. caninum, 137
  A. duodenale, 137, 139
Angiostrongyliasis, 85–86
Angiostrongylus cantonensis, 85
Anopheles spp. 213, 214, 226
  A. darlingi, 189
  A. funestus, 189
  A. gambiae, 189
  A. punctulatus, 189
Anthrax, 158–159
Arthropod-borne infections, 161–227
Ascariasis, 46, 77–79, 263
Ascaris lumbricoides, 46, 77
  A. suis, 78
Average values, 16
  mean, 16
  median, 16
  mode, 16

Bacillus anthracis, 158
Bacillus thurigiensis, 224
Balantidiasis, 74–75
Balantidium coli, 74
Bartonella bacilliformis, 188
Bartonellosis, 188–189

BCG vaccination, 144, 241, 294
  'direct', 242
  isoniazid resistant, 242
  and leprosy, 132
  of newborns, 242, 294
Bilharziasis, 145
Biological control, 227
Bitot's spot, 266, 267
Bolivian haemorrhagic fever, 159
Bordetella parapertussis, 253
  B. pertussis, 252
Borrelia duttoni, 185, 187
  B. recurrentis, 185, 187
Breast feeding, 48, 56, 57, 61, 186, 259, 262, 292
Brill's disease, 175, 176
Bronchopneumonia, 245
Brucellosis, 63–65
Brugia malayi, 213, 216
Buruli ulcer, 143–144

Campylobacter enteritis, 57
Candida albicans, 134
Candidiasis, 133–134
  in newborn, 134
Carriers, 11, 31, 229
  amoebiasis, 70
  cholera, 60
  diphtheria, 254, 255
  hepatitis, 52
  meningococcus, 248
  mumps, 233
  psittocosis, 234
  Streptococcus pneumoniae, 245
  S. pyogenes, 251
  typhoid fever, 53, 54, 55, 60, 63
Chagas' disease, 162, 202–203
Chemoprophylaxis, 39
  gastrointestinal infections, 47
  leprosy, 132
  loiasis, 220
  malaria, 193–195, 296
  meningococcal meningitis, 249
  plague, 184
  pneumococcal pneumonia, 246
  streptococcal infection, 251
  trypanosomiasis, 201, 202
  tuberculosis, 230, 242
Chickenpox, 102, 106–107, 228
  compared to smallpox, 106

Chiclero ulcer, 208
Chikungunia, fever, 195
  virus, 165
Child care, 259, 280, 288, 293–296
  indicators, 298
  mental, 337
Chilomastix mesnili, 72
Chlamydia trachomatis, 108
Chlorination, 308–309
Cholera, 59–63
Chrysops spp. 214, 219
Classification of diseases and causes of
  death, 21, 22
Clonorchiasis, 96–97
Clonorchis sinensis, 54, 96, 97, 100
Clostridium perfringens, 68
  C. tetani, 140
  C. welchii, 68
Cluster tracing, 113
'Cold chain', 250, 295, 296
Coliform count, 310
Colorado tick fever, 164
'Common cold', 236
Community participation
  mental health, 336
  primary health care, 285
Conjunctivitis,
  bacterial, 108
  inclusion, 110
Contact infections, 32, 102–136
Corynebacterium diphtheriae, 229, 253
  type gravis, 254
    intermedius, 254
    mitis, 254
Coxiella burnetii, 175, 180, 238
Crimean haemorrhagic fever, 159
Culex pipiens fatigans, 214, 215, 218
  C. tritaeniohynchus, 172
Culicoides spp. 165, 214, 224
  C. austini, 224
  C. grahami, 224
Cyclops, 83, 87
  and *Diphillobothrium latum*, 90
    Dracunculus medinensis, 83
    Gnasthostoma spinigerum, 86
Cysticercosis, 87, 89
Cysticercus bovis, 88
  C. cellulosae, 88

Dark field microscopy, 120, 122, 125, 152,
  187
Data,
  analysis and presentation, 13, 16
  collection, 6, 24, 25
  defects, 12

epidemiological, 29
  graphic representation of, 16–19
  sources, 6–13, 20, 40
  tabulation, 16
Death, certification, 10, 22–24
  rates, 13, 14, 15, 21
  registration, 10
Dengue fever, 159, 166, 172
  viruses, 165, 171
Dermacentor andersoni, 164
Diagram,
  bar, 16, 17
  pie, 16, 17, 18
Diarrhoeal diseases, 48
  control, 100
  prevention, 311, 314
Dientamoeba fragilis, 72
Diphtheria, 142, 253–256
Diphyllobothriasis, 90–91
Diphyllobothrium latum, 90
Dirofilaria conjunctivae, 224
  D. louisanensis, 224
  D. magalhaesi, 224
  D. repens, 224
Dirofilariasis, 224–225
Disease,
  distribution of, 26
  notification of, 10, 11
  surveillance of, 39
Disinfection, current, 318
  terminal, 318
Donovania granulomatis, 116
Dracontiasis, 83–84
Dracunculus medinensis, 83
Drepanidotaemia lanceolata, 91
Dysentery, amoebic, 70, 71
  bacillary, 58–59
  schistosomal, 144

Ebola virus disease, 160
Echinococcus granulosus, 92
  E. multilocularis, 92
  E. oligaettas, 92
Elephantiasis, 114, 214, 217
  of legs, 214
  vulvar, 114
ELISA test, 147, 192, 222
Encephalitis, 161
  California complex, 165
  equine, eastern, 165
    venezuelian, 165
    western, 165
  Japanese B, 165, 166, 172, 173
  Murray Valley, 165, 166
  Post-measles, 230

vaccinal, 294
Tick-borne, 165
rabies, 153
West Nile, 166
Endemic goitre, 267–269
Endolimax nana, 72
Entamoeba spp.,
  E. coli, 72
  E. fragilis, 72
  E. hartmanni, 70
  E. histolytica, 44, 69–72, 308
Enteric fevers, 53–55
Enteritis necroticans, 68
Enterobiasis, 81–82
  adhesive tape swab, 82
Enterobius vermicularis, 81
Enterotoxins, 56, 57
  Escherichia coli, 56
  Staphylococcus, 67
Environmental health, 303–319
Environmental sanitation, 274, 290, 303–319
  schools, 299–300
Eosinophilic meningitis,
  in angiostrongyliasis, 85
  in gnathostomiasis, 86
Epidemiology, 26–43
  analytical, 28
  communicable diseases, 30–36
  definition of, 26
  descriptive, 28
  experimental, 29
  methods, 27–30
  non-communicable diseases of, 41, 42
Epidemiological
  approach, 42, 43
  methods, 27–30
  surveys, 6
Epidermophyton, 132
Escherichia coli, 56, 310
Espundia, 209–210

Family health, 288–302
  organisation of services, 297–298
Family planning, 288, 292, 296–297
Fasciola gigantica, 98
  F. hepatica, 98
Fascioliasis, 98–99
Fasciolopsiasis, 99–100
Fasciolopsis buski, 99
Filariasis, 212
  Bancroftian, 213, 219
  Malayan, 213
Filtration, 308, 318
Food handlers, 51, 66, 67, 68, 70, 71, 243,
    300, 318
Food hygiene, 318
Food poisoning, bacterial, 65–69
  Clostridium welchii, 68, 69
  Salmonella, 65, 66
  Staphylococcus, 67, 68
Frei test, 114
Frequency distribution, 16

Gastro-enteritis, 56–57, 263
  bottle feeding, 261
  non-bacterial, 48
Gastro-intestinal tract infections control, 47
Genetic counselling, 333
Genetic disorders, 329–333
  G-6-PD deficiency, 329, 332
  haemoglobinopathies, 329, 331–332
  mental, 335
  Rh-negative gene, 332–333
  thalassaemia, 332
'German measles', 232–233
Ghon focus, 239
Giardia lamblia, 72
Giardiasis, 72
Glossina morsitans, 163, 197
  G. pallipides, 197
  G. palpalis, 197
  G. swinertoni, 197
  G. tachinoides, 163, 197
Glucose-6-PD deficiency, 192, 329, 332
Gnathostoma hispidum, 87
  G. spinigerum, 86
Gnathostomiasis, 86–87
Gonorrhoea, 102, 103, 116–118
Granuloma inguinale, 116
Graph, 16, 17, 19
Growth chart, 261, 293
Guinea worm, 83, 162, 307

Haemagogus spp. 167
Haemaphysalis spinigera, 173
Haemoglobin levels, 264
Haemoglobinopathies,
  high risk children, 296
  malaria, 192, 329–332
Haemophilus ducreyi, 115
  H. influenzae, 228, 246
  H. pertussis, 228
Haemorrhagic fever
  Chikungunia, 172
  Dengue, 172
  South-east Asian, 166, 172
Health education, 285, 290–291, 293, 320–323
  food hygiene, 318

Health education (*contd.*)
  school, 298, 299, 323
  workers, 342
Health services,
  community participation, 285–287
  components, 272–276
  coverage, 276, 287, 298
  curative, 272–274
  evaluation, 272, 287
  health education, 276
  impact, 276
  levels of care, 276–282
  management, 284
  organisation, 270–287
  personnel, 283–284
  planning, 287
  preventive, 274
  resources, 282–283
  special, 274–275
  statistics, 275–276
  supervision, 284
  tasks, 270–272
Height at school entry, 259
  of pre-schoolers, 259
Helminthic infections, 77–101
Hepatitis, viral, 51–53
  A, 51
  B, 52
  Non-A: Non-B, 52
  passive immunisation, 53
Herpangina, 48
Herpes zoster, 107
Heterophyiasis, 100
Heterophyes heterophyes, 100
Hippelates pallipes, 122
Histogram, 16–18
Histoplasma capsulatum, 210, 228
Histoplasmosis, 256–257
Hookworm, 102, 137–140
Host, factors, 33, 46, 47
Housing, 316–318
  labour migration, 338
Hydatid disease, 92–94
Hydrocoele, 214, 217
Hymenolepiasis, 91–92
Hymenolepis diminuta, 91, 92
  H. nana, 91, 92

Iceberg phenomenon, 20
Immunisation,
  active, 36, 230
  expanded programme of, 142, 242
  in childhood, 142
  passive, 36, 230
  schedule, 294–295
  specific, 47, 230

Immunity, 33–36
  acquired, 34
  age, 34
  factors affecting, 34–35
  genetic, 33
  herd, 35
  nutrition, 35
  pregnancy, 34
  racial, 192
  specific, 33, 46, 47, 229
  trauma and fatigue, 35
Immunoglobulins, 47, 52, 53, 142, 192, 231, 233
Inclusion conjunctivitis, 102, 110
  of adults, 110
  of neonates, 109, 110
Incubation period, 35
  extrinsic, 161
Infectious mononucleosis, 237–238
Influenza, 235–236, 246
Information feedback, 12
Insecticides, 225–227
  knock down, 225
  methods of application, 225
  residual, 225
  resistance to, 226
  toxicity, 226
International health regulations, 324–326
International organisations, other, 328
Intracytoplasmatic inclusion bodies, 108
Iodamoeba butschlii, 72
Isolation of patients, 38, 159, 170, 183, 231, 233, 253, 325
Isospora, 75
  I. belli, 73
  I. hominis, 73
Isosporiasis, 73

Kala-azar, 204, 207
KAP studies, 321
Klebsiella pneumoniae, 246
Koplik spots, 230
Kwashiorkor, 231, 260, 262
Kyasanur Forest fever, 159, 166, 173

Larva migrans,
  cutaneous, 137
  visceral, 79
Larvicides, 174, 195, 223, 226
Lassa fever, 159
Latrine, 311–314
Leishmania aethiopica, 205
  L. amazonensis, 205
  L. braziliensis, 205
  L. chagesi, 204
  L. donovani, 204

L. *infantum*, 204
L. *major*, 205
L. *mexicana*, 205
L. *minor*, 204
L. *penemensis*, 205
L. *pifanoi*, 205
L. *tropica*, 204, 205
Leishman-Donovan body, 206
Leishmaniasis, 204-212
  cutaneous, 207-209
  Ethiopian, 209
  lupoid, 209
  mucocutaneous, 209-210
  tegumentaria diffusa, 209
  visceral, 207
Lepromin test, 127
Leprosy, 125-132, 209
Leptospira bovis, 152
  L. *canicola*, 152
  L. *icterohaemorrhagica*, 152
  L. *pomona*, 152
Leptospirosis, 102, 137, 152-153
Link-host, 167
Loa loa, 214, 219
Loiasis, 219
Lymphogranuloma venereum, 113-114
Lysozyme, 229

Malabsorption, 72
Malaria, 161, 162, 163, 189-196, 249, 307
  erythrocytic cycle, 190
  haemoglobinopathies, 330-333
  in pregnancy, 196
  quartan, 190
  stable, 190
  subtertian, 190
  tertian, 190
  unstable, 190
Mallassezia furfur, 132
Malnutrition, 4, 26, 139, 187, 231, 241
  control of, 258-260
  mental disorder, 335
Mansonella ozzardi, 214, 224, 225
Mansonia spp. 213, 214, 215, 216
  M. *annulatus*, 214
  M. *longipalpis*, 214
Mantoux test, 240
Marasmus, 260, 262
Marburg virus disease, 160
Marisa cornuarietis, 151
Mastomys natalensis, 159
Maternal care, 259, 280, 288
  antenatal care, 289-292
  delivery services, 292
  post-natal care, 292

Measles, 142, 230-232, 240, 241, 246, 263, 266
Meningitis, aseptic, 161
  bacterial, 228
  'belt', 248
  eosinophilic, 85
  meningococcal, 248
  pyogenic, 248, 249
  tuberculous, 239
  viral, 48
Meningococcal infection, 248-250
  sulphonamide resistance, 249
Meningo-encephalitis,
  infectious mononucleosis, 237
  mumps, 233
  necrotising, 72
Mental health, 333-338
Metagonimiosis, 100
Metagonimus yokogawai, 100
Microfilaria, Timor, 215
Microsporon canis, 132
Monkey pox, 104
Montenegro reaction, 208, 209, 211
Morbidity, 6
  analysis, 19, 20
  statistics, 19
Multilocular hydatid cyst, 93
Mumps, 233-234
Mycobacterium audouini, 132, 133
  M. *leprae*, 125
  M. *tuberculosis*, 228, 229, 239
  M. *ulcerans*, 143
Mycoplasma pneumoniae, 242

Naegleria fowleri, 72
Necator americanus, 137, 139
Negri bodies, 154-155
Neisseria catarrhalis, 248
  N. *gonorrhoeae*, 116, 117
  N. *meningitidis*, 248
Non-infectious diseases,
  aetiology, 41, 42
  epidemiological investigation, 41, 42
  risk factors, 41, 42
Notification of disease, 10, 11, 37, 107, 117, 244, 245, 254, 342
  improvement of, 11
  international, 11, 37, 60, 171, 183, 324, 325
Nutritional disorders, 258-269

Occupational health, 338-342
Onchocerca volvulus, 214, 220
Onchocerciasis, 220-225, 307
  Control Programme, 220, 223

Ophthalmia neonatorum,
  chlamydia, 108
  gonococcal, 111, 117, 118
Opisthorchiasis, 97–98
Opisthorchis felineus, 97
  O. viverrini, 97
Oral rehydration, 62, 100, 263, 296
Oriental sore, 208
Ornithodorus moubata, 185
  O. rudis, 185
Oroya fever, 188

Paragonimiasis, 94–96
Paragonimus africanus, 94
  P. heterotremus, 94
  P. siamensis, 94
  P. westermani, 94
Paratyphoid fevers, 55
Pasteurisation, 64, 67, 181, 238, 243, 251,
  318
Pediculus humenus, 175, 187
Pertussis, 142, 252–253, 263
Phlebotomus, spp. 164, 173, 188, 204–205
  P. papatasii, 173
Pigbel, 68
Pila, 86
Pinta, 118, 123–124
Plague, 162, 177, 182–184, 325
  'blocked fleas', 182
Plasmodium falciparum, 189, 190, 191
  and sickle cell gene, 330–331
  P. malariae, 189, 190
  P. ovale, 189, 190
  P. vivax, 189, 190, 192
Pneumonia,
  ascariasis, 77
  atypical, 247–248
  other bacterial, 246
  plague, 183
  pneumococcal, 245–246
  psittacosis, 234
  Q fever, 238
  tuberculous, 239
Poliomyelitis, 47–51, 142
  immunisation interference, 48, 50
PPD, 240
Pregnancy, 288
  amoebiasis, 70
  anaemia, 263, 265, 291
  endemic goitre, 267
  haemoglobin, 264, 331
  health care, 289–292
  infectious hepatitis, 51
  malaria, 196, 291
  monitoring, 291

nutrition, 259
  education, 262, 290
  PEM, 260
Primary health care, 276–282
  Alma-Ata declaration, 278–281
Protein-energy malnutrition, 231, 260–263
  and infection, 260
  foetal, 260
  infant, 260
  in pregnancy, 260
Psittacosis, 234–235
Public Health, laws, 329
  other aspects, 324–342
  significance, 273

Q fever, 175, 180–181, 238
Quarantine, 36, 38, 60, 61, 62, 171, 183,
  234, 324, 329
'Q' flag, 325

Rabies, 137, 153–157
Rates,
  birth, 297
  case fatality, 21
  child death, 15, 260, 288, 293, 299
  crude, 13
  crude birth, 13
  crude death, 13
  fatality, 21
  fertility, 14
  incidence, 20, 21, 27
  mortality—
    infant, 14, 15, 288, 298
    maternal, 14, 263, 288
    neonatal, 14, 15, 298
    perinatal, 14, 260, 298
    post-neonatal, 14, 15
  natural increase, 13
  point, 21
  prevalence, 21, 27
  specific, 13, 14
    age, 14, 15, 259
    sex, 14
  standardised, 14
  stillbirth, 14
Reduviid bugs, 202–203
  gen. *Panstrongylus*, 202
  gen. *Rhodnius*, 202
  gen. *Triatoma*, 202
Registration, births, 10, 329
  deaths, 10, 329
  medical personnel, 329
  schools, 329
Relapsing fevers, 185–188
  louse-borne, 162, 185

in neonates, 186
tick-borne, 185–186
Reservoir of infection,
elimination of, 38
in animals, 32
in man, 31
in non-living things, 32
Rheumatic fever, 251–255
Rickettsia akari, 175
  R. australis, 175
  R. burnetii, 175, 238
  R. conori, 175
  R. mooseri, 175, 177
  R. orientalis, 177
  R. prowazekii, 175
  R. quintana, 175
  R. rickettsii, 175
  R. siberica, 175
  R. tsutsugamushi, 175, 177–178
Rickettsial diseases, 174–181
Rift Valley fever, 159, 174
Risk factors, 289
  high risk groups, 288, 296
Rubella, 232–233

Saccharomyces, 134
Salmonella spp. 53, 65, 66
  S. paratyphi, 53
  S. typhi, 53
  S. typhimurium, 65, 188
Sandfly fever, 164, 173
Sarcoptes mange, 136
  S. scabiei, 135, 136
Scabies, 103, 135–136
Schick test, 254
Schistosoma bovis, 146, 147
  S. haematobium, 144–152
  S. intercalatum, 146, 147
  S. japonicum, 144–152
  S. mansoni, 54, 144–152
  S. mattheei, 146, 152
Schistosomiasis, 102, 137, 144–152, 307
School health, 298–302
  mental, 337
Seaport health services, 324–325
Sexual behaviour, 111–113
  promiscuity, 111
  prostitution, 121
Sexually transmitted diseases, 103, 110–122
Simulium, spp. 214, 220
  S. callidium, 220
  S. damnosum, 220
  S. metallicum, 220
  S. ochraceum, 220

Smallpox, 103, 104–105, 159, 228
  vaccination, 105
Snail, intermediate hosts,
  Achatina fulica, 86
  Biomphallaria, 146
  B. glabrata, 151
  Bithynia, 96, 97
  Bulinus, 146
  Limnea, 98
  Melania spp. 86, 95
    M. malayanus, 86
  Oncomelania, 146
  Pirinella connica, 100
  Segmentina, 99
  Semisulcospira, 100
Social welfare, 326
Soft chancre, 114–115
Splenomegaly,
  hepato-, *S. mansoni*, 333
  infectious mononucleosis, 237
  malaria, 189
Standard deviation, 16
Staphylococcus aureus, 246
  enterotoxic, 67
Streptococcus pneumoniae, 228, 245
  S. pyogenes, 250
Summer grippe, 48
Surveillance, 36, 39, 40, 184
Syphilis, 102, 103, 104, 118–122
  non-venereal, 119
  congenital, 119
  venereal, 118–122

Taeniasis, 87–90
Taenia saginata, 87
  T. solium, 87, 89
Test,
  observer variation, 30
  repeatability, 30
  results, erroneous, 30
  sensitivity, 29
  specificity, 29
Tetanus, 102, 137, 140–142, 253, 255, 295
  cryptogenic, 141
  neonatorum, 141, 142
  post-ebortal, 141
  -puerperal, 141
  -surgical, 141
  -traumatic, 141
Tetrapetalonema perstans, 214, 224, 225
  T. streptocerca, 214, 224, 225
Tinea capitis, 103, 132
  T. tonsurans, 132
  T. versicolor, 132

Toxocara canis, 79
T. cati, 76
Toxocariasis, 79–80
Toxoplasma gondii, 75
Toxoplasmosis, 75–76
Trachoma, 102, 107–109, 307
Traditional birth attendant, 292
Transmission,
  interruption of, 39
  modes of—
    biological, 162
    contact, 32
    faeco-oral, 45
    infectious, 33
    inhalation, 33
    mechanical, 162
    penetration of skin, 32
    transplacental, 33
Treponema carateum, 125
T. pallidum, 118, 119, 122
T. pertenue, 122
Treponematoses, 118–125
  nonvenereal, 122–125
  venereal, 118–122
TRIC agent, 108, 110
Trichinella spiralis, 84
Trichinosis, 84–85
Trichomonas hominis, 72, 73
T. vaginalis, 73, 135
Trichomoniasis, 73, 134–135
Trichophyton, 132
Trichuriasis, 80–81
Trichuris trichiura, 80
Triple antigen, 142, 253, 255, 294
Trombicula akamushi, 178
T. deliensis, 178
T. pallida, 178
T. scutellaris, 178
Trypanosoma b. gambiense, 197–202
T. b. rhodesiense, 197, 202
T. cruzi, 203
T. rangeli, 203
Trypanosomiasis, 197–204
  African, 197–202
  American, 202–203
Tuberculin reaction, 143, 240
  cross sensitivity, 240
Tuberculosis, 239–244
  bovine, 243, 244
Typhoid fever, 4, 46, 53–55
  schistosomiasis and, 53, 54
Typhus, African tick, 175
  epidemic, 175–177, 186
  murine, 177
  scrub, 177

Typhus, flea-borne, 177, 181
  louse-borne, 175–177, 181
  mite-borne, 177, 181
  tick-borne, 175

United Nations Agencies, 328
Urethritis,
  chlomydia, 108
  gonococcal, 118
  trichomonas, 134
Uta, 209

Vaccines,
  BCG, 144, 241
  brucellosis, 65
  cholera, 62, 63
  diphtheria, 255
  enteritis necroticans, 68
  influenza, 236
  leprosy, 132
  malaria, 195
  measles, 231
  meningococcal meningitis, 249
  mumps, 232
  pertussis, 253
  plague, 184
  pneumococcus, 246
  poliomyelitis, 50
  Q fever, 181
  smallpox, 105
  tetanus, 142
  triple antigen, 295
  typhoid fever, 55
  typhus, 176
  yellow fever, 171
Vaccination certificate, 63, 171, 324
Verruca peruana, 188
Vesicular stomatitis, 48
  virus, 165
Viruses,
  arbo, 161, 164–174
    alphaviruses, 164–165
    bunyaviruses, 173
    flaviviruses, 165–173
  atypical pneumonia, 228
  Bunyamwera group, 173
  chickenpox, 228
  common cold, 228
  dengue, 165, 171
  Ebola, 159
  enteroviruses, 47, 236
    Coxsackie, 47
    Echo, 47
    Reo, 47
    Rota, 47

hepatitis, 51, 52
influenza, 228
Junin, 159
Lassa, 159
lymphogranuloma venereum, 114
Marburg, 159
measles, 230, 231
mumps, 228
Phlebotomus fever group, 173–174
PLT group, 108, 228, 234
poliomyelitis, 48
rabies, 154
rhinoviruses, 236
Rift Valley fever, 174
rubella, 228
smallpox, 228
varicella-zoster, 106
variola, 105
West Nile, 166
Yellow fever, 166
Vitamin A deficiency, 265–267

Wastes, disposal, 310–316
industrial, 316
refuse, 314–316
sewage, 311–314
Water associated diseases, 307
purification, 307
quality, 309–310
sources, 304–307
supplies, 304
uses, 304
Weight at birth, 259
low, 260, 263
chart, 261
for age, 259, 261
for height, 261, 262
reference, 261
Weil-Felix reaction, 176, 177, 178, 179, 238
World Health Organisation (WHO) 327–328
Wuchereria bancrofti, 213

Xenopsylla, 177
X. cheopis, 182
Xerophthalmia, 265–267

Yaws, 104, 118, 122–123
Yellow fever, 159, 162, 164, 166–171, 295, 325
Yersinia pestis, 182, 183

Zoonoses,
anthrax, 158
arbo-viruses, 164
brucellosis, 63
campilobacter, 57
cysticercosis, 89
definition, 32
encephalitis, equine, 165
Japanese B. 172
fascioliasis, 98
fasciolopsiasis, 99
filariasis, Malayan, 213
histoplasmosis, 256
hydatid disease, 92
Kyasanur Forest fever, 173
Lassa fever, 173
leishmaniasis, cutaneous, 207
mucocutaneous, 209
visceral, 206
leptospirosis, 152
plague, 182
psittacosis, 234
Q fever, 181, 238
rabies, 153
reservoir elimination, 38
Rift Valley fever, 174
salmonellosis, 65
Schistosomiasis japonicum, 147
taeniasis, 87
tick-borne relapsing fever, 185
toxocariasis, 79
toxoplasmosis, 75
trichinosis, 84
Trypanosomiasis b. rhodesiense, 198
T. b. gambiense, 198
tuberculosis, bovine, 241
typhus, African tick-borne, 180
louse-borne, 175
mite-borne, 178
murine, 177
yellow fever